W9-APB-204

DISCARD

ALSO BY JONNY STEINBERG

Midlands
The Number

Sizwe's Test

A Young Man's Journey
Through Africa's AIDS Epidemic

Jonny Steinberg

SIMON & SCHUSTER
New York   London   Toronto   Sydney

Simon & Schuster
1230 Avenue of the Americas
New York, NY 10020

Copyright © 2008 by Jonny Steinberg

All rights reserved, including the right to reproduce this book or
portions thereof in any form whatsoever. For information address
Simon & Schuster Subsidiary Rights Department,
1230 Avenue of the Americas, New York, NY 10020

First Simon & Schuster hardcover edition February 2008

SIMON & SCHUSTER and colophon are registered trademarks
of Simon & Schuster, Inc.

For information about special discounts for bulk purchases,
please contact Simon & Schuster Special Sales at
1-800-456-6798 or business@simonandschuster.com

Designed by Davina Mock-Maniscalco

Manufactured in the United States of America

1   3   5   7   9   10   8   6   4   2

Library of Congress Cataloging-in-Publication Data
Steinberg, Jonny, date.
Sizwe's test : a young man's journey through Africa's AIDS epidemic / Jonny Steinberg.
p.   cm.
1. Magadla, Sizwe—Health. 2. AIDS (Disease)—South Africa. I. Title.
RA643.86.S62S74   2008
362.196'979200968—dc22   2007029672
ISBN-13: 978-1-4165-5269-7 (hardcover)
ISBN-10:   1-4165-5269-3

R06009 02054

Contents

PART THREE

A Note on Terminology and Names

Dispersed among the pages that follow is some of the language of traditional healing, which, in the absence of a brief explanation, may prove confusing to the uninitiated.

An *inyanga* is an herbalist, but has no clairvoyance, only a deep knowledge of the medicinal properties of herbs and plants.

Igqira is the Xhosa word for a diviner-healer. She is the interface between living people and their ancestors; through communication with her spirit-guide, she interprets the cause of illness where the cause is either ancestral displeasure or witchcraft. Plural: amagqira.

Sangoma is the Zulu word for diviner-healer, but is used throughout South Africa in all of its languages.

Muthi literally means "tree" in Zulu. The proximate English translation is "medicine," but that is inadequate. An *inyanga*'s herbs are *muthi,* as are the medicines used to protect people from occult attack. But the murderous substances that witches and wizards deploy are also *muthi,* and often conceal demons that come to life in your body once you have ingested them. *Muthi* has also made its way into the colloquial English and Afrikaans spoken by white South Africans; here it refers to allopathic medicine.

The names of Ithanga residents and of Kate Marrandi's patients have been changed. Andrew Rutland is a pseudonym. No other names have been changed.

List of Illustrations

Sizwe's Test

Preface

I came upon the idea of this book sometime during the afternoon of April 9, 2005, while reading Edwin Cameron's book, *Witness to AIDS.*

In that book, Cameron tells a ghastly story one does not easily forget.

Knowing that up to a third of its population had HIV or AIDS, and that about one hundred thousand people were in urgent need of drugs, the government of Botswana announced in 2001 that it would offer free antiretroviral treatment to every citizen with AIDS. It was a dramatic declaration of intent, unprecedented in sub-Saharan Africa. By the time the drugs had hit the shelves and health personnel were ready to administer treatment, just about every soul in Botswana knew of it.

And yet, on the last day of 2003, more than two years after the launch of the program, only about fifteen thousand people had come forward for treatment. The rest—over eighty-five thousand people—had stayed at home. The majority would now be dead.

Why did they not go to get the drugs?

"Stigma," is Cameron's answer. "People are too scared—too ashamed—to come forward and claim what their government is now affording them: . . . the right to stay alive . . . In some horrifically constrained sense, they are 'choosing' to die, rather than face the stigma of AIDS and find treatment."

Does this foreshadow an entire region's response to AIDS? When the history of this great epidemic is written, will it be said that an untold number of people died, not because the plague was unstoppable, but because they were mortally ashamed? Will it be said that several successive generations of southern Africans were decimated by a sense of disgrace?

About 2.1 million people died of AIDS in sub-Saharan Africa in 2006. Another 25 million are living with HIV. In South Africa, where I was born and bred, nearly 6 million in a population of 46 million are HIV-positive: more than one in eight people. Some eight hundred South Africans die of AIDS on an average day. And the epidemic is spreading at a rate of more than a thousand new infections a day in South Africa. That death could keep accumulating on this scale despite the presence of lifesaving medicines is chilling beyond description.

A certain intellectual temperament greets such spectacles with excited fascination. The moral of Cameron's story, it may be tempting to conclude, is that human lives are not sunny and progressive projects, but the sites of blunt, blind tragedy. Not just the world, but even our own natures are indifferent to our programs of betterment.

I am not one of those fascinated souls. When I read a story like Cameron's, my gut response is that something is wrong, something that might be fixed. This is not to say I subscribe to the proposition that, at core, our natures are healing and life-giving. There is a surfeit of shame and envy and destruction within us, quite enough to go around. But it seems to me that what becomes of this darkness is not a question of fate but of politics. When people die en masse within walking distance of treatment, my inclination is to believe that there must be a mistake somewhere, a miscalibration between institutions and people. This book is a quest to discover whether I am right.

———————————

WHEN I FINISHED reading Cameron's book I began to look for the most successful antiretroviral treatment program in South Africa. I wanted to find a place where poor villagers lived within walking distance of well-administered drugs, and where nobody need die for lack of medical care. I wanted to go there and find people who were staying at home and dying, and I wanted to know why they were doing so.

The closest thing I found to what I was looking for was the rural district of Lusikisiki in Eastern Cape province. It is not quite true that everybody there lives within walking distance of antiretroviral (ARV) treatment, or that nobody need die for lack of medical care. It is a chronically poor place, where people have been dying for want of decent care since long before the HIV virus. But extraordinary work was being done there. The international nongovernmental organization Médecins Sans Frontières (MSF, and called in English, Doctors Without Borders), in partnership with the Eastern Cape Department of Health, was using the district's rickety and neglected primary health-care clinics to administer antiretroviral treatment. When MSF arrived in 2002, nearly one in three pregnant women was testing HIV-positive. At least one person a day was dying of AIDS at the hospital on the outskirts of town. Most of those infected with the virus were still asymptomatic; in the absence of a medical intervention, an avalanche of death was to come.

MSF was putting out very good news indeed. Staffed by a cohort of laypeople and ordinary government nurses, the clinics were up and running, the organization said. Thousands of villagers were cramming the waiting rooms to test for HIV. And the shelves were stocked with drugs. By the time I made contact with MSF in mid-2005, a thousand people were on ARVs.

The program was run by an MSF doctor called Hermann Reuter. He is to occupy quite a few of the pages that follow. Reuter's guiding proposition was quite simple: If you provide treatment that works, people will come and get it. If you provide poor treatment, make people stand in lines, or shunt them from one institution to another, they will look elsewhere for succor, or they will stay at home and die. His work was that of a medical missionary: he wanted to show that you could provide decent AIDS treatment anywhere, even in places that had long ago been routed, and that if you did so, people would come forward.

I went to Lusikisiki deeply skeptical of Reuter's evangelical simplicity. While I wanted to resist the stance of the morbidly fascinated, I suspected that things in Lusikisiki were a lot more complicated than he made out. And it did not take long to find people who lived close to a clinic staying at home and dying. The question was why.

IF THE BROCHURES produced by the area's negligible tourist industry are to be believed, Lusikisiki owes its name to the sound of the wind moving through reeds. According to locals, the word does not mean anything, or if it once did, its meaning is lost to memory. In any case, they say, *Lusikisiki* refers to two things: the town center with its commercial street and its smattering of suburban-like homes, and the thirty-six or so villages scattered around it in a forty-mile radius.

It is not an easy place to describe. Were you to read its economic data off a spreadsheet without seeing it in the flesh you might think it was a depressed inner-city zone. The majority of adults are un- or underemployed, and most households get their income either by cheap, unskilled labor, or survivalist self-employment, or government grants.

And yet its physical setting is anything but urban. Lusikisiki's 150,000-odd people live in about three dozen villages spread liberally over a spirited, temperamental landscape. Streams and rivers run through villages flanked by wild forests; cows, horses, and goats graze off deep green grassland; the villages along the seaboard stand on high cliffs and command breathtaking views of the ocean. Wandering through this place, it takes dogged labor to remind oneself that its political economy is no longer rural, that almost everyone you meet is either unemployed, or in a job that earns less than a thousand rand a month (roughly equivalent to 140 U.S. dollars), or is the recipient of a grant.

You know it, however, when you leave the villages and make your way to Lusikisiki's town center. There you see what transpires when a single market street becomes the focal point for 150,000 residents of a rural district who must come to one central throughway to purchase everything in their lives, from the food in their stomachs to the tin roofs over their heads. There is no place to move—not in a car, not on foot, not inside the massive warehouse stores. The rows of hawkers push the pedestrians off the pavements and into the streets, leaving a narrow tunnel for the cars. And there are too many cars. Five days a week, eight hours a day, the street is dense with people, metal, noise, and a cloud of carbon. By seven in the evening it is quiet and empty.

At first I thought that this anomaly between the rural landscape and the urban profile was simply a symptom of my outsider's incomprehension. Yet I soon discovered that the villagers were as confused as I was, that they themselves felt the place to be in a painful and extended interregnum, and that it was this state of affairs that shaped the meaning of the AIDS epidemic.

More than a century ago, Lusikisiki was the capital of Eastern Pondoland, the last independent black polity in these parts to surrender its independence to the British. Political defeat spawned economic defeat; its economy hobbled by its political impotence, the men of Eastern Pondoland began working nine or ten months a year in Johannesburg's gold mines some six hundred miles away, beginning a pattern of circular migration that would persist throughout the twentieth century.

The kingdom's subjugation took a new and cynical form in 1963, when it was incorporated into the northeastern reaches of the Transkei, one of apartheid's notorious old bantustans, the separate "homelands" in which black South Africans could claim citizenship and whose sovereignty was recognized only by South Africa and its most credulous allies. Until the early 1990s, the Transkei was run by a succession of small-time dictators, among them callous and expedient men, their regimes heavily underwritten by the apartheid government.

As a reservoir of cheap labor for Johannesburg's gold mines and a dumping ground on the margins of South Africa's economy, Transkei districts such as Lusikisiki are no strangers to chronic illness. For the last eighty years, at least three out of four residents have incubated the tuberculosis bacillus, a disease that plagued South Africa's gold mine workers and their rural families throughout the twentieth century. Yet during the final decade of apartheid, the annual maintenance and operating costs of the whites-only Johannesburg General Hospital exceeded the combined health budgets of all seven of South Africa's bantustans, home to a population of several million people, among whom the modern diseases of poverty were legion.

So, while AIDS is without doubt the largest catastrophe Lusikisiki has experienced in living memory, the district is painfully familiar with chronic disease, early death, and wretched health care.

And yet, paradoxically perhaps, the villages of Lusikisiki represent something else entirely. Through much of the twentieth century, they constituted home ground, a way of life to defend and cherish, the site of a rearguard battle against a corrosive economic order. The men may have spent much of each year away from home at the gold mines, but they did so to gather the resources that nourished a way of life back home. In the villages of Lusikisiki, they were proprietors of peasant homesteads and they were patriarchs. This sense of command and continuity made up the kernel of their identities. They lived alongside the graves of their forebears, they paid bridewealth to marry, and they sired children who bore their names. The villages and the productive fields were thus the site of their quest to leave a legacy in this world after their deaths, the site of their humanity.

It is a cruel irony that by the time apartheid was defeated and the Transkei incorporated into a democratic South Africa, the twin foundations of this world—work in the gold mines and a peasant economy at home—were both in a state of irreversible decline. And with it, so was a way of life based on the land. On the town's main street, pedestrians exchange idioms about plows and hoes and harvests, as if the land were still productive, its inhabitants still rural proprietors. The place, its people, and the words that issue from their tongues are steeped in a way of life that is no more.

An epidemic that kills young adults in droves spawns difficult politics. How does a society absorb the death of its young? Whom does it blame?

When the dying is transmitted by sex, the politics get more difficult still. And when the dead were voters in a brand-new democracy, sons and daughters of a people just liberated from a white dictatorship, the spectacle appears cynical in the extreme, as if guided by an evil hand.

A new democracy is an era of resurging life. Sex is the most life-giving of activities. That a new nation's citizens are dying from sex seems to be an attack both on ordinary people's and a nation's generative capacities, an insult too ghastly to stomach. AIDS has given rise to accusation. Nowhere is this more evident than in the politics of South Africa's president, Thabo Mbeki, who questioned with bitterness whether the dying was caused by a sexually transmitted virus after all, and who asked caustically whether antiretroviral drugs were for the benefit of Africans or pharmaceutical companies.

Rage like Mbeki's is all over Lusikisiki. Where there is AIDS, there is blame. It is said in the villages that the virus was hatched in laboratories, to be let loose on blacks until whites become an electoral majority. And the accusations are not only racial, not only overtly political. The ill are accused of having murdered loved ones by their promiscuity. Neighbors are blamed for using magic to infect the beautiful and the successful. The accusations expressed in national politics are also stitched into village life, and, indeed, into individual consciousness. On one level, this book is an exploration of the place of blame and resentment in one man's decision whether to test his blood for HIV.

I VISITED LUSIKISIKI periodically over a period of eighteen months. After meeting many people—nurses and patients, traditional healers and treatment activists—I decided to research much of the book that follows by sitting on the proverbial shoulder of a man I shall call Sizwe Magadla. He was almost thirty years old when I met him. His child was growing in his lover's womb, his family was negotiating bridewealth with hers, and he was preoccupied with imagining the course of the remainder of his life.

On the day I clapped eyes on him, Sizwe was healthy and strong and had never tested for HIV, which puts him in a category shared by most South African men his age. That is why I chose him. In this narrow sense, and no more, he was an Everyman, and it was his perspective on the antiretroviral program that I wanted to understand.

The MSF project run by Hermann Reuter has only a peripheral place in Part One of this book. That may seem odd, given my motivations for writing it. The reason is that I wanted to approach antiretroviral medicine from Sizwe's vantage point, and when I met him, it was no more than a distant presence for him, one that cast a troubling shadow over the very edges of his world. The meaning of AIDS in his life had a good deal more to do with being a son, a prospective husband, and a shopkeeper than living in a district that administered antiretroviral drugs. I needed to show how the treatment program entered his life and wrestled with his other preoccupations.

As we began touring Lusikisiki's clinics, Sizwe came alive to the sheer scale of the illness that he had been seeing around him for some years. The more he witnessed, the more the prospect of testing his own blood for HIV frightened him. That he saw people taking pills and getting well did little to alleviate his fear. What follows is a chronicle and an exploration of that fear.

I have given him and his village pseudonyms and tried to disguise them both. That is a crucial feature of this book. A story about shame is also about privacy, for who wants others to witness their shame? And yet precisely what privacy means in the midst of an epidemic of shame is far more complicated than I ever imagined.

PART ONE

Sizwe

I met Sizwe Magadla in the spring of 2005. I was looking for him because I hoped to meet his father. Some weeks earlier, I had put out word that I wanted to get to know an *igqira*, a diviner-healer, from one of the remoter villages of Lusikisiki. Someone had told me that there was a young man from a village called Ithanga with a spaza shop—a ubiquitous presence in rural South Africa, where customers buy everything from headache powder and baby food to cold beer— and that his father was an igqira.

When we finally met, it was, ironically, on the premises of one of Sizwe's competitors. There is a spaza shop some distance from the edge of Ithanga, about fifty yards before the gravel road ends. It is about the only building in the vicinity of the village that one can access by public road. I went there accompanied by a man called Luyanda, whom I had hired as a translator and a guide. He was in his late forties, had been coming to the Lusikisiki area since he was a child, but had never before set foot in Ithanga.

We parked our car, walked in, and asked for Sizwe by the description I had been given: the young man with dreadlocks who owns a spaza shop and whose father is an igqira. The woman behind the counter nodded. She called over a small child and instructed her to go into the village to call him. The child dawdled out of the shop reluctantly, scraping her bare feet against the floor, and made a slow journey into the village.

We waited. Opposite us was a group of young men. There were seven of them. Four sat languorously on the chest-high shop counter. The other three stood leaning against the wall. They had about them an aura of short-tempered proprietorship, as if they were waiting to be entertained but were very hard to please. For the hour or so we inhabited the same space, they managed both to take much interest in us and to ignore us.

After waiting for some time, we decided to stretch our legs. Out in the sunshine, I told Luyanda that if the spaza shop man did not show up soon, we should leave. I would come back alone the following day, ask for directions to his shop, and make my way into the village on foot.

"Please don't do that," he said. "Not alone. Those boys . . . You will be carrying a bag. They will want your bag."

I shrugged. "I'll leave my bag in the car."

"Please," he said. "I know boys like those. They have spent time in Durban or Port Elizabeth. They have guns. When they come back to the rural areas they feel they can do anything. They are feared."

And so my first impression of Sizwe's village was of these sullen young men idling dangerously through empty time, of souls with unknowable futures and great, wide stretches of the here and now to be filled. I was to learn that they were indeed feared, not least by those who had known them since they were infants.

SIZWE APPEARED JUST as we were about to leave. At first he did not see us. He came into the shop, walked past us, stopped, turned around, and looked at us inquiringly.

He was strikingly beautiful. He had a wide face, his cheekbones high and carved, his mouth thick and full. He took us in with eyes that suggested he inhabits his own skin, that he has no urge to drift or to wander. His hair was braided into thick dreadlocks that fell off the sides of his face over his ears and onto his shoulders.

He shook our hands solemnly, took three plastic chairs from the shop, and put them out in the sun. We sat, and I told him my business: that I was writing a book on AIDS, that I wanted to meet his father and get his views on the virus, that I sought to ask his father if I could watch him work.

When I had finished speaking he held out his forearm and shaped his hand to hold an imaginary syringe. "I have not tested," he said. "My girlfriend is pregnant and she went to the clinic to test. She's negative. Do you think that means I'm definitely negative?"

I was taken aback by his openness.

"If you want to know, you must test," I said.

"I know," he replied. "But I'm scared."

He smiled at me and laughed, got up, motioned for us to get up, too, and took our three chairs back inside.

I met him the following day at the same place, and we walked into the village together. At first he was somewhat stiff; the previous day's levity appeared to have abandoned him. Sometimes we spoke, sometimes there was silence. At some point I noticed a subtle change in his gait and his footsteps. He was beginning to relax. As he did so, he began to ask me one question after another: why I was writing this book, what precisely it was I wanted to learn. His interest in me was neither watchful nor suspicious; I had arrived from a world he knew little about, and he wanted to imagine the place I had come from. By the time we reached his parents' homestead I liked him. He possessed a curiosity both rare and distinctive; one recognizes it the moment one sees it. It is the curiosity of a person who has no interest in confusing the boundaries between himself and others, who does not identify or envy too much.

I SPENT THE following two days with Buyisile, Sizwe's father. He was over six feet tall, with the taut, muscled body of a man less than half his age and a temperament capricious enough to make me uneasy. He was a great performer; when he spoke he possessed the space and the people around him. He told story after story, entertaining both himself and the adults and children who wandered through his household. And then, without warning, his face would drop, he would grow silent, and he would begin to sulk. As with his stories, his dark moods took up space: they suggested that he had both disappeared deep within himself and wanted to take those around him with him.

Throughout the two days I spent with Buyisile, Sizwe was quietly present. When I took his father to see a patient an hour's car journey away, Sizwe was in the backseat. When I sat in Buyisile's great rondavel listening to his stories, Sizwe would sit next to me. He seldom spoke. He would bow his head and allow his dreadlocks to fall over the sides of his face and cover his eyes. It was difficult to know what he was thinking. He was, it seemed, in another's space, that of his father; his thoughts, I imagined, must remain private here.

I listened to Buyisile's stories, recorded them faithfully, and learned a great deal. But I wanted to move on. He had, I imagined, a limited stock of tales, and beyond them he was impenetrable to me; his words seemed a thick buttress, one I feared I would never skirt.

At the end of our second afternoon together, we were sitting in Buyisile's rondavel, about half a dozen of us, listening to him talk of the forests and the medicines it harbored. He told us of how, when he was a boy, his own father would take him into the forest and teach him about herbs, how his father's mother had done the same, how his knowledge of Ithanga's forests was the inherited knowledge of several generations.

Sizwe and I were sitting close to each other on a bench. I asked him if he too would one day take his unborn child to the forest to teach him about herbs.

"I am not sure how much longer I can live here in Ithanga," he said quietly.

I looked at him, my surprise at his sudden declaration clearly showing in my face.

"Where do you want to live?" I asked.

"Somewhere I am not known. Where you are known, you cannot run a business. People see you through your parents and your grand-parents and they judge you. They ask how a man can be successful when his parents are poor."

"You want to come to Johannesburg?"

"No. People go to the city and they live in shacks alongside strang-ers and they come home sick. I am not going to the city."

"Where then?"

"In Lusikisiki, but another village: somewhere I am not known."

"What are you afraid of? What is it you think people might do to you?"

"There have been things happening in my sleep," he said, looking down at the floor. "Twice now, I have woken up in the morning and I have been wet and sticky. I am twenty-nine. Wet dreams are for boys, for when you are maybe thirteen or fourteen. I have Nwabisa sleeping next to me. I am a man."

"So what is happening to you when you sleep?"

"Some people have maybe sent a demon to have sex with me: a demon with HIV. That is why I am scared to test. I think I will test positive."

At the time of this conversation with Sizwe, I was taken aback by what appeared either to be a confessional outburst or a moment of exhibitionism. I couldn't decide which. I asked him immediately whether I could write about him. He told me he would think about it; it took him more than a month to say yes.

Ithanga

Pondoland is a place of abrupt changes, of moods you have not expected: the spirit of the place is hard to pin down. It is not just its short-tempered, unstable weather. It is also a question of topography. As you drive away from the Umzimvubu River, the world outside your window is close and intimate. The horizon is seldom far, yet between yourself and the end of what you can see the land buckles and drops way below you and climbs to heights far above. The result is a sense of worlds on top of one another, instead of side by side. Looking out to the horizon, you are accosted by the feeling that your horizontal gaze is misguided or out of focus, that you are missing almost everything in between. Turn a corner or climb a hill and you find yourself in a village or a pasture of which the view from your window did not warn.

And so it is with Ithanga, the village in which the last five generations of Sizwe Magadla's paternal forebears were born and bred. There is no vantage point from which to see it; it is a place you first witness from close range. You take one of the dirt roads from Lusikisiki's center and drive for about twenty miles through a varied landscape of thick forest and naked hills. From the summits of the tallest hills you can glimpse the ocean. After some time, the trees disappear and the land flattens. You turn a bend and suddenly you can go no farther. In front of you there is a barbed-wire fence, and on your left a very steep, rutted road. Unless you have a four-by-four, you must leave your car and climb it on foot, about three hundred yards. It is arduous; when you reach the top there is sweat on your brow and you are breathing heavily. I always associate the sight of Ithanga with the sound of my own breath in my ears.

It appears quite suddenly and unexpectedly: a deep valley surrounded by green hills, clusters of round mud huts and square, tin-roofed structures at the summits, a river flowing through the basin. The river bisects the village. To visit a neighbor you take off your socks and shoes and you wade. Cows and goats and pigs graze on the slopes and come down to the valley bottom to drink. The hills make of the valley an acoustic amphitheater. You cannot always see children, but you always hear them, exclaiming and shouting and crying, as if somebody has piped a recording of a crowded school ground into the village and plays it over and over.

SIZWE LIVES ON a perch near the top of one of Ithanga's highest hills, about a half mile from his father's place. Standing at his front door, you tower above the village, the horses and cows in the valley basin mere stick figures. He built much of his house with his own hands, using wood from the forest, mud from the riverbed, several dozen bags of concrete from town, and corrugated iron for the roof. He erected the frame, put on the roof, and then grew bored with the work and hired a man called Stars to finish it. He did not like Stars's craftsmanship. Every day he watched Stars work he grew angry, but said nothing.

"What can I do?" he said to me. "In this place, you must not be quick to fight. Stars comes and works for me. Stars fucks off. I greet him every day, but I never use him again."

This is indeed a place where one must not be quick to fight. There are only seven hundred souls here and one sees most of them every day.

"Do you know each person in this village?" I ask Sizwe.

"Everyone," he replies.

"By name, by sight?"

"By everything. By their parents, their grandparents, their cousins. Maybe someone new comes and for a while I don't know them. For a week, maybe. Then I know them. And I know how they fit in."

And everyone else, of course, knows Sizwe, and has his own sense of how Sizwe fits in. Among the things everyone knows is that when he was a boy his family grew very poor, that he was once lean and quite literally hungry. They know too that Sizwe is no longer poor; he owns a spaza shop at the age of twenty-nine, and in this village that is no mean achievement. It puts him head and shoulders above just about all his peers. That is not something that courts unalloyed joy. The path from poverty to success is watched and noted, and not always with generous eyes. More than most residents of this place, Sizwe must not be quick to fight.

HIS HOUSE HAS two rooms. He and Nwabisa, his lover and the mother of his unborn child, live in one of them. It has a double bed, a wardrobe, and an interminable collection of kitchen utensils. It also contains two very large books that lie on top of each other on the windowsill: a comprehensive edition of the *Roberts' Birds of Southern Africa,* and an Oxford dictionary for second-language English speakers.

Sizwe's English is sound, but some of it he learned alone, in the small hours by paraffin light. His speech sometimes oscillates between the colloquial and the technical, as when he speaks of a neighbor who was kicked by a horse in the testes. English is a weapon he sharpens nightly; he knows that Ithanga and the fate of its people are connected to the larger world, and that he must confront it appropriately armed if he is not to get hurt. Yet he also believes English to be dangerous. Five generations of family lie beneath the ground of this village, and to drift from them would be to drift from himself. Embodied in the vocabulary of this language, he thinks, is a force of great corrosive power, one that has been eating away at the substance of his family since his grandfather's times. Sometimes he believes that in studying English too well he will imbibe its destructiveness, that too much learnedness in the head of an Mpondo man will quite literally drive him insane.

The other room in his house is his spaza shop. A chest-high counter runs across the length of one side, and behind the counter there are shelves from floor to ceiling. They display an eclectic assortment of wares: headache powder, baby food, breakfast cereal, potato crisps, washing detergents, loaves of bread, matches, candles, tins of pilchards and baked beans, a rack of chickens. Everything is tightly packed in an ordered flamboyance.

On the floor, wedged between the shelves and the counter, is a large fridge. It is filled with bottles of beer. It accounts for more than half of Sizwe's income and most of his trouble.

"I am a person who must deal with the difficult side of people," he tells me. "That is my job. That is how I make a living."

Most households in Ithanga are supported either by the state pension of an elderly person, or the meagre wage of a family member working in the tourist industry on the coastline or in the state forests. Those with money to spend are, disproportionately, people in their sixties, seventies, and eighties, since they are the only Ithangans guaranteed an income, courtesy of the state. Old men and women shuffle into Sizwe's spaza shop in the midafternoon, sit on stools drinking stout and listening to Maskanda, a modern form of Zulu folk music, on his hi-fi, then drift away after sunset.

He keeps a hard-backed ledger behind the counter, with the name of a client on the top of each page. The old people buy steadily on credit during the course of the month. On pension payday, each must settle his debt. Some customers drink far too much. They are old and tired and have lived difficult lives, and they come to Sizwe's place to relax. They are not always counting their pennies, and so Sizwe counts for them. He knows each customer, the size of her income and her credit, the number of people her pension supports, whether there is food on her table. For each customer, Sizwe has a credit threshold in his head, a point beyond which he knows she will not be able to pay the debts that she owes him. He tries to pace his customers. He warns them a few days before they reach their limit. He talks them through a plan to stagger their buying. And then he refuses to sell to them.

It is an awkward task. Controlling an elder's purse strings, as if he were a mere child, is a delicate matter. It is particularly delicate if you are young, have stylish dreadlocks, and are wealthier than most of the people who walk through your door. Among the most important tools in Sizwe's repertoire are his mildness, his deference, and his timing: his intuition for extending an act of generosity at the most unexpected times.

His younger customers are more troubling and more difficult to manage, but that is another story.

THERE IS NO electricity here. The fridge in which Sizwe keeps his beer runs on gas. His hi-fi is in fact an old-fashioned car tape player attached to a large battery. He wants to buy another battery, a much larger one, large enough to run a television set. If he did so, his would be the only television in Ithanga. He would have to build a much larger spaza shop to accommodate his customers, he tells me, because everybody would come to watch television. Thus far it is just a thought, and he is reluctant to give it life. If everybody came here, if the young and the old of Ithanga were crammed into a single room, all drinking beer, he would, he believes, be courting disaster. The television set is a thought animated by great ambition. It would make him rich in a matter of months. But in sober moments, he fears he would be inviting catastrophe.

There is also no waterborne sewerage or running water in Ithanga. Fetching water from the river is a woman's job. Sizwe's sister, Lindiwe, does it once every three days. It takes her much of the morning to carry it from the valley basin to Sizwe's hilltop perch; she fills a bucket holding over six gallons and balances it on her head.

Most important, from Sizwe's perspective, is that there are no roads in Ithanga, just scarred and rutted paths that heavily laden four-by-fours negotiate in dry weather. Twice a week, he hires a pickup and is driven to the town center of Lusikisiki about twenty miles away. He goes to the massive wholesale stores on the main street, buys as many goods as can be piled into the back of the pickup, and is driven home. When the ground is hard and dry, the pickup ventures into Ithanga, crosses the river at its lowest point, and makes a slow and perilous journey up the hill to Sizwe's shop. When the ground is wet, the pickup is offloaded at the end of the road on the outskirts of the village; a posse of schoolboys is waiting, and each of them carries Sizwe's wares into the village on his back.

A few months after I met Sizwe it rained for more than a week without respite. The river grew deeper, the current menacing. By the third day, it was not possible to carry anything heavy across the torrent, not even on the backs of schoolboys. The stock on his shelves began to thin. His customers grew irritated. When walking through the village with Sizwe, both of us wearing shin-high Wellingtons and long, shapeless raincoats, his customers would stand in the doorways of their homes and reprimand him.

"Where are my candles?" a woman's voice called through the rain. "Are you trying to humiliate me, making me eat my supper in the dark?"

Sizwe kept his head down. "For you, Granny," he replied dryly, "I will swim to town and back."

Sizwe and Jake

Sizwe is twenty-nine years old. He began growing his hair shortly after his twenty-first birthday. He is not, by my reckoning, a vain person: he is mild and contained—within himself. Yet he has invested a great deal in his dreadlocks and it is common cause that they are beautiful; they are his signature.

"Tell me about your hair," I say. "Tell me a story which says something about what your hair means."

I am driving us away from Ithanga; he is in the passenger seat of my car. He swipes a sideways glance at me and smiles cautiously. I am playing, and he likes to play, but the question is a little invasive: his hair is to be admired, not interrogated. He takes a moment to decide whether to partake in this game. He chooses not to. He chuckles and turns his head away from me and stares out the window into the forest.

He does answer me eventually, though; he does tell me something about the meaning of his hair. Not today, but a few weeks later. And not in response to this question, but to another.

We have been talking about HIV in Ithanga. I ask him whether somebody close to him has died of AIDS.

Again, we are driving, this time back to Ithanga. My voice recorder is on. He takes the microphone and holds it close to his mouth, hunches his shoulders, and grows very serious. He begins to tell me about Jake.

Jake and Sizwe grew up a few hundred yards from each other. They must have played together from their earliest times, yet Jake is strangely absent from the stories Sizwe tells about his boyhood. Jake only begins to appear in Sizwe's stories of his late teens or early twenties, in the mid-1990s.

It was a lean, difficult time for Sizwe, the only time in his life when there were days he went hungry. At their mother's insistence, he and his younger brother, Mfundo, had taken themselves off to school. But the effort they expended to stay there was truly Herculean. Buyisile, their father, was in the midst of his seemingly interminable training to become an igqira, a diviner-healer. Buyisile had no income. School was some twelve miles from home, and the family did not have money for public transportation. On Sundays, Sizwe and Mfundo would dig for sweet potatoes and potatoes and mealies (Indian corn) from their parents' garden until they had filled a sack. They would wake at two o'clock Monday morning and begin the long walk through the forest to school, arriving at daylight.

During the week they lived together in a bare room close to their school on the property of some distant relatives. They would stay there until their mealies and potatoes and sweet potatoes ran out, and then they would walk home to collect more food.

It is into this life that Jake makes his entrance. He does not go to school, but he sometimes arrives outside Sizwe's classroom unannounced. He is there waiting when the school day ends. Jake and Sizwe spend the afternoons and the early evenings hunting for girls. Jake arrives at school prepared; he has done sufficient reconnaissance to keep them busy the rest of the day and night. There is an athletics meeting at Palmerton, and the girls from Dubana will all be there. There is a girl in Malangeni who has invited them over.

Sizwe is not a man to boast of his sexual prowess, but he has agreed to tell me his story, and in the interests of testimony he tells me that he could not possibly count the number of girls he and Jake slept with during that time.

"You were not a shy boy," I say.

"I am very shy," he replies mildly. "I was always very shy. Especially with girls. If the teacher asked me to read in front of the class, I could not do it. If somebody asked my opinion in a room full of girls, I would want to run away."

He is right. There are times I have watched him try to disappear, times he has closed his shoulders together and shrunk.

"But when it came to sex," I say, "you were not shy."

"It's funny," he says. "When you are young, things don't make sense. I was making big sacrifices to go to school. I experienced big pain to stay in school. And I knew why. I knew from early on what it meant to be uneducated. But when I was at school, all I could think of was girls. I was no good at schoolwork. I was confused."

It is 1995, perhaps 1996, and Jake hears some exciting and unexpected news. Ithanga is three miles from the ocean. On the sea cliffs there is a cluster of cottages where rich white people take their holidays. Among them is the wife of a senior executive at a gold mining company. Jake hears that she has arranged for a hundred people from the area to be employed at a mine up in Johannesburg.

It is a gesture filled with pathos. For four generations, the men of Pondoland worked in the gold mines. There is barely a man here over the age of forty who did not spend a considerable period of his life six hundred miles from home in the single-sex hostels on the Witwatersrand. But in the 1980s, the gold mines began to retrench. By the time democracy came to South Africa, the industry's labor force was almost half the size it had been in its heyday. Few of Ithanga's young men go to the mines now. Many find no work at all.

The woman at the holiday cottage is perhaps signaling her acknowledgment that a long history has ended badly. On her vacations, the sea is in front of her, the mud-brick huts of the black people behind her. They once lived off the wages paid by her husband's company. Now young men spend listless afternoons sitting outside the spaza shops. They cover their eyes with cheap sunglasses and they drink one quart of beer after another.

"When Jake heard the news," Sizwe tells me, "the first thing he did, he borrowed a bicycle, went to my parents' house, and told them he wanted to fetch me so that I could register and go to the mines with him. There were people coming from all over the place to be registered. People were coming from as far as Port Saint Johns. The taxis from town were full. Not everyone was going to be employed. You would be lucky to be employed. My mom said no. She said Sizwe must stay in school. No matter we don't have anything, he must stay in school."

Her decisiveness is a story in itself. Hers is a home with barely two coins to rub together. At the mines, Sizwe would earn as much as two thousand rand per month, an income that would bring her family considerable relief. And yet, despite the fact that her grandfather, her father, and her husband chose migrant work over school when they were young, she has read the meaning of the changing times, and her son must stay in school.

Jake goes to the mines alone, and they do not hear from him for nine months. And then, out of the blue, Sizwe and his brother Mfundo arrive home at Ithanga from school one weekend, and he is there. He is smiling from ear to ear. He is very pleased with himself. He is clearly happy. They spend the weekend together, talking through Friday and Saturday night, and he tells them they must miss school on Monday. They must accompany him to town. They demur. They must go to school, they say. No, Jake replies. He is excited. He cannot contain himself. They must accompany him to town.

"So we went to town with him," Sizwe recalls, "and Jake had money because he had been working for nine months, and he went from shop to shop buying things for me and Mfundo."

"What sort of things did he buy you?" I ask.

"All sorts of things. Canned soup and potatoes. A tape recorder. A pair of trousers. Lots and lots of things. All these things were just gifts. He wanted nothing from us. He was working and we were very poor, and he wanted to share. I am so sorry that I did not repay him."

The second time Jake comes home from the mines, he is sick. What started as severe lesions in his crotch has spread to his genitals; they are scarred and they itch incessantly. He has been to see a doctor at the mines. The doctor has prescribed medicine and it had worked for a while and then stopped working. Jake goes to see Buyisile, Sizwe's father. He is a diviner-healer. His father and grandmother were also healers, and they specialized in sexually transmitted infections. Buyisile treats Jake. His medicine helps a little. The scar stops growing. But it does not go away, either.

"The next time he came home," Sizwe recalls, "the scar had started to grow again. And that is how he died. It spread to cover his whole penis, and then his whole crotch. The skin from his penis was peeling off. And in his pubic area, where there should be hairs, there were no hairs. As a black person, he was dark like this." Sizwe holds up his forearm for me to see. "But in his private parts," he continues, pointing at my forearm, "he was white like that."

I try to get Sizwe to mold a chronological narrative, a sequence of symptoms. He begins telling me of the time Jake spent in the hospital, but he has no enthusiasm for my question and soon loses interest in the story he is telling. He is not thinking of sequences. He is thinking of a single moment.

"How did you know it was AIDS?" I ask.

"The whole village thought his uncle had bewitched him," he replies. "Jake had money and could be generous with people. His uncle had no money and could not be generous. He was jealous. And the rash in the crotch—it is a common means of witchcraft. The jealous one slips the *muthi* into Jake's girlfriend's food. The next time Jake has sex with her, he gets the poison. It is especially for him.

"One day, when Jake was very ill, he confided in me. He had gone to a doctor in Port Elizabeth who had taken his blood and told him that he had tested HIV-positive. But the way Jake put it to me was to say that the doctors do not know what is wrong: 'they are saying I am HIV-positive.' He was denying it even while he was saying it."

"How did you respond to this?" I asked.

"He was in big pain. He was crying from the pain. All I could do was calm him. And during the times the pain went away, we would talk about other things, things to take him away from his pain.

"Then there was one time, I think it was a few months before he died, when he finally admitted what was wrong with him. But he did it in a very strange way, in a very sad way. I was sitting and he was lying and he started staring at my hair. There was a different pain in his eyes. Not from his body, but from his mind.

"He said to me, 'You are a rasta. Look at your hair. You are a rasta.'

"I said, 'Yes, I have dreadlocks.'

" 'You are a rasta,' he said. 'Nowadays, the times are bad. Your dreadlocks talk. They say you are looking for girls. They say you are beautiful and you want girls. This hair of yours is attracting girls because you are looking beautiful.'

"I understood what he was saying. He was in trouble. In his mind, his trouble was becoming my trouble. He was so angry. He was so upset. He was looking at me and crying. He was desperate to protect me. He pleaded with me to cut my hair."

"He wanted you to be ugly?"

"He wanted me to be very ugly, to be so ugly that the girls would not want to look at me."

"What did you think of what he said?"

"I felt sad for him. I knew from my side that whether I have beautiful hair or whether I have no hair, if I sleep with girls it is because I have chosen to. And if I don't, it is because I have chosen not to."

A HAPPIER MOMENT in my car. We are driving to or from Ithanga, I don't remember which. This time, the mood is light. There is giggling and laughter. We are giving a lift to a young woman called Phumza. I am practicing my Xhosa on the two locals, particularly the words whose meanings have changed over time, the words that no longer mean what they did in the early-twentieth-century ethnographies I have been reading.

"If I call a middle-aged woman *idikazi*," I say, "will I be insulting her?"

They shriek with laughter. "It will be a very big insult. You will be accusing her of stealing other women's husbands. It is almost like you are saying she is a prostitute."

There is silence for a while. Sizwe is happy. When he is happy, he is playful.

"Do you know the word *isishumane*?" he asks.

"No."

"If I tell you I am *isishumane*," he says, "do you know what I am saying about myself?"

Phumza giggles. "He is insulting himself," she says. "He is saying he has no girlfriend, or maybe just one. He is saying he is too frightened to look for more girlfriends. It is as much an insult for a man to be *isishumane* as for a woman to be *idikazi*."

"I am *isishumane*," Sizwe says. "And I am very proud."

More than five years have passed since Jake died. Sizwe is about to marry. His lover is pregnant with his child. He sleeps with no one else. When Jake was dying he looked into Sizwe's face and saw his own death transported into his friend's body. Sizwe looked into Jake's dying face and saw himself. For a moment in that room, the boundaries between the two men dissolved. Who lay on the bed and who stood up healthy and strong was merely a question of chance. It was an unusual moment, one that embodied an attitude to AIDS that Sizwe would struggle to re-create in time to come. For it is not an easy thing identifying with the dying and the dead. Among our deepest responses to them is an unacknowledged feeling of triumph.

"I did not cut my hair," Sizwe tells me. "But I have been true to Jake. I have tried to cash in on my luck. I hope I am lucky. I hope there is no virus in me."

It sounds clean and simple when he says it, but it is just the beginning of the story. Why he does not know whether the virus is in him is a large tale, a tale about so much.

Testing Day

Jake died in 2000. By the end of 2004, the people of Ithanga had, in whispers and behind closed doors, attributed five other deaths among their ranks to the virus.

"How did you recognize that these people had AIDS?" I asked Sizwe.

"The pimples on the body. The person getting thin. The diarrhea. There is always diarrhea but the stomach is never sore. It runs and it does not stop."

Notably absent from this list are the symptoms of tuberculosis, pneumonia, and cryptococcal meningitis, the most common causes of death among AIDS sufferers in these parts. Ithanga did not yet have sufficient knowledge of the epidemic to recognize it, for many of its symptoms were identical to illnesses the village had known for many generations to be the work of witchcraft. A person who contracted cryptococcal meningitis or suffered from AIDS dementia was said to have had a demon sent to him by an enemy. A person suffering from shingles—a common opportunistic infection triggered by immunodeficiency—was said to have had a witch's snake crawl over her skin while she slept. It was only much later, when people with shingles went to the clinics and the nurses diagnosed their condition as an AIDS-related infection and treated them successfully, that the definition of AIDS in Ithanga began to expand.

Besides, the figure of six deaths surely becomes three or four, or eleven or twelve, depending on one's vantage point. Whether an Ithangan believed that someone had AIDS depended a great deal on his proximity to the sick one. Sizwe knew that Jake had AIDS because they were intimate. Most people in the village believed Jake had been bewitched by his uncle. I would imagine that many AIDS deaths in Ithanga were characterized by similar uncertainties.

THE SIX DEATHS Sizwe had identified remained his formative experience of AIDS until a Saturday morning in early February 2005. On that morning, the Médecins Sans Frontières treatment program came to Ithanga for the first time. By late afternoon, the meaning of the virus in Ithanga had changed forever.

Ithanga is an outlying village, among the most peripheral in Lusikisiki. The nearest clinic is an arduous nine-mile journey. Dr. Hermann Reuter and his staff at the Médecins Sans Frontières office in Lusikisiki's town center believed that the village had been sorely neglected. The program was more than two years old, yet the people of Ithanga knew little about it. A group of MSF counselors visited the local chief to ask his permission to set up a mobile HIV testing center at Ithanga's school. The chief reluctantly gave his consent. MSF lay workers then spread word across the village that they would be staffing a testing center at the school for the duration of the following Saturday. The idea was to bring news of antiretroviral treatment to Ithanga.

This is not the way Sizwe understood what happened that day. When he gave me his account he mentioned neither MSF nor ARVs. Indeed, he studiously refused to discuss ARVs with me until we had known each other a long time. For him, that Saturday had little to do with medicine; it was about shame and fear.

"The whole village knew that people would be coming to test," he told me. "The previous week, the young counselors had been all around the village telling everyone.

"They came the next Saturday to set up their testing center at the school. Many, many people came to test, young people and not such young people. And to know who was positive and who was negative, you just had to stand and watch."

"For what?"

"For how long the people stay. You see, there is counseling before the test, and counseling after the test. The counseling before the test, it's the same for everybody: a few minutes. But the counseling after the test, for some it lasts two minutes, for others, it is a long, long time. They don't come out for maybe half an hour, even an hour. And then you know."

"By the time the day ended, the whole village knew who had tested HIV-positive?"

"The whole village."

"You went to the school to watch, not to test? You went to see who was HIV-positive?"

"No. Not to watch. They said that you could come and learn without being tested. There was a room on the side, and if you went there, somebody would answer all your questions, but you would not have to be tested. That is what I did. I stayed in that room for maybe an hour."

The following morning, the people of Ithanga awoke to a different village. In the course of a few hours, eight or nine healthy, ordinary-looking villagers, most of them young women, had been marked with death.

Such information is not easily absorbed. In the weeks and months that followed, those who had tested positive were silently separated from the rest of the village. They were watched. Nobody told them that they were being watched. Nobody said to their faces that their status was common knowledge. But everything about them was observed in meticulous detail: whether they coughed, or lost weight, or stayed at home ill; whether they boarded a taxi, and if so, whether that taxi was going to the clinic; above all, with whom they slept. These observations were not generous; they issued from a gallery of silent jeerers.

"Not everyone scorns the ones who are HIV-positive," Sizwe pointed out. "Some say they don't care. They say it is the people's disease, just like there is the cattle disease. It is here to kill us, whether we use condoms or not. So let's just live. Everyone must just live until the disease kills us all."

"But others are scornful?" I asked.

"It is a disgrace to be HIV-positive."

"Why?"

We were walking from his father's place to his shop. He stopped in his tracks and glanced at me anxiously. The look in his face was one of acute embarrassment, as if he and his entire milieu had been caught doing something shameful and nasty.

"Is it not a disgrace where you come from?"

"It was considered a disgrace from the very first," I said. "A part of my research is to ask why it is such a disgrace everywhere."

He sighed with relief and started walking again. "Yo! It is very difficult to explain. I am not sure I know how . . . It will come. It is something that will come with your questions. You will see.

"But maybe you can help me," he continues. "We are confused. Is there a cure? Some say there is a cure in Durban. Others say down south."

"To my knowledge there is no cure," I replied. "To my knowledge, the best medicine available is the one they told you about on the day they came to test: antiretrovirals."

He looked at me queryingly. "Yes?"

"They do not cure you of HIV," I continued. "But they stop the virus from multiplying. They keep you reasonably healthy. You need to take the pills twice a day forever, for the rest of your life."

I felt strange giving him this brief. We were having this discussion because MSF had come to Ithanga. He had gone to see the counselors and had spoken with them for a long time. He had clearly heard a great deal about ARVs, yet he acted as if he knew nothing of them.

"Some people say there is a cure in Durban," he said. "But it is a long way to go, and sometimes people talk rubbish."

I tried to swing the discussion back to ARVs. He would not go there. He delicately changed the subject.

It was only much later, when we had known each other a long time, and I had pushed him relentlessly on it, that he told me what he thought of the MSF counselors who came to Ithanga that Saturday morning.

"They reminded me of those religious cults," he said, "of the prophet who comes to the village and says he has seen the light and you must follow him.

"This is how the counselors sounded to me." He stood up and donned the plaintive, high-pitched voice of a Sunday preacher. "I am living with this virus," he said in his shrill, insistent voice. "I am living with this virus and I am healthy, I am strong. With these pills, the virus is dormant inside me. It cannot hurt me now. It cannot make me sick."

He regarded them, not only as a cult, but as a dangerous one. For what they were asking him to do was reveal his HIV status in the public arena of Ithanga.

"What did testing day mean to you?" I asked. "What have you learned from it?"

"That I must never test for HIV in my own village. If I test positive, I would be destroyed."

"How?"

"It would be the end of my business, the end of my future. It would be the same as if my enemies tied me to a chair in front of my shop, and forced me to watch while they took it apart brick by brick, and carried away my merchandise item by item. That is what would happen."

"I HAVE NEVER told you," Sizwe tells me a few days later, "that Jake's family is one day going to lose another son. Last year, Jake's older brother, Xolela, went to test. But he was scared to test here for the same reason I am. He went to a clinic on the other side of Lusikisiki where nobody knows him. He tested positive. He told me and maybe two other people."

"Did they do a CD4 count [a test of the level of immunity in his body]? Does he know when he must start taking drugs?"

"He has not discussed that with me."

"Is he sick?"

"He is often sick."

"Has he been back to the clinic? Will he take drugs?"

"We do not discuss it. But I don't think he went back to the clinic."

"Even when he was sick?"

"We don't discuss it."

A surge of anger bolts from my stomach to my chest, taking me utterly by surprise. I feel my cheeks flush. "You know," I say, "you live in one of the few rural areas in this country where you do not need to die of AIDS. At the clinic, Jake's brother could start attending a support group, he could have his blood tested every six months, and when the time is right, he could start taking drugs. Why don't you discuss this with him? It is a question of life and death."

He does not reply. We are sitting under a tree in an empty field. My car is parked some distance away.

His silence makes me feel foolish. Until now, I have studiously replicated his muteness on the question of treatment. I do not know what it is he refuses to express, and I fear that if I begin to preach, he will forever censor himself in my presence. My outburst is a mistake. I have shut off a channel between us.

His Father's Child

It was not until I learned of the circumstances of Sizwe's childhood that I began to appreciate what an unlikely achievement his spaza shop signified. From the age of six or seven, the odds of him ever learning to read or write, or perform the arithmetic necessary to run a business, began stacking heavily against him. He has lived his current life in defiance of all he could ever have expected. In a place such as Ithanga, such a life is noted and observed, often with envy. A person is not easily forgiven for exceeding meagre expectations.

Once I began to see the visible current of envy that Sizwe saw trailing him in his village, I began to understand his horror at the prospect of testing HIV-positive under the gaze of his peers and neighbors.

SIZWE'S PARENTS HAVE long forgotten precisely when in 1975 he was born; both had little schooling, and Ithanga, then even more than now, resided on the margins of official recordkeeping. He has settled on December 1 as his birthday since his mother tells him she is confident it was in the early summer.

He is the third of five children who survived childhood. The remains of his three siblings who died as infants and toddlers lie in unmarked graves in the corner of his parents' mealie garden, about fifty yards from their kitchen. We pass the three mounds of earth every time we visit Sizwe's parents, and he refers to them in a soft voice as his sisters and his brother. When Buyisile addresses his senior ancestors, he expresses his hope that his three dead children are well cared for and at peace.

Of his living siblings, it is the first of his younger brothers, Mfundo, who dominates his memories of childhood, for the two boys shared the same life and the same fate.

Foremost among the eccentricities they shared was their father, Buyisile. He was unusual primarily because he was there, all the time, throughout the year. In contrast to most of his peers, he stopped mine work after a single spell in Johannesburg, long before Sizwe and Mfundo were born. "Too much alcohol, too many men, too much fighting," Buyisile told me. By profession he was for most of Sizwe's childhood an *inyanga,* an herbalist, following in the tradition of his father and his grandmother. He specialized in treating barrenness in women, sterility in men, and later, in sexually transmitted infections. But his work as an herbalist never earned enough to feed the family, and seldom accounted for the bulk of his time. Around Ithanga, he was known for his physical strength, his deftness with an ox and a plow, and his unsurpassed skill at building homes from mud, cement, and wood.

Here and now, at the beginning of the twenty-first century, South Africa's social diagnosticians have identified the crumbling of the family as our most poisonous legacy. Many would smile benignly at the unusual image of two Mpondo boys and their parents living under the same roof in the early 1980s. The boys occasionally saw it this way, too. But in equal measure, they sometimes wondered whether they had not been cursed.

WHEN THEY FIRST tried to go to school, Sizwe was eight, Mfundo six. It didn't work. From the moment the first seeds were planted in October to the day the last crop was harvested in May, Buyisile's cattle had to be tended. He did not allow his boys to go to school until early winter, almost halfway into the academic year. And then he took them out again just before end-of-year exams because the plowing season had begun and the cattle had to be tended again.

"The teachers knew us," Sizwe recalls. "They knew us as the boys who arrived in May. Everyone else had been in school from January. We were way behind. There was no time to catch up. We must do what the others are doing. And then when it was time to plow, we had to leave again.

"Partly it was because we were quick learners, and partly it was because there were some teachers who were sympathetic, but often, for tests, we were given ten out of ten, when some other children were getting four or five. But there was this other teacher at that time, an old fat mama. When she was handing our test results back, she got to my paper and to Mfundo's, and she stopped and looked at us, and in front of the whole class she said: 'You have done very well in your test, you two boys. But am I proud of you? No. Because when it is time to write exams, you will be gone. It makes me sad to see these good results, because they are going to go to waste.'

"She said this in front of all the other children, and it hurt. But she was talking the truth. We were making this effort to go to school, but why? We would never be able to pass grade one.

"We knew this. We knew our time at school would not last, but it so happened that the way we left was directly because of our father. It was a day in October. My father came to look for us in school. He walked into the classroom, and he said he needed his boys, his boys must come now, there is work for them to do in the fields. After that day, I did not see a classroom again for maybe seven years."

———————————

THE DECISIONS BUYISILE made about his sons were not out of the ordinary for an Mpondo man of his times and circumstances. When he became a young father, a debate had been raging for several generations about what it meant to be an Mpondo in a land ruled by white Christians. And the question of the education of boys lay at the heart of this debate.

During the course of the nineteenth century, in response to the growing presence of Christian missionaries in black society, a new binary opposition arose in the Xhosa and Mpondo languages: the ochre people and the dressed people. The ochre people were so-called because they donned the traditional blankets of the Xhosa and smeared ochre clay on their skins. (They were also known as the *am-*

aqaba, literally, "the smearers.") The "dressed people" abandoned their blankets for European clothes. They were also known as the *amagqo-bhoka,* people who have been pierced through the heart, since their hearts had been pierced by Christianity: they were converts.

The dressed people were vectors of European civilization. Their children were educated in mission schools, and were strictly barred from attending the formal activities of the ochre people's children. They were taught Victorian sexual morality, railed against what they regarded as the scandalous sexual practices of the ochre people's teenagers, and were married by priests. They built rectangular houses, rather than mud huts, and bought European furniture.

For generations, the dressed people's children were made acutely aware of the distinction between themselves and the ochre people. Writing about Pondoland in the early 1930s, the anthropologist Monica Hunter observes: "If when the dogs bark as someone goes past and a child is asked by its parents, who passes, a Christian child will say, if it be a Christian who has passed: '*Ngumntu*' (It is a person); if a pagan: '*Liqaba*' [a smearer of ochre] . . ."

Sizwe's parents both hail from ochre families. Ochre people's sons seldom went to school for longer than two or three years. By the second or third grade, they had abandoned the classroom for their father's fields and for the traditional children and youth associations. These associations were to fascinate anthropologists and historians, primarily because of their autonomy. No adults were present at youth association meetings. Older children inducted younger ones into work, play, fighting, and sexual conduct. Yet, despite the absence of an adult censor, they were remarkably conservative organizations. "The values they preach and largely practise," the anthropologists Iona and Philip Mayer marveled, "are basically the same as their parents' values; they include respect for seniority, preference for 'law' over brute force, and avoidance of pregnancy before marriage. The picture is therefore in sharp contrast to the alleged 'generation gap' of many contemporary cultures."

When Buyisile was a child, to join the youth association was almost synonymous with being an *iqaba* boy in a peasant community. Leaving school and joining the association was not simply an expression of poverty, or a lack of resources. It was an affirmation of a way of life. A boy who attended the association had a narrative of his adulthood carved out for him. He would imbibe Mpondo culture from his youth-elders; meet his future wife at a weekend association party; inherit fields and cattle from his father; begin to run a homestead of productive land; and settle into the life of a peasant patriarch. He would spend much of his adulthood migrating to the mines and thereby earning wages that would be invested in his plow and his livestock. He would live and die on the land of his ancestors; he would sacrifice goats and cows to attend to their well-being; and he would live under their protection.

SIZWE IS DEEPLY invested in living the life of an Mpondo. But when he sees the sort of man into which his father almost made him, he shudders with fear. For by the time he was a boy, the *iqaba* path to adulthood Buyisile had imagined for his sons was dying. The two pillars on which a youth association boy's future rested—mine work and a peasant homestead—were being eroded. Men more forward-looking than Buyisile, men better than he at reading the changing times, were sending their children to school. They knew that in the late twentieth century, an Mpondo boy who could not read and write was doomed.

By the early 1980s, youth associations, once proud bastions of *amaqaba* values, were hollowed out and rotting. The boys who peopled them were drifting into empty and hopeless futures.

"They were wasting their time," Sizwe says when he recalls what the youth associations had become by the time he was old enough to remember them. "They didn't know what they are doing . . . They walked all day to a party of another association in a far away area, and then they fought and died. Maybe they were something better in earlier times. But not when I was a boy. Their life was to walk, to fight, and to die."

If Buyisile had had his way and kept his sons out of school, that is the fate he would have bequeathed to them. It was their mother who saved Sizwe and Mfundo.

A Mother's Boys

In the autumn of 1991, when his elder sons were fifteen and thirteen respectively, Buyisile was offered a job some thirty miles from Ithanga. He would be going to live on site, he told his family, and he would only return home about once a month. The job was to last for between two and three years.

Ironically, his work would consist of building a school and then maintaining it.

Buyisile packed his bag and departed in the early winter of 1991. It was May or June; Sizwe does not remember which.

"The day he left," Sizwe recalls, "my mom came to me and Mfundo and she said: 'You must go to school now.' We refused. It was the middle of the school year. We had bad memories of arriving halfway through the year. But my mom was firm. She said: 'No. You must go. And you must go now. Today. I want you to go to school today.' She forced us, and we went that very day, and we found straightaway that we remembered everything we had learned, even though we had not been in school maybe seven years: it all came back very quickly. And so after a few days we were promoted into the next grade."

That they were older than most of the students in their class did not bother them much; it was not unheard of in Pondoland to find teenagers in the second or third grade. The greater source of embarrassment was that they had neither school uniforms nor shoes. Sizwe had not put on a pair of shoes in his life.

"Twice when I was a boy," he recalls, "I was bitten on the sole of the foot by a night adder. But my feet were hard like shoes. A herd boy does not bathe. He only swims in the ocean. Feet that have walked everywhere and are not softened by washing are hard, hard, hard. The snakes could not bite through the skin. They bit me, but I was okay."

In the first two years after returning to school, the boys spent their afternoons doing the three-mile walk from Ithanga to the ocean, catching crayfish and selling them to the stream of white backpackers who hiked the Pondoland coastline in the summer. With the money they saved, they bought school uniforms, and then shoes. A foot that has never been crammed into a shoe is adorned with impressively splayed toes. Both boys battled to get their feet into size twelves. It took two years before Sizwe's foot would fit into the shoe size he now takes: a nine.

Mfundo's toes never did compact like Sizwe's. He still takes a size twelve. He is shorter than his older brother, his hair cropped close to his skull, his face plain, its expression often a little diffident. The brothers agree today that during their school days Mfundo was the more shy of the two. It was Sizwe who faced the world, with Mfundo following cautiously in his wake.

"Who looked after your dad's cattle while you were at school?" I ask.

"Many different things came together," he replies. "For one, with my dad gone, people no longer brought their cattle to us to be yoked. So there were only his cattle to look after. Sometimes we would swap. Mfundo would go to school one day, and I would herd. The next day I would go to school and he would herd. When we reached standard five [the seventh grade] there was no school for us near Ithanga so we had to go and live somewhere else. That was when my mom started helping herd the cattle. It is not something you see a married woman do, herding cattle, but she would help, so we could go to school. She would run the house, and tend to her vegetable gardens, and she would still find time to help us herd the cattle. She worked herself very, very hard so that she could help us."

"So your dad knows now it was a mistake to choose cattle over education?"

"I don't think so. I don't think he can see that he made a mistake.

When the school-building job was finished and he came to live with us again he thought he had sent us to school. He didn't think my mom had sent us. He thought he had let us. He doesn't understand that we know how we went to school."

So BEGAN SIZWE and Mfundo's time as hungry commuters, the period during which Jake was to appear in the story Sizwe tells of his boyhood: Jake waiting outside the school grounds in the afternoon, having plotted the course of their next seduction; Jake with money in his pockets, taking the penniless boys to town to buy clothes and food.

These were very lean times indeed. Once, walking through the center of Lusikisiki with Sizwe, we came across a woman he had not seen since school. She looked at him with wide eyes: "I hardly recognized you," she said. "You're so fat. When did you become rich?"

He is broad-shouldered and sturdy, but he is not by any reckoning fat. Once the woman had left, I wondered aloud what he had looked like at school.

He laughed: "Mfundo and I were so thin. If I pulled up my shirt and tried to grab some of my stomach in my fist, there would be nothing. There was nothing to grab."

Sizwe and Mfundo must have been among the last of the Mpondos to live almost entirely off what their family grew. If Sizwe is right, Buyisile brought little home from his school-building job. What provisions his mother did buy with Buyisile's remittances were soon spent on the people at home. The way Sizwe remembers it, he and his brother were utterly penniless. When they ran out of food, they walked twelve miles home through the forest, picked the vegetables their mother grew in her garden, and walked through the night back to school.

It is hard to put together a crisp image of Sizwe during this time. He is an assemblage of paradoxes. Staying in school took monomaniacal determination. The boys may have resented spending the summer months chained to their father's cattle, but compared to their days as schoolboys, the time in the fields must have seemed luxurious. Their schoolboy lives were stripped bare.

Sizwe endured years of privation to stay in school, but he did not especially enjoy the work. He was shy, refused to talk in class, and claims that he struggled with his homework. Most of his energy he funneled into sexual conquests. The way he describes it, he and Jake were utterly relentless.

"Mfundo was shy with girls," he recalls. "He never had his own girlfriends. But if you were going to spend time with me and Jake, then life had to be about girlfriends, no matter that you did not have your own. So Mfundo would spend his time finding me girls. That was his job."

One thing that stays with him from this period is this: his young man's testosterone dragged him across the countryside at the very time the HIV virus was invisibly banking itself in the blood of Lusikisiki's sexually active population. What strikes him now is how much pain he suffered to educate himself, and thus how much he sacrificed for the future, and yet, too, how close he unwittingly came to dying young. Jake's wasting away is the undeniable evidence of his own brush with death.

Igqira

B uyisile stayed away for three years. Shortly after he returned, he gathered his wife and children in his rondavel and made an announcement that was to change their lives. He was not well, he said. And he had not been well for a long time. Since early adulthood, he had been afflicted by a combination of physical ailments and dreams. Sometimes the pain was in his head, sometimes it moved to his shoulders, but always, unrelentingly, there was pain in his leg. The more he tried to treat it, the worse it became.

He has known the cause of his illness for some years now: his father's ancestors have been calling him to mediate between themselves and the living, to become an igqira, a diviner. He is by no means the first in his family to receive the calling. His father was called, and used the black medicine to ward off the calling, and both his mother and his mother's father were called, and they all fought it. But he can no longer struggle against it. It is making him ill. He will soon be unable to work. He knows that if he does nothing about it he will die. He must surrender to it. He must begin the extended period of training: he must become an igqira.

The family was bewildered. This had come from out of the blue; they had never known Buyisile to be ill. They spent the following days trying to absorb what he had told them, and when the consequences of his decision had sunk in, they walked silently around the homestead as if in mourning. It was nothing short of a disaster.

The story Buyisile sat his family down to hear was not unfamiliar to them, for it has many of the classic elements of an igqira's tale. The one who is called usually experiences bodily pain. There are no determinate symptoms, but often the sufferer experiences pain in the shoulders, or the sides, or the upper back. The sickness sent by the ancestors is called *inkathazo*, which literally means "trouble." It is pretty much standard that the one who is called will deny that he or she has "trouble," will run from it, will use the "black medicine" to weaken it. Sometimes she will spar with it for many years and eventually shrug it off. For to become an igqira is a burden most do not want. The training is arduous and horribly expensive. And the life of an igqira is not an easy one: you give over your days to an unfathomably complicated array of avoidance rituals, for much of the taken-for-granted detail of daily life is polluting for an igqira and must be skirted. Moreover, your body is no longer entirely your own; it is a receptacle for messages from the departed: you are often sick and drained.

Aside from physical ailment, *inkathazo* is also associated with, although never reducible to, nervous disorder. Most of the *amagqira* I spoke to in the Lusikisiki area told me one can usually recognize the calling in a person by his behavior. Pointing to her trainee, who was sitting alongside her, an igqira from the village of Ntambalala described her novice's behavior when she met him.

"It was most obvious at parties or celebrations," she told me. "He would be sitting in a room where there is entertainment—singing and dancing—and he would go into deep depression. At times he would wander outside and pick things from the dustbin to eat. At other times, you would address him and he would not hear you. He was somewhere else."

This "somewhere else" was somewhere specific. It is understood that these drifting people, present in body but not in spirit, are listening to the *imilozi*—the voices—of their ancestors, "a strange, whistling kind of language," writes the historian Jeff Peires, "that only the privileged [can] understand."

Among the many reasons Buyisile's family was shocked by his announcement is that he never, to their knowledge, displayed any of the symptoms of one who has been called.

"I didn't understand," Sizwe told me. "I didn't understand because he was healthy. He was strong. He was working. He kept on telling us he was sick, but he didn't look sick. He said he was always suffering with his legs, but he was working, riding horses, walking. It did not make sense."

"And his behavior?" I ask. "He was never crazy or . . ."

"No, he was never crazy. But who knows? You never know when somebody becomes crazy. But, no, he never acted crazy."

UPON ACCEPTING THE call, the initiate begins a long process of instruction at the home of an igqira. His training is meant to accomplish two things. The first is the restoration of the initiate's health. The longer he has avoided the call, the more severe are the physical ailments of which he must be cured. Buyisile claimed to have been ducking the call since he was a small boy. He was now in his mid-fifties. The other task of training is to teach the initiate to interpret his spirit-guide well, and to learn to withstand the guide's presence in his body and his mind without going mad. For as a diviner his very being will become a receptacle for the voice of his spirit. To learn to interpret what he is saying is one thing, to keep intact the receptacle one's being has become is another.

From the very beginning, Buyisile's training was troublesome and complicated. He fought with and abandoned one tutor after another. It was to take five years, and a good deal of expense, before his *thwasa*, his coming out. The problem was one of credibility.

"My ancestor had told me I must go through the river," he says, "but my first tutor did not take me to the river, nor the second. You see, there are a lot of charlatans out there. They could not take me through the river because they had not been themselves. They were pretenders. If you have standard six [eighth grade], you cannot take people through matric [twelfth grade] science. That is what some of these people were trying to do to me. I had to go through a lot of things on my own. Luckily, the spirit working with me was clear. I could follow him. I could learn from him without worrying about the charlatans."

Nonetheless, even if he would learn nothing from the "charlatans," he was to invest the better part of his earthly possessions in his training. The average period of instruction is two or three years. The trainee is away from home much of that time, living with and paying his tutor. It is thus a financial and a family ordeal. The initiate sees his family only intermittently, spends a great deal of its resources, and earns none. There are also several ritual sacrifices to be made to the ancestors during training. An initiate can generally expect to slaughter a goat and between two and four cows, the accumulative cost of which can exceed twenty thousand rand.

Between the various tutors Buyisile abandoned, his training lasted five years, and the cattle he was to sacrifice finally numbered six. Throughout their high school careers Mfundo and Sizwe saw their father only fitfully, and usually in the company of groups of *amagqira* and their trainees, who would camp out in their home and live off its meagre resources. They also watched their homestead grow poorer. Very little money was coming in. The stock of cattle that they had sacrificed their schooling to tend to, shrank with each passing year. Finally, on the brink of his graduation, what was left of Buyisile's herd was struck by disease. By the time of his *thwasa* in 2000 he had two head of cattle and no income.

Sizwe and Mfundo began their final year of school in January 2001. Sizwe was twenty-five, Mfundo twenty-three. They came home for the April holidays to find their household battling to put food on its table. Together with their parents, they decided it best that they not return to school. They needed to go out and earn some money. Neither of them would ever complete secondary school.

SIZWE'S RECOLLECTIONS OF how he felt about his father during this period are not what you might expect. He certainly despaired as he watched his family's assets disappear, and he was devastated to be robbed of his final year of school. But these are not the first things that come to mind when he recalls observing his father become an igqira.

"Yes, we were worried about what would happen to us," he says. "But our main worry was him. We were ashamed for him. We did not know what life would be like for him. It is not just that he was going to be a very poor man. When you are training to be an igqira you become like a woman or a child. You do all the things that are supposed to be done by a woman, no matter that you are a man. You have to collect water from the river. That is a woman's job. You have to fetch firewood. That is another woman's job. During your training, you wear a skirt like a woman, and you sit on a mat like a woman. Sometimes you see the novices walking from place to place in their skirts, and carrying their mats under their arms. And when a novice speaks to someone he must kneel down; he must not stand. That is how he shows that he is serving the ancestors. He must kneel down even when he talks to somebody young enough to be his son."

ONE NIGHT, SIZWE and I find ourselves among a group of young people around a fire. The conversation is light and is interspersed with laughter. Someone I have never met before is talking of men who have been ruined by bewitchment, men whose families have descended into penury because a demon has gotten inside their heads and caused them to drift and wonder and lose the capacity to make money and to hold on to family assets.

"The best way to ruin a man," the stranger says at one point, "is to have a demon disguise itself as his ancestor and pretend he is being called. Then he spends all the family's money on his *thwasa* all for nothing. The family is ruined."

I examine Sizwe's face in the firelight. He is expressionless. He does not return my gaze. I cannot help but wonder what he is thinking; he is a son who found his father's ancestral calling inexplicable, and who subsequently watched himself and the rest of his family fall into poverty. The resemblance between his family and the imaginary family in the fireside tale is uncanny.

I do not raise the matter with him, and I am thus not sure whether he identified the story the stranger told as his own. But whether he does or doesn't, the point remains that the tale of how he came to be educated is one in which somebody is vanquished, and the victor must live with the consequences. In the first version, an incompetent patriarch had to be deceived; his wife and children sidestepped his wishes while his back was turned. The achievements of the educated one are thus inseparable from the defeat of his father.

The other version is that Buyisile was bewitched. There is perhaps some virtue in attributing your father's psychological complexities to a malevolent, outside agency. For you close ranks around loved ones; the anger you feel is deflected away from your family. It is far easier to love a bewitched than a failed father.

But there is a price to be paid, and a heavy one at that. If Buyisile's behavior is to be explained by a surreptitious attack against him, then Sizwe himself is equally under attack. For the aim of the conspiracy is not to destroy Buyisile, but his family. And if this is the case, Sizwe's unexpected and unlikely success as a businessman is not a boon, nor a piece of good fortune; it is an act of defiance, a provisional victory in a battle not yet won.

The day the counselors came to Ithanga to test the people for HIV in 2005 was a new event in an old history. The prospect of testing HIV-positive under the gaze of one's neighbors was to hand old foes a new and potent weapon.

A Grandson

Sizwe does not want to live his father's life; he has spent his early adulthood by turns skirting and ruing the obstacles Buyisile has thrown in his path. But that is not to say that he aspires to cast off and forget all that has been passed down to him. On the contrary: he believes his family landed in trouble because it lost touch with the spirits of its forebears. Buyisile's problem was not one of rigid rootedness, but the opposite: he was, Sizwe fears, cast adrift from those who preceded him.

There is a story the Magadlas tell about Sizwe's paternal grandfather, Buyisile's father. His name was Vuyani. He died when Sizwe was eleven or twelve. It is not so much a story as a set piece, told over and again at mealtimes in the family rondavel. And it is not so much about a man with his own character and quiddity as a commentary on the history and fortunes of a family.

The tale is of Vuyani's death and its aftermath. The old man had been ailing for some time; his family had taken him to hospital three times in the preceding months. Finally, he announced that there were to be no more hospitals and no more herbalists. He instructed that he was to be taken to his home; it was understood that he had decided to begin preparing for his death.

Vuyani was a patriarch among patriarchs. He was the oldest of three brothers, husband to five wives, and father of more than a dozen

children. He thus stood at the apex of the Ithanga Magadlas. He was
the one who rooted the family to this piece of ground; he was the
channel through which it sought appeasement and protection from its
forebears. When any Ithanga Magadla reached one of the four transitional points of life that requires ancestral communication—birth, initiation into adulthood, marriage, and death—Vuyani presided over the
sacrificial ritual.

And so the story of the old man's death began well. For a family
leader's passing should not come as a surprise. That he called off the
trips to the hospital, instructed that he be carried to his deathbed:
these things signaled that the patriarch was in control, that he was
laying the ground for the delicate period of transition that would
begin with his demise.

On his first night at home he was struck by fits and convulsions
that came in successive waves until dawn. When his body finally
calmed the family found to its horror that he was speechless. The
whole of the following morning, children, wives, grandchildren, and
neighbors came to his bedside to try to induce him to utter something,
or, at very least, to delay the moment of his death until his voice returned.

At about midday, without warning, the old man suddenly broke
into speech. He summoned his firstborn son to his bedside, and those
assembled around him shook their heads and had to tell him that his
son was not in Ithanga: he was in Natal. Next he called for his firstborn grandson, and was again told that the man in question was not
present.

Knowing that death was approaching fast, and with no family
leader in sight, the old man turned to Buyisile, firstborn son of his
third wife, a very poor substitute indeed for a family leader.

"As from today," he told his son, "you and your siblings are no
longer children. You are old now. At this home you must be united as
my children. If you are united, nothing will get between you. If you are
not united, there is nothing you can solve. My time now is finished."

Buyisile left his father's bedside and walked alone into the countryside to weep. When he returned, he was informed that the patriarch
was dead.

The calling of the firstborn son and the grandson must have been
placed in the deathbed scene retrospectively. For everybody knew that
Vuyani's heirs were not in Pondoland. Both had been lured north to

KwaZulu by the *ama-Nazaretha,* the great Zionist church movement founded in the early twentieth century by the Zulu prophet Isaiah Shembe. Shembe's people believed that their prophet and his successors had been instructed in the ways of purity by Jehovah himself; they lived in exclusive villages of the faithful, and believed the rest of the world to be fatally polluted. Indeed, Nazarethites have at times refused to shake the hands of outsiders, for fear of contamination.

As far as Vuyani the old Mpondo patriarch was concerned, his firstborn son and grandson had torn themselves from their roots; they had no interest in their home ground, and had lost the knowledge required for ritual communication with their ancestors. When the old man died, the community of living Magadlas was left without a family leader and was thus cast adrift to wander alone, unseen and unprotected by the dead.

Vuyani was buried in the absence of his firstborn. The trouble began before his corpse had settled into its grave. Minutes after the body had been lowered into the ground, the older of Vuyani's two younger brothers collapsed in a fit of uncontrollable coughing. He was rushed to hospital, stabilized, and taken home. Days later, he fell ill once more, and the family hired a car to take him to Kokstad, site of the best hospital in the region. He died the following week.

A year later, Vuyani's first wife, the mother of the very man who should have been leading the family but was praying with Shembe's people, fell ill. She too went to the hospital, back and forth, back and forth, and finally died some months later. Her son came back from Shembe's place to bury her, his first appearance in Ithanga since his father had been alive.

The following year, the younger of Vuyani's brothers fell ill and died. Some twenty months had passed since the patriarch's death, and his entire generation but one had been wiped from the planet. The only person left among his brothers and wives was Buyisile's mother, a sharp-tongued and bad-tempered old woman who still lives today.

"My grandfather predicted that this would happen," Sizwe tells me. "He said that when he dies they will follow him."

"That makes their deaths all the more mysterious," I comment. "It means that his anger and his spite may have been the cause of their deaths."

"That's not impossible. It can happen that he grabbed them as he went. When someone dies, you are never sure why. There are many possible reasons. But the interpretation the family has settled on is that they died because my grandfather was the only one who could appease the ancestors. He was the only one who understood how to do the ritual sacrifices properly. When he died, the family was left unprotected."

"You say that is the family's interpretation," I reply. "Is it yours, too?"

He does not answer for some time. We are at the summit of one of Ithanga's highest hills, looking down into the village. He plucks a blade of long, straw-colored grass and twirls it around his fingers.

"When my father was making some very difficult decisions in his life," he says, "decisions that affected us all, I wonder: Was my grandfather there? Was he advising? Or was his spirit no longer in this village? I cannot answer those questions. I don't know."

A Gangster

That a person makes his own luck is both jarringly clichéd and largely right. The origin of Sizwe's success was undoubtedly a smile from the gods, but what he did with that smile was marked with his character.

Some two or three years before I met him, Sizwe heard that a group of serious bird-watchers had hired a cluster of cottages on the coast some two hours' walk from Ithanga. He set out before dawn one morning, found them at home eating breakfast, asked them which birds they were looking for, and told them he knew Pondoland's forests and its animals as well as a human being can.

They hired him, and within the few hours it took to correlate the Xhosa names of birds against their Latin classifications, they were seduced. He had in his head a taxonomy of every bird in the forest. He could identify each by its colorings, its call, and by its feeding and nesting. He had never opened a bird book in his life. The party of birders believed they had found themselves in Eden with Adam as their guide.

During their many hours together, the enchanting young man spoke of his plans. He said he had hopes of running a taxi one day, or maybe opening a spaza shop. He was as smitten with the bird-watchers as they were with him. This was the closest he had ever been to white people. Among all the things whites meant to him, they were members of a foreign culture and thus represented the breadth of the world. He could fire question after question at them about their lives, and they replied with enthusiasm.

They returned to the Pondoland coastline a year later with a hardback copy of the latest *Roberts' Birds* guide, and with another, much larger gift. They had clubbed together and raised money, a lot of money, enough to build an extension to his home, and to fill its shelves with goods. Their gift was nothing less than the beginnings of a spaza shop. He returned to their cottage each day for several days, and together they wrote a business plan and discussed how best to reinvest profits, how to avoid debt.

He has his mother to thank. It is due to her that he is literate and numerate, and thus capable of running a shop at all. But he also has his own intuition to thank: his certain knowledge that his father was facing backward, that his future would always lie with reading and writing and a knowledge of English, with engagement with the world outside.

There was a final piece of luck, and it was less of his making. For all the joblessness in Ithanga, the absence of roads, lights, and running water, it remains true that Sizwe was fortunate to come of age during the infancy of his country's democracy. In 1999, South Africa's five-year-old government began plowing money into social welfare grants and old-age pensions, and this is precisely the money that found its way to the plastic box behind his counter. I doubt he could have started his shop in the mid- or late 1990s: the village could hardly have supported it.

———————

IT IS AN unseasonably cold and very wet morning in mid-November 2005. A regular customer of Sizwe's died during the week: it is necessary that he attend the funeral. He has lent me his spare raincoat and Wellingtons, and we are making a slow, mud-churned course to the burial site.

The dead man is from a village six miles away, a place entirely devoid of modern infrastructure. At about eight o'clock the previous night, a hearse delivered the dead man's body to the end of the public road on the outskirts of Ithanga. Four men were waiting to receive it in the howling rain. They transferred the coffin from the hearse to a sled, strung the sled across the backs of two oxen, and began making their way through the pitch dark, up and down ridges and over a stream, to the dead man's home. They arrived at their destination long after midnight.

Now, the following morning, we retrace the corpse's journey, and the mood is light. We are among a party of some dozen or so Ithangans, most of whom drink at Sizwe's shop. The group has split into twos and threes, and we are followed by the sounds of the conversation of those behind us. I have brought along a stranger, a young woman named Nomalanga from a village some distance away, whom I have employed as an interpreter.

We arrive at the bank of a normally shallow stream, but the hours of unremitting rain have brought it to life. We sit on the bank, pull our Wellingtons off our feet, and roll our trousers halfway up our thighs. Sizwe is lazy. He has taken off only one Wellington and is hopping across the stream on one leg. He loses his balance, his clothed leg is suddenly thigh-deep in water, and he stands there foolishly in the middle of the stream cursing under his breath. From the bank, I chuckle unapologetically. He looks around in surprise. He is wounded; he has not expected anyone to see slapstick in his misfortune.

It is now my turn to cross the stream, and Sizwe and Nomalanga make for an ungenerous audience on the far bank. She is talking to him about me in Xhosa. "People think I am his wife," she says. "I feel so watched and so judged I want to crawl under a bush."

I have understood her, and I smile to myself, and Sizwe watches me smiling to myself.

"You are *imenemene*," he shouts from the bank. "Do you know what is *imenemene*?"

I shake my head.

"There is no word for *imenemene* in English," he continues. "Maybe the closest word is *spy*. But *spy* is still not right. *Imenemene* is one who pretends not to understand, but he does. And then he goes and uses that information at your expense. Or he laughs at you privately." He looks down at his wet foot and his dry foot and grins broadly. "I have caught you being *imenemene*."

I look at his face closely to see whether there is any ambiguity there; given what I am doing here in his life, his observation is not uncomplicated. But there is nothing in his expression, just pleasure. He is smiling generously and happily; he is enjoying strolling through the rain and getting wet; he is on his way to pay his respects to a man who walked twelve miles every day to drink his beer.

THE FUNERAL IS held under the shelter of a large tent, and is dominated by a man who is the archetype of the fervent lay preacher. He wears an old, stained suit and speaks in sharp bursts, a limitless pile of thin parables volleyed at his audience in quick succession.

"A man who becomes sanguine about his dogs will be bitten," he shouts in Xhosa. "The dog of a complacent man will be faithful for five years and then turn around and bite."

After the service, the congregation files into a large, windowless rondavel, and in the semidarkness we are served plates of meat and beans, and buckets of maize beer. Sizwe's youngest sister, Yandiswa, lives in this village, and she has given him her six-month-old son to hold. The boy is entranced by the dancing of Sizwe's dreadlocks. He swipes at them with clumsy fists each time they flash past his nose, and, eventually, he gets his timing right: he finds his fist full of locks and he pulls for all he's worth. As Sizwe's face draws closer to his, he shrieks and lets go. Sizwe keeps his face close and giggles. "*Mubi wena*," he says. "You are ugly."

My eyes meet those of a young man sitting halfway across the room. Momentarily, we are locked in one another's gaze. He smiles at me and doffs his cloth cap. I am immediately aware that I am to write about him, for he carries himself with a charisma so extraordinary that he appears for a moment to be the only living being in the room, the remainder mere cardboard figures or stage props, there to round out his presence.

When he leaves the rondavel, I follow him, introduce myself, and hold out my hand.

"I know you," he laughs. "I have seen you walking around with your friend Sizwe. I am also from Ithanga. My name is Simlindile."

"I'm surprised I've never seen you," I say.

"I live on the other side of Ithanga," he says, laughing once more. "So it is not so strange that I have seen you while you have not seen me. In any case, I am a native; I blend in. You," he chuckles, "you are . . . well, you stick out."

His English is polished, his accent not of this place. It is not just urban, it is middle class: it belongs to a man in a good suit and a tie.

He is wearing a dull tweed jacket over a black turtleneck sweater. His jacket is fastened, and there is a button missing, in its place a thick safety pin. On his face and in his demeanor there is something I recognize, something I have seen many times before. It is a time-honed screen that bars you from the thoughts he is thinking about you. You are not to know whether you hold any interest to him, but you do know that he has done the necessary calculations: he is not a man given to bouts of spontaneity.

We are joined by Sizwe and others, and it is soon time to leave. We do so in a large party, perhaps thirty in all, including Sizwe's mother, and as we begin walking I notice that Simlindile is not among us.

"How old is he?" I ask Sizwe.

"He is younger than me. Twenty-four maybe. Perhaps twenty-five."

"Where did he learn his English?"

"He worked at a big tourist resort down south," he replied, "far south, out of Pondoland. He was there I think four years. He knows whites very well. He can make them feel comfortable."

"What does he do now?" I ask.

He shrugs and smiles at me. "What do people do in Ithanga?"

THE FOLLOWING DAY, a Sunday, Sizwe and I spend the afternoon in town. We return to Ithanga in the twilight. Two taxis are unloading their passengers at the end of the public road, and the early evening is filled with figures making slow progress up the hill into the village. Sizwe approaches an elderly woman. She is negotiating with a taxi driver, two suitcases beside her and a large bundle over her shoulder.

"You must visit us often," Sizwe says enthusiastically. He is warm and attentive. "We are going to miss you. I do not want to bump into you in town. I want to see you here. You must come."

She laughs and thanks him and says she will miss him, too. We say good-bye and begin climbing the hill into the village. It is very beautiful at this time of day. The hilltops catch the dying light and are crisp and well formed. But the valley bottom shimmers and blurs; one cannot make out distinct objects, only color: it is yellow and orange, and there are still traces of the late afternoon's warm beige.

"Who is the old woman?" I ask.

"She is a customer of mine. She has been coming to drink since the day I opened."

"Why is she leaving?"

"Because of the gangsters. She has been robbed twice."

He points to a hilltop on our right. It is among the highest in the village and is particularly steep. A solitary round hut sits incongruously near the summit. It appears as if its inhabitants might open their front door, step outside, and roll down the hill.

"That is her home. It is very isolated at night. Twice, on the night after pension day, very late, maybe one in the morning, they have knocked on her door, and when she opened they pointed a gun at her. After the second time, she said enough is enough. She has gone to live with relatives in Holy Cross."

"It was boys from Ithanga?" I ask.

"Yes."

"She knows them?"

"Yes. She won't say who they are. She is afraid they will shoot her if she says who they are."

I think of what he has said for a while. We are walking along the side of the valley basin now, and Sizwe's home is high above us.

"But, really," I say, "the whole village must know who these boys are. They are surely boys who have grown up here, who peed in the river when they were children."

"Yes," he says.

"And their fathers cannot stop them?"

He laughs dryly. "Tomorrow I will take you around the village. We will go to each homestead and see who is doing building extensions. At the end, you will read me your list, and I will tell you that the son of each person on your list is a gangster."

"Are you scared of them?" I ask.

"I am very scared. But so far they only go for old women, for women pensioners who live alone."

WE ARRIVE AT Sizwe's place, take two chairs from his room, and sit in front of his small house, watching the early evening life in the valley below us. I have known Sizwe for six weeks now, and I have still not met

Nwabisa, his wife-to-be. She works some two hours' walk from here—cleaning and house maintenance in the very cottages where Sizwe met his birders—and she leaves at dawn each morning and returns after dusk. This weekend she has gone to visit her family in a village some distance away, and is only returning tomorrow morning.

I am still thinking of our conversation on our journey from the public road.

"The man I met at the funeral," I ask. "What does he do for a living?"

"Who?"

"Simlindile."

He smiles at me broadly. "Do you know what Simlindile said to me about you last night? He said he thinks your shoes are very expensive. That is what he noticed about you."

"He's . . ."

"He is the biggest gangster in Ithanga. It is him who is responsible for my customer running away. He would not have done it himself. He would have sent some younger boys. He would have lent them a gun."

"He does the bigger stuff," I suggest.

"He knows criminals from all around the area. And he knows big criminals from Durban. He has spent time there. A spaza shop like mine, he can tell criminals from Durban, show them where to go. They come at night with their guns, shortly before the shop is closing. They tell all the customers to get down. Then they go to the owner and they demand money. If he resists, they shoot him."

I ask if this has happened before in Ithanga, and he says no, never in Ithanga, but in other villages around here, and that it is a question of time.

"Your place is very exposed," I say. "There is no fence, no entrance."

"I need a gun," he replies. "If people walk in while I am behind the counter, there is nothing I can do. But if somebody knocks on the door at midnight after pension day, while I am sleeping, then a gun is useful. Then I can protect myself. I am scared to buy one: if the police come and find I have no license for it I will go to jail. In the meantime, what I do is, a customer of mine has an old shotgun. I borrow it from him every pension day, and then I give it back to him after I have put my money in the bank. It only takes one bullet at a time. It is very slow."

He pauses and looks at me severely. Quite spontaneously, we both begin to laugh. We have, I believe, the same image in our heads, of Sizwe taking an old and unwieldy gun and blowing a hole through his front door into the empty night.

I turn from the view into the valley, which is almost dark now, and look at Sizwe's home. In the context of our discussion, it now has an air of vulnerability about it. It is not just its humble size. In a broader sense, it is a place of transition, a kind of no-man's-land. With Sizwe no longer in his parents' homestead and not yet in a homestead of his own, his two-roomed mud house—his "flat," as he calls it—is the most visible sign of his transitory status. In a few years, his business will have taken solid root, there will be children about the place, and he will have built a rondavel and another bedroom. But for now that is just a trajectory, an imagined future. His two simple rooms index the fact that he has not yet arrived.

What comes to me as I look at his home is not so much an image as a sense, a feeling under the skin. It is the night after pension day, I imagine. Under his roof lies several thousand rand in cash that he has collected from his customers during the course of the day, waiting to be banked the following morning. He bolts the door, turns off the light, and he and Nwabisa settle into bed. But they are uneasy. They do not sleep well.

Those they fear are familiar to them: people they see every day, people, indeed, with whom Sizwe has shared a life since childhood. What frightens them is not just the gun that may be pointed in their faces, but the intent of the one with his finger on the trigger. To be held up at gunpoint by someone you know, or on the instruction of someone you know, is to be invaded in the most exquisitely intimate fashion. Your perpetrator wants more than the money under your bed. He wants something more personal than that. He envies you, resents you; he wants to ruin you.

It strikes me that Sizwe's tale is as much metaphoric as literal. He does of course have a specific fear that a specific villager will orchestrate an armed robbery at his home on the night after pension day. But Simlindile stands in for all the watching eyes he believes envy him, and the gun for all the countless instruments of destruction envy may deploy. He fears that he has broken a silent rule: becoming a success in the midst of a generation that is failing has been disallowed.

Fears such as these, I am thinking, lie in a border zone. It is difficult to judge how much they are the product of an objective assess-

ment of an external threat, and how much they are generated by
internal demons. As I am thinking these thoughts, Sizwe begins to tell
me a story. He began building his flat about a year ago, he says. He
rented a wheelbarrow, handed it to a group of children, and paid them
to collect mud from the river. With the mud, he started building bricks.
During the same period, Simlindile announced that he too would
begin construction on a flat; he marked out a space next to his father's
homestead at the other end of Ithanga.

Around this time of flat building, one of the bird-watchers who
had given Sizwe his wonderful gift, a man named Graeme, appeared in
Ithanga brimming with his own ideas about construction. He wanted
to build a cluster of cottages right here, just outside the village. No
roads, no electricity, no one about except unobtrusive black villagers:
there is a pedigree of tourist, he said, who would pay dearly for that.
He wanted Sizwe to manage the cottages in exchange for a share—a
large share—of the earnings.

"He came and he spoke," Sizwe tells me, "and then he came back
again with a builder, a colored man called Terence who we in Ithanga
knew. Graeme came with Terence, and all the people in the village saw
him walking to my place, and everyone, including Simlindile, gathered
around. Whites don't understand that you must not talk about things
in front of people, and he started talking about his plans.

"Simlindile came up to Graeme and introduced himself. He was
very charming. He spoke perfect English. He said he had a car. He said
he could run a service bringing the tourists from Port Saint Johns, or
from the airport at Mthatha. Graeme was very impressed. I said nothing. But I watched Terence, the builder, and he watched me, and we
were both thinking the same thing. Terence knows Simlindile.

"Graeme did not come back so much after that. I'm sure that as
soon as they walked off together, Terence told Graeme all about Simlindile. Graeme never said he had changed his mind, but he had. Because he had learned about the gangster boys in Ithanga, and he knew
this was not a place where you can build cottages.

"In any case, Graeme came that day with Terence, and the very
next morning Simlindile came to me and he said: 'With this Graeme
helping you, you do not need your bricks.' I said to him, 'No, you are
talking nonsense, you cannot have my bricks.' He kept on speaking
about it for a long time. And then he stopped speaking about it. After
that, my bricks started to disappear. I went to talk to Simlindile's father

about it. I went to talk to the headman about it. The bricks kept disappearing. Then I thought, no, if I am going to build my own place, and if I'm going to run a spaza shop, I need proper protection. That is when I did a very long trip, to a famous man who lives near East London, to buy muthi, traditional medicine, to protect my place."

Listening to Sizwe, I marvel at the clarity and the simplicity of his relationship with Simlindile. Sizwe begins building a new life outside his father's homestead, and Simlindile literally steals the bricks. The prospect of a business venture comes Sizwe's way, and Simlindile destroys it. In the narrative Sizwe weaves, Simlindile is not merely a greedy man, not merely an obstructive man: he is pure envy; he sniffs out budding success in the village, and he destroys it.

Another Shop

Very early one morning in April 2006, I set off from the room I had rented in Lusikisiki and headed for Ithanga. On the outskirts of the village, my mind having wandered far away, the voices on the car radio long expelled from my consciousness, I came across a scene so out of the ordinary I slowed down and watched. Some fifty paces from the side of the dust road, a procession of a dozen or so people had assembled at the base of a steep hill, and were preparing to make an ascent. They were solemn and stony-faced. One or two turned their heads briefly to look at my car and then ignored me. The postdawn light lent the scene an exaggerated stillness, as if the landscape itself had prepared for the occasion.

At the center of the group was a man who was clearly very ill. He was swathed in blankets and could not stand on his own feet. Two young men supported him, his armpits hitched over their respective shoulders. As the procession moved, opening a gap through which I could see the threesome unobstructed, it was apparent that they were in fact carrying him; his feet did not touch the ground. One of the young men carrying the sick one was Simlindile. His brow was creased, the expression on his face entirely blank. I also recognized Charlie, Simlindile's father, whom I had met only once before.

At the rear of the procession were an old man and a goat. The animal was reluctant. It strained at the rope around its neck. The old man heaved, throwing his entire body into the task, and the goat, like the sick man, was carted up the hill.

OVER BREAKFAST, I described to Sizwe what I had seen.

"It is a ritual for Simlindile's cousin," he explained. "He lives in East London. They have especially brought him back to Ithanga, to his ancestors, to perform this ritual for him. They are slaughtering a goat up on the hill."

"What is the matter with him?"

"It is believed that the problem is his late wife. She died last year. No sacrifice was made for her after she died. He went on to a new wife, and made no sacrifice for his old wife. There is a belief that if no sacrifice is made for the dead one, her spirit remains trapped. She cannot go to the other world. She possesses her husband and makes him ill."

"What are his symptoms?" I asked.

"I saw him yesterday when he arrived. I know that this man has AIDS. I can see it in the way he is sick. His stomach is running all the time. It does not stop. And there is no pain in the stomach. And he has lost too much weight. He is going to die any day from now.

"Brian has no father. His uncle, Charlie, Simlindile's father, he is the one who must make decisions about Brian's treatment. Charlie says nothing about AIDS. I think he knows, but he says nothing. I do not think it is right. They must talk about what's really the matter."

BRIAN DIED IN his home in East London some three weeks after the ceremony on the hill. His body was brought back to Ithanga in a trailer, attached to a hired four-by-four. He was buried on the grounds of his ancestral homestead.

The hired vehicle that brought his remains back to Ithanga also carried his wife. She too was very ill, so much so that she was unable to return home after the funeral. A sickbed was made for her in Charlie's house, and she stayed some ten days, until Charlie finally took her back to East London. I followed these proceedings vaguely and from a distance; I was not at all close to the family, and knew no more than anyone in Ithanga might.

In late June, some nine weeks after Brian's death, I returned to Ithanga after a month's absence. I parked my car where the road ends, and climbed the hill into the village. A new structure stood in the right-hand corner of the clearing at the top of the hill. It was a simple wooden hut, no bigger than a child's treehouse. The front façade had neither a window nor a door, but a large rectangular hole, beginning at waist height and extending across the breadth of the hut, like the space through which a mobile ice cream vendor serves his customers.

As I walked closer, it became apparent that the hut was indeed a shop. A kwaito song—kwaito being South Africa's homegrown equivalent of hip hop—blared from poor speakers, the sound grating and tinny. Clusters of people were dispersed around, some leaning against the wall, others sitting on the grass, most clutching bottles of beer.

A joyous voice shouted my name, and an arm waved furiously at me from inside the hut. As I approached, I saw that it was Simlindile. He threw his hands above his head, clamped them onto something outside my line of vision, hoisted himself through the hole in his front façade, and dropped lightly onto the grass outside.

He put his arm around me. His heart was beating fast and he smelled of fresh sweat.

"Check out my new place, boet [brother]," he shouted, turning me to face his hut squarely. "And check out the people. This is business. Your friend Simlindile is a businessman, a serious businessman."

His performance had attracted the attention of his customers, and people glanced at us and laughed. He laughed back, took his arm off my shoulder, pushed himself away from me, grabbed the roof of his hut, and launched himself back over the counter.

The watchful and deliberate man I had met at the funeral some months earlier had been transformed into something utterly different. He was ebullient, outside his skin, drenched in an uncontained celebration.

It was a chilly, midwinter day, but he wore jeans and a vest, as if his powerful shoulders were part of the prize, as if they went with the new spaza shop.

He leaned on his counter, pointed to a piece of flat ground some hundred yards away where two small children were playing, and whistled to them.

"My children! My children!" he declared with mock earnestness.

"They *are* his children," a woman standing next to me commented. "Their mother was one of his girlfriends until last year."

"My children!" Simlindile cried out again. "Everywhere I look, my children!"

"How many do you have?" I asked.

"In Ithanga he has three," the woman replied on his behalf.

"Three?" Simlindile laughed. "No, man, not just three! I am a playboy. I play without condoms. A playboy does not have three children." He jumped onto his counter and poked his head out, scanning the entire village with his gaze. "My children are everywhere."

"WHAT DO YOU think of the new competition?" I asked Sizwe cautiously when I saw him.

"It is not competition," he replied dryly. "None of my customers come from that side of the village. In any case, the danger is to you, not me. I would not advise you to spend too much time at that shop. Something terrible is going to happen there."

"Why?"

"There are two reasons. First, because that hut was built by a man called Stars, and the things he builds fall down."

I looked carefully at the wall on my right, which Stars had erected after Sizwe grew tired of building his own house. It seemed quite stable.

"And the second," he continued, "is that the spirit of Brian is going to do something horrible to that shop. The spirit of Brian is very angry with that shop."

Brian, I discovered during the course of the day, was the third spaza shop owner in this story. Only his shop in East London was far grander than anything Sizwe or Simlindile could ever hope for. He drove a BMW and lived in a four-roomed house.

When Charlie took Brian's ailing widow home, Simlindile went with him. The two of them moved into the dead man's house and began selling off his assets one by one. They began with his car, and then moved on to the stock on his shelves. The winding up took less than a week. They left Brian's widow with some cash, took the difference back with them to Ithanga, and used it to open Simlindile's spaza shop. A fine inheritance indeed.

"Brian had two small children," Sizwe told me, "children who will soon be orphans. Whether they are being looked after, I don't know. Did Charlie make sure they are still in school and in a good home? I don't know. I think that Brian's spirit is very, very angry."

Brian's story was the first I heard, and perhaps the first Sizwe heard, too, of a rich Ithanga man dying of AIDS. His family jostled to be the ones closest to him at the time of his death. And then the flesh on his corpse was there for the eating.

WALKING INTO ITHANGA the following morning I heard a child's light footfalls and panting breath on the path behind me. I turned to find I was being tailed by a young boy. He closed the distance between us and danced around me on swift feet, his eyes trained on the ground, guiding his bare soles from the sharp-edged stones and half-submerged rocks that littered the path.

"Why do you come here?" he asked in English. His voice was surprisingly deep, his accent so thick I had trouble understanding him.

"What?"

"What are you doing here?"

"I'm coming to visit Sizwe Magadla," I said.

"I know. But why? Are you the owner of his shop?"

His eyes still glued to the path, there was in the tone of his questions a doggedness, a single-minded urgency.

"No," I replied. "I'm here doing research. I'm writing a book."

"But you are here to see that Sizwe is running your shop nice and proper," he persisted.

"No."

"So you do not own the shop?"

"No."

He stopped dancing and fell in step with me, his neck bowed, his eyes watching his feet. We walked this way in silence for some time.

"It's not yours?" he asked.

"No."

He veered off the path, turned around, and walked slowly back to where we had come from.

WHEN I ARRIVED at his home, I told Sizwe of my encounter.

"What did you say?" he asked eagerly. "Did you say it was your shop?"

"I didn't."

He smiled with resignation. His disappointment was as palpable as its expression was polite.

"You like people to think the shop is mine?" I asked.

"Of course I like. It means they think I'm not such a big man. They think I'm just a stupid someone working for the rich *umlungu*."

"I should have told them I pay you nine hundred rand a month," I said.

"You should have said seven hundred and fifty rand. Even less than the old-age pensioners."

"How long have you known about this rumor?"

"A month, maybe. Three weeks. It is a big rumor." He waved an arm in the direction from which I'd come. "Everybody from that part of the village, from where you park your car right up to the river, they are suspecting that I work for you."

LATER THAT WEEK, as I drove away from Ithanga in the early evening, Simlindile's father, Charlie, flagged me down and asked me for a lift to the next village.

I did not know how to deal with Charlie. I had met him just once before. He was not much younger than my father, yet he called me "baas" and cocked his head solicitously when I spoke. The manner of the high apartheid houseboy is bizarrely out of place here; I stared at him incredulously, made my excuses, and walked away.

"*Ninjane, Tata?*" I asked now. "How are you, father?"

"Not good, not good," he replied in English. "Last month, we buried my nephew from East London. We buried him up there at his late father's place."

"I heard," I said. "I'm sorry."

"There were seven of them in that family: seven brothers and sisters. Now they are three. Three left out of seven. It is terrible. Three left out of seven."

I began to say something, but his volley of words was uninterruptible.

"It was AIDS. And his wife is sick, also with AIDS. We will be burying her also, her also, not so long from now. With AIDS, you must talk early. Then they can help you. If you talk early. He did not. He said nothing. He should have known, if it is AIDS, you talk early, and then they can help you. But he said nothing. We could not help him."

Thandeka

I arrive at Sizwe's place early on a mid-December morning with a proposition. It is shortly before Christmas 2005, some six or seven months before Simlindile is to acquire his spaza shop. I have told Sizwe on the phone that I am coming, that I am making a special trip to Lusikisiki to ask something of him. When I arrive he is standing outside his front door waiting for me, his arms stiffly folded, his expression serious. He invites me inside, ushers me into a chair, sits opposite me, and waits for me to speak. The bed is freshly made, the room quiet. Once again, Nwabisa is not here; she left for work nearly an hour before I arrived.

During the course of the next year, I plan to visit several of Lusikisiki's clinics to write about Médecins Sans Frontières's antiretroviral treatment program. I ask Sizwe to accompany me. I want to employ him as my interpreter. I could use someone else, I tell him, but I want him for a specific reason: he is, if he agrees to it, to be something of an interpreter-subject. He has already agreed that I write about him and the place of AIDS in his life. Now I am proposing that I write something of a travelogue, a story about him and me discovering the treatment program together. I tell him that I will pay him a daily rate for his time, and that we will be traveling together for about sixty days over the course of the year.

"I don't know if you can afford the time away from your business," I say, "but I guess that's something for you to judge."

He replies the instant I have finished speaking: "I will do it."

"That was quick. You're sure you don't . . ."

"Yes, I'm sure. I will worry about my business when I am with you; my sister is not very good at looking after it alone. But the benefit to my business is greater. I will invest the money I get from working with you in the business. It will be good for my business."

"And how do you feel about the fact that you will be more than an interpreter, that I will be writing about the things you think and say about the treatment program?"

"You are already writing about what I think about AIDS," he replies.

I am trying to grasp the source of his decisiveness. He watches me closely and appears to sense what I am thinking.

"I have personal reasons for wanting to do this," he says. "There is a cousin of my father's from Durban. He is very sick."

"How will your going to the clinics with me help him?"

He begins to say something, then stops. He is silent for a while.

"There is a secret," he says, "a secret most members of my family, including my father, do not know about. A few months ago, my niece Thandeka tested HIV-positive."

"Where does she live?"

"In the next village. You have met her, but you don't remember her."

"She is not yet sick?"

"No."

"She tested here?"

"Yes."

"They would have taken her CD4 count, to know how soon to start with the drugs."

He shrugs.

"Has she been back to the clinic?" I ask.

"No. I don't know. She has told me and my mom, and no one else. Now I must help her decide what to do. I am trying to urge her to tell her mother. She does not want to. I must respect her. I must help them both decide what to do."

"Why did she test?"

"She went to the clinic for other reasons. When she got to the clinic, she was encouraged to test. But now it is for me to help her to decide what to do. So I am happy to come with you to the clinic. It will help me."

"Are you close to Thandeka?"

"Very close. I describe her to you as my niece, but really she is more like a daughter, or a young sister. I am the one who has been caring for her. Until just before I met you, she lived at my place."

"Why?" I ask. "What is her story?"

"She is the daughter of my older sister, Nosipho. When Nosipho was seventeen, maybe eighteen, she married a man near here. They split up after two, maybe three years. I am not sure what was the cause. Nosipho now had no husband's home, and her own father's home was very poor, so she went up to KwaZulu-Natal to look for work. Instead of work, she found a Zulu man. That is the story of many women from around here. They go to Durban or Pietermaritzburg to look for work. There is no work; they only find a man who will pay for them.

"This man's house was next to his parents' homestead. I do not remember exactly where in Natal it is: somewhere north of Durban. This man of Nosipho's, he had another girlfriend when Nosipho arrived. There was tension between the two women. The old girlfriend had to leave, and she left her baby behind. Her baby was Thandeka. Nosipho became Thandeka's mother.

"That boyfriend of hers was a tyrant. He beat her. He did not allow her to travel back to Ithanga to visit her parents. She was a prisoner in her own home.

"After she had been there some time, my father decided to perform the initiation ceremony for all of his daughters. Somebody sent word to Nosipho that she was needed at home. She escaped. She came home. The boyfriend chased after her and arrived in Ithanga. My father was very angry with him. He instructed that man to go home and fetch Thandeka; he said Nosipho and Thandeka would be living here with us.

"They have now been here three years. Nosipho is married to a man from Ithanga. Thandeka, she is meant to live with my father, because a child born out of wedlock is the responsibility of her mother's homestead. But my father is a very difficult man to live with, so she came to live with me and Nwabisa. She is not my blood but it is the same as if she was my daughter, or my young sister. I paid her school fees. I put food on her plate every day. She left my place because she found work in the next village. She is staying with family there."

In the coming months, I will meet Thandeka two or three times. But my encounters with her are frustrating. She is not to know that I know of the virus in her blood, and I can ask her nothing. She is shy. I struggle to get more than a greeting out of her.

"You want to come with me to the clinics because you must assess the options," I say to Sizwe. "What are the other options?"

"There is a lady near Mthatha," Sizwe replies. "My father had a patient with AIDS. He went to get muthi from this lady near Mthatha. He got better. Then he tested again for HIV and he was negative."

I have heard a great deal about the lady from Mthatha. She is spoken of in every Lusikisiki village I have visited. She is, in fact, a fifteen- or sixteen-year-old girl, and she is said to possess extraordinary healing powers. Her practice is managed by her mother; one buys medicines from the mother, not the girl; very rarely do people get to see the girl herself. It is said that her mother is sheltering her from the world, wants her to have a normal adolescence, wants to protect her gift from corruption and misuse.

"She is your first option," I suggest. "The clinics is your last option."

He nods. "A cure is better."

"Is that the problem with the clinics? They don't offer a cure?"

"I have three problems with antiretrovirals," he replies crisply. "First, people do not know about them. We don't know them here. Second, it seems you must get sick before they give you the antiretrovirals. You must wait until you are sick. I do not like that. Why must you get sick first?"

He has been staring at his hands as he speaks. Now he lifts his head and looks me in the face.

"The third reason is the biggest reason. I feel terrible for the people living with this disease inside of them. It is there for their whole lives. I think of Thandeka living with this disease inside her for the rest of her life, and I feel so sorry for her, I wonder whether she can cope with that, whether anyone can cope with that. A cure is much better."

"We will go together," I say, "to the girl from Mthatha and to the clinics. At the clinics you will meet the doctor who runs the ARV program. You will ask him everything you want to know. His name is Hermann Reuter."

His head jolts as if he has been slapped. It is momentary. He recovers his composure in an instant.

"You know Dr. Hermann?" he asks.

"Yes," I say. "He has given me permission to come with him when he visits the clinics. You seem to know him, too."

"No," he replies. He is calm now, nonchalant. "I just saw his name somewhere. Maybe in a pamphlet I picked up. It was written by him. I read his name."

He will not tell me what it is I saw in his face when I mentioned Hermann Reuter, and I do not press it further. But there is clearly a story to tell.

We talk about other things, mainly Thandeka. She has a three-year-old child, Sizwe tells me. He was conceived back in Natal. The father was a trainee *sangoma*. He came to Thandeka's village to stay with a training sangoma, and while he was there, he had an affair with Thandeka. Her Zulu family was very angry. The trainee sangoma was banished in shame.

I ask if she has a current boyfriend. Yes, he replies. Her boyfriend is from here. He lives at the bottom of the valley. They have been together two years.

"Did she tell him about her test?"

"She told him, and he was very angry. He shouted at her, and then he refused to talk to her for a long time. He said he does not want to know about these things.

"He is angry, and he does not want to know, but he is sick. Every second day, he is coming to my shop to buy painkillers for his stomach and his chest and his head."

I struggle to concentrate on his words, for my mind keeps drifting; I am wondering what it is he has chosen to conceal about Hermann Reuter.

PART TWO

Garden and Home

C an I ask you a personal question?" inquires Dr. Hermann Reuter, head of the Médecins Sans Frontières project in Lusikisiki.

"You can ask what you like," I reply.

"Have you had sex with women ever?"

We are sitting in a garden outside a house; it is not clear from what he has said whether the house is his, but it appears that it might be. It stands on high ground, about a mile and a quarter from the center of Lusikisiki, and we are looking across a valley onto a straggle of dusk-lit hilltops.

I consider his question and begin to answer it, but he interrupts me.

"I'm not interested," he giggles. "I am asking because I want to know how do you understand the word *impotence*."

I hesitate, fearing that I am about to answer a trick question: "To the best of my knowledge," I say cautiously, "it refers to a man's inability to have or sustain an erection during a sexual encounter."

"That's my understanding also. But it is not the understanding of many young men in Lusikisiki."

"How do you mean?"

"You know, when I first arrived here, I used to do things like talk to groups of young people about sexuality. I stopped doing it because I'm shy. It makes me feel uncomfortable. I should be doing it still. But I don't."

It takes me a while to understand that he is no longer talking about impotence, or not yet, anyhow. I will learn over time that he has a habit of beginning with an unannounced aside, sometimes several.

"Anyway," he continues, "young men sometimes come to me and tell me they have a problem: there is something wrong with my penis, they say; it isn't working properly . . . I ask them what do they mean it's not working properly, and they say they can't give a girl an orgasm. And I say to them, 'Hold on, hold on: can I ask you something? How many times a night do you ejaculate?' And they say, 'Maybe six times.' And I say, 'Six times! I've never done that in my life. Can I explain to you something about the female orgasm maybe?'"

He pauses and laughs. "This is why I ask if you have slept with women ever."

I nod, a little exasperated at the route he has chosen to arrive at this point. But I am appreciative. In his bluffing, elaborately opaque manner, he has assembled an image that imprints itself vividly in the mind: so much invested in sexual performance, in potency, and yet the performance itself so fraughtly autistic, so swallowed up in itself, that it must fail.

It is a refreshing antidote to the careless proposition that in poor communities young people fuck each other all the time because there is nothing else to do. As if desire is a function of boredom. On the contrary, Hermann seems to suggest, when there is nothing else to do, when, for instance, one cannot give expression to one's manhood by becoming a household patriarch or careerist, the whole of manhood becomes endowed in sexual performance. It is made to do too much work; it is a source of anxiety.

"Yes," I say. "Sexual morality—"

"Something I have noticed," he interrupts, "is that for poor people sexual morality is Father Christmas mostly."

He says nothing more, and I sigh deeply, preparing for the volley of questions it will take to tease his thoughts from him.

He senses my irritation and continues. "For the poor, it is difficult for sex to be a private thing. Too many people live in one household. It is something that is seen and heard, by children, by the household. So this severe sexual morality people preach, it is like Father Christmas. It is something it is nice to believe. Or maybe a better way of putting it, it is like the starch poor people put on their clothes. Everyone knows the shirt is old and worn. But you must still put the starch on it, it is still very important, even though it does not hide very much usually."

Earlier in the day, Hermann had taken me around the garden next to the house that may or may not be his. He has planted several indigenous trees during his two-and-a-half-year stay in Lusikisiki. He took me from one sapling to another, pronouncing the name of each very slowly and asking if I knew of it. I shook my head every time.

"I know little about trees," I said apologetically. "I can recognize a willow, an oak, or a poplar, maybe a baobab. But that's about it. And bluegums and wattles, of course."

He ignored me. At each new sapling, he asked again whether I knew the name of the tree. I shrugged.

He was explaining to me which trees would grow tall and which were mere shrubs, which would die in a few years and which would live the span of countless human generations. In midsentence he stopped, shouted with delight, plunged into the tall grass next to his trees, and emerged holding what seemed to be a locust or a grasshopper.

"Food for my snakes," he said, showing it to me carefully. "Please help me look for some more. My snakes need food."

And so I imitated him, putting my eyes to the ground, scanning for insects. It had never dawned on me before that snakes might eat insects. Perhaps they don't. We slowly drifted to opposite ends of his garden.

"So," I shouted across the saplings and the tall grass, "is this or isn't this your house?"

"I don't know," he shrugged, head down, unwilling to interrupt the insect hunt.

"It is the sort of question," I said neutrally, "to which one usually expects a reasonably straightforward answer."

He smiled to himself and kept looking for grasshoppers or locusts.

"I used to live here," he said finally, "but it is not clear if it is still mine anymore. I moved to a house in the middle of town, but I didn't want to give this one up. I had an idea to make it into a youth center. I got some other people to live here for me so that it wouldn't stand empty in the meantime. Then the lady who owns the house heard that I wasn't living here anymore and she thought it was standing empty, and she got very, very cross. There are still some of my possessions in there and I don't know whether I'll ever be able to get them."

He shrugged and laughed, as if to say: "I am eccentric: see how even the simple things I make difficult."

He is in his late thirties, on his youthful face a thin beard that suggests either country doctor or Guevaran revolutionary. His hair is light brown and thick and stands up straight on his head. "It is usually much longer than this," he tells me. "What you are seeing is unusual." He has a thick German accent; he is a son of old South West African stock.

Properly told, the story of his presence here begins nine years ago, in July 1996, half a world away, in Vancouver, Canada. There, AIDS clinician David Ho and colleagues made what would soon be recognized as the most significant announcement in the brief history of AIDS medicine. An antiretroviral treatment program dubbed "highly active antiretroviral therapy" (HAART), a cocktail of three classes of drugs taken twice daily, had been shown in a series of clinical trials to halt the replication of the HIV virus. By late 1996, reports in the *New York Times* and *Sydney Morning Herald* were talking of the Lazarus effect, of the mortally ill rising from their deathbeds, putting on their coats and ties, and reporting for work. The most optimistic virologists hoped aloud that halting the replication of the virus would kill it, that HAART was a cure for AIDS.

By late 1997, it was clear that the news was not quite as good as that. In the vast majority of patients, the virus remained latent for as long as twice-daily treatment continued. Going off the drugs for a period of time was certain to court a return of serious illness. The drugs themselves were pretty toxic. Most of the side effects were confined to the first months of treatment, but for a minority the illnesses associated with taking the drugs were chronic or episodic and required permanent management. And those on ARVs still remained far more vulnerable to infectious disease than HIV-negative people. The lives of people on treatment would thus be a good deal more fragile and probably shorter than those of their peers.

Nonetheless, a large cohort of people who in mid-1996 had been destined to die were back at work and living normal lives by January of the following year. In cities such as Sydney, San Francisco, and New York, where the most visible gay populations on earth had been decimated, scores of young men faced the bewildering dilemma of what to do with the futures they assumed had been stolen from them. The celebrated gay writer Edmund White wrote in a late-1990s essay of the resumption of New York dinner parties after a decade-long interval; for dessert, the assembled guests would communally swallow their cocktail of pills.

Médecins Sans Frontières began its South African antiretroviral work in 1999. By then, middle-class people throughout the world who contracted AIDS could expect to begin a lifelong drug regimen as a matter of course. The largest unresolved matter about AIDS treatment had shifted to the heartland of the epidemic: sub-Saharan Africa. The question was whether HAART could be delivered to poor people in underdeveloped states. In fact, there were three questions. The first was cost. A global campaign to set aside patents on antiretroviral drugs, thus making them affordable to the health departments of developing countries, was under way. This campaign achieved a significant victory less than two years after MSF's arrival in South Africa: in February 2001 an Indian manufacturer offered to sell generic, unpatented HAART drugs for 350 U.S. dollars per person per year.

There were two further questions: one was whether third-world health departments had the capacity to manage and deliver treatment in the context of a widespread plague. A middle-class New Yorker who falls ill can expect to attended to by a personal physician, and a battery of nutritionists. He also shares his city with fine virologists and infectious disease specialists, and several tertiary health-care institutions built to study and manage chronic illness. A person who falls ill with AIDS in a poor African village is more likely to be attended to by a single nurse. She is treating dozens of cases every day, trying desperately to manage her workload. If one of her patients should fall ill with TB or pneumonia, will the drugs he needs find their way to the nurse's shelves? And if he requires intensive care, is there a hospital close by, one not so swamped by the epidemic's casualties that it has a bed for him to lie in and the spirit and the means to care for him?

A third question concerned poor people themselves and whether they would adhere to lifelong treatment. A notorious comment made in 2001 by the head of the U.S. Agency for International Development, Andrew Natsios, became the abiding emblem of the debate. He cautioned against investing too much in a therapy that required taking pills at strict twelve-hour intervals. In Africa, he said, "people do not know what watches and clocks are. They do not use Western means for telling time. They use the sun."

In 1999, when MSF began its South African work, it was entirely unknown whether the country's public health system could deliver ARV medicine to the poor. Treatment had been administered by private physicians to middle-class people on health insurance, and in clinical trials at academic hospitals. Hermann scoffs when I mention clinical trials.

"You have four or five doctors," he says, "all of them with highly specialized training, hovering around one patient. Four or five doctors to a patient: how can you deal with an epidemic that way? How many doctors will you need to put a million people on treatment?"

When MSF came to South Africa to begin an antiretroviral pilot project, it went to the only South African province that would cooperate with it: Western Cape. It chose as its initial site Khayelitsha, a poor and crowded ghetto of more than half a million people on the outskirts of Cape Town. One in three of its adult residents was unemployed, and one in five was HIV-positive. Hermann was among those who pioneered the project. Its aim was to show that it was possible to deliver quality ARV treatment en masse to the poor.

The underlying approach of the Khayelitsha project was really a leap of faith, a piece of outcome-based reasoning. The epidemic was pervasive. Millions of its victims were poor and without access to decent health care. Doctors, nurses, technology, and infrastructure were all scarce where they lived. If AIDS medicine were to remain the preserve of specialists at academic hospitals, it would never reach poor people; the overwhelming majority of the epidemic's victims would simply die.

So MSF and like-minded organizations stood up and declared, by simple fiat, that it was not complicated medicine, that the knowledge required to make it successful could be condensed into simple codes and distributed among nurses, laypeople, and ARV users themselves. They declared, too, that stagnant and ill-functioning health-care systems would be brought to life when ARV medicine became popular medicine, and ordinary people began demanding it.

"In the twentieth century," Hermann was to tell me some time later, "the medical intervention that saved the most lives was oral rehydration fluid. A liter of water, half a teaspoon salt, eight teaspoons of sugar, saved millions from dying of diarrhea. ARVs are the most significant intervention since then. And it's also a primary health-care intervention. No fancy machines, no organ transplants. You just need a nurse. And frankly, you don't even need that."

MSF's Khayelitsha project did not quite live up to Hermann's ideal of nurse-administered medicine. The treatment sites in Khayelitsha were run by doctors—Hermann and his colleague Eric Goemaere. But in other respects, the project did begin to cultivate some of the flavors of popular grassroots medicine that MSF insisted was the only way to bring AIDS treatment to the poor.

Among the ingredients of the project's success, for instance, was the recruitment of a cohort of laypeople into support functions. Laypeople were trained to perform voluntary counseling and testing, establish support groups for antiretroviral users, and monitor adherence to treatment. Antiretroviral users themselves played a significant role, tracing people who did not turn up to get new batches of pills, recruiting others to test, and giving treatment a public face. In the course of managing their own treatment, users became highly conversant in the causes of illness, the pharmaceutical actions of the drugs they took, and the politics of public health.

In short, the project's assumption was that treatment would only work if animated by a social movement of laypeople and antiretroviral users. And indeed, through its work in Khayelitsha, MSF soon found itself in a natural alliance with the Treatment Action Campaign (TAC), the vanguard of South Africa's social movement for AIDS treatment. Founded in 1998 by the former antiapartheid militant Zackie Achmat, it borrowed from an eclectic array of traditions, from the direct action tactics of American groups such as ACT UP to the spirit and culture of South Africa's antiapartheid movement.

For a time, Achmat was the face of South Africa's treatment movement. His signature t-shirt, white with the letters *HIV* emblazoned in bright purple, was inspired by the legendary Danish practice of wearing the Star of David during the Nazi occupation in order to make Jews indistinguishable from the general population. However, Achmat is indeed HIV-positive, and not merely in solidarity with those who are. In the late 1990s, he announced that he would not start antiretroviral treatment until it was available to all South Africans. Under pressure from colleagues, he finally began treatment in 2002, becoming the best known South African on ARVs.

Hermann Reuter and Achmat go back a long way. Both were

Trotskyist militants during the apartheid years, way to the left of the mainstream antiapartheid movement. Indeed, Hermann began his AIDS work on the payroll of the organization Achmat founded; he was employed by the Treatment Action Campaign as an organizer shortly after it began. He knew next to nothing about MSF before the organization began AIDS work in South Africa.

MSF began administering HAART in Khayelitsha in 2001. Within three years, more than a thousand Khayelitsha residents had begun treatment. The rate of patients' adherence to their regimens appeared to be as good as, if not better than, in the affluent and literate gay communities of first-world cities. By the mid-2000s, the project's lessons had spread well beyond Khayelitsha: nurse-managed government clinics across the Cape Peninsula were administering ARV treatment as a matter of course. The project had been a resounding success.

"Our victory brought its own problems," Hermann tells me. "A line started coming out about MSF's success in Khayelitsha.

"Everybody started saying, 'Ja, you can do it in Cape Town, but Cape Town is not the rest of South Africa. Cape Town has a lot of academic doctors. If there are complications, there is Groote Schuur and Tygerberg hospitals, two of the best hospitals in the country, just around the corner. Why don't you go somewhere where the drug supplies arrive once every three months when you are lucky? Go somewhere where there are no doctors and half the nurses' posts are unfilled. See if you can put people on ARVs there.'

"So we came to Lusikisiki."

That was in early 2003. By the time I met Hermann in late 2005, MSF had put out word that it had made fools of the skeptics. It had got the Eastern Cape's wounded primary health-care system, with its vacant nurses' posts and battered infrastructure, to deliver antiretroviral treatment to one of the most destitute and densely populated rural districts in South Africa. There were more than one thousand people on treatment, and adherence rates were even higher than in Khayelitsha.

When I met the head of MSF South Africa, Eric Goemaere, in his office in Khayelitsha, he painted Hermann as a maniacal hero.

"When we first visited the Lusikisiki clinics," he tells me, "there was no paracetamol on the shelves. The TB drugs had been out of stock for several months. We thought, Shit, this isn't going to work. We're going to have to fix the entire primary health-care system. You need someone crazy and idealistic like Hermann. He basically went in and fixed the primary health-care system. There are drugs on the shelves. The place works. All in all it is a miracle."

Goemaere's pride is double-edged. MSF wound up its Lusikisiki project less than a year after I interviewed him, leaving ARV treatment there in the hands of the provincial health department and the district municipality. Its intervention was always meant to be temporary; its goal, after all, was to show that ordinary nurses, not rich international NGOs, could administer a treatment program. What happens to ARV treatment after the heroic Hermann Reuter's departure? And if it takes a crazy idealist like him, what of the dozens of rural districts staffed only by plodding, workaday managers?

IT IS GROWING dark now, too dark to look for insects in long grass. We leave the garden and cross the yard next to the empty house, its windows reflecting the last of the dusk back at us. There might be a sliver of an allegory buried somewhere in Hermann's maddeningly cryptic story of this house. He has dedicated his life to health-care activism, moving from place to place, burying body and soul in work. His presence, here and elsewhere, is by its nature transitory. And yet he rented a house with a garden and planted young trees, and he makes an extravagant performance of how difficult it is for a man with no permanent abode to care for the things he plants.

I tell him about Sizwe: his village, his shop, the secret illness in his family, his inscrutable silence about ARVs. I tell him that I want to write a book that tracks and interprets Sizwe's perspective.

He responds with visible irritation. "I do not think that his story will reflect what is happening in this place," he says. "It will not give a picture of what this program is about."

Sizwe's apparent hostility to ARVs, he tells me, is exceptional. And the fact that he lives in Ithanga is also of concern. Ithanga is unusually remote, a difficult nine-mile journey from the nearest clinic. Hermann believes that whether a person embraces a health-care service is determined primarily by the accessibility of that service. Of course a young man from Ithanga will be unusually circumspect. If he lived five or ten miles south of where he does, he would be telling a different story.

Hermann has introduced me to people about whom he would like me to write, HIV-positive people who began antiretroviral treatment in the early days of the program, people who now devote their lives to treatment activism in Lusikisiki.

I am not sure, however, that those who have become treatment missionaries are necessarily the best people to write about. Perhaps there is a more interesting tale to be told about those beyond the margins of the ARV program, those who are skeptical and unsure. I tell Hermann of Sizwe's haunted account of the day the mobile testing unit came to Ithanga: the pairs of eyes that note who goes into the makeshift testing center and how long their post-test counseling lasts; the whispering and the silent scorn.

"Nothing you are saying is new to me," he replies curtly. "In fact, I think that what you have described is a good thing. We in MSF have a very different attitude to confidentiality compared to the health department. The health department was saying you must not write on people's clinic cards that they are HIV-positive. Everything must be a big secret. We are saying, unless people disclose they are not going to deal with AIDS. If it's a big secret you are trying to hide from everybody, you will not be able to deal with it.

"Your friend Sizwe, if he goes to test and he tests positive, then yes, the people in his community will know, and he will make some enemies. But the friends he makes will be more important than the enemies. The people testing positive develop meaningful relationships, the sort of relationships they have never had. Before, they were sitting around and doing nothing. Now, their lives become meaningful."

At first, his comment jars. I mistake him for saying that being chronically ill is better for the soul than being healthy; that those on ARVs have been granted the privilege of living lives somehow more human and more substantial than those of their peers. I imagine a secular church, fervent and dogmatic, scouring the countryside for converts. The history of the Transkei is littered with faith healers and prophets and their bands of followers. The thought that this program, which wields drugs rather than magic, nonetheless takes its place in an old story, is an intriguing one.

But this is not, I learn with time, what Hermann is saying. He is saying that a mass treatment program will fail if secrecy and shame predominate, that a medical assault on a plague will only work when animated by the people it serves. And I will discover, as I meet more and more people on ARVs, that to embrace indefinite treatment is indeed to recalibrate one's relation to the world, and that the primary tool of recalibration is dialogue. There are networks of ARV takers in many of Lusikisiki's villages, and they talk. Their talk is about far more than drugs: it encompasses sex and love and work and the course of life; it is about the relation between all these things to one's body. As public talk, it is by definition political and ideological: it carves out friends and enemies, it scorns and it praises and it excludes. But it is not a church. It is contradictory and messy and often wildly eccentric, and its content varies from village to village.

Of course Hermann is irritated that I am writing a book about a skeptical man on the margins of his program; for it is surely to be a book about the limitations of his work.

Magic Pills

Between the day Hermann Reuter came to Lusikisiki in early 2003 and the day I met him in October 2005, the meaning of his work had changed a great deal. In early 2003, President Thabo Mbeki's infamous doubts about the link between HIV and AIDS still formed the bedrock of national health policy. Antiretroviral treatment was emerging in pockets around the public health system, largely as a result of spontaneous local efforts. The government was administering an ARV program to prevent the transmission of HIV from mothers to children, but only because the Constitutional Court had ordered it to. Mbeki and his health minister still refused to roll out an ARV program accessible to everyone with AIDS.

The South African president's heterodox position on AIDS has many roots. One of them, ironically, is his perceptiveness. Any serious student of the AIDS epidemic is compelled to answer a difficult question: Why Africa? Why has the epidemic been uniquely terrible here? The answer Mbeki found in established social and medical science was, simply, that Africans had too much sex, that they could not control their carnal appetites, even when their libidos were literally killing them. That is the assumption, Mbeki thought, underlying the hegemonic idea that the answer to the AIDS epidemic was sexual behavior modification. It suggested that the epidemic was uniquely terrible here because sexual appetite was uniquely voracious here, that taming the epidemic required taming African men.

Established medical science, Mbeki believed, had been blinded by the racism of its practitioners. It had suspended a piece of knowledge that ought to be workaday for epidemiologists: that among the cofactors of the vast majority of epidemics in history is poverty, that any explanation for why AIDS has been so ghastly here must surely absorb the fact that Africa is underdeveloped and poor. Indeed, the diseases of poverty, he argued, incubated by malnourished bodies, endemic parasites, lack of fresh water, and wretched working lives, have been legion in Africa for generations. Surely AIDS is one of them.

It was in this state of disillusionment and anger that Mbeki became aware of groups of dissident scientists, long ago dismissed by orthodox science, who questioned whether HIV was the primary cause of the AIDS epidemic. By 2000, Mbeki firmly believed these outliers and supported them. They were not so much dissidents, he wrote in a letter that was to become infamous, as heretics, questioners of established dogma. Stitched together with poor science and racist prejudice, this pernicious dogma's centerpiece was that sexually transmitted HIV was the sole cause of the African AIDS epidemic.

And the greatest champion of this dogma, Mbeki believed, was the immensely powerful pharmaceutical industry, its research budgets larger than those of most developing nations, its marketers scouring the globe for consumers of the antiretroviral medicines it manufactured. The received wisdom that Africa's epidemic of immunodeficiency was caused by HIV, Mbeki believed, was sustained by one of the most powerful commercial interests on the planet. Antiretrovirals were toxins quite literally forced down Africa's throat.

So what Hermann Reuter regarded as the most important healthcare intervention in fifty years, Mbeki regarded as a package of racial and pharmacological poison. Hermann is an African-born white Marxist, Mbeki a black third-world nationalist. In another era, they would have been allies.

MBEKI'S IDEAS ON AIDS were always complicated and never clearly articulated. By the time they filtered down to provincial ANC strongholds such as Eastern Cape, they had become a cocktail of nativism, ersatz epidemiology, and anti-imperialism: the drugs are toxic; the West is dumping poisons on Africa; the problem is poverty and ARVs cannot help someone with an empty stomach.

MSF was invited to Eastern Cape by one section of a fractious and ambivalent health department. When Hermann met with the provincial health minister, Dr. Bevan Goqwana, in May 2003, the minister appeared to discover only there and then that MSF was in his province to administer ARV treatment. Irritated and surprised, he told Hermann that the drug program would have to be put on hold. When Hermann replied that he would continue to provide ARV treatment with or without the minister's consent, Goqwana lost his temper. He compared Hermann's threat of defiance with the warmongering of Angola's Jonas Savimbi, and so implied that he would fight him as a patriotic soldier fights a counterrevolutionary.

If the minister's outburst was a little mad, it nonetheless captures the besieged and aggressive nativism that greeted the arrival of AIDS medicine in South Africa: ARVs were cloaked in suspicion and conspiracy; they had been brought to our shores by people bent on deceiving us, people bent on robbing us of something.

By October 2005, much had changed. Two years earlier, Mbeki had capitulated to a rebellion in his cabinet and had agreed to a universal ARV rollout. It was an unsettling spectacle: a reluctant administration, defeated by a broad range of political opponents inside and outside the ANC, begrudgingly rolling out the most ambitious health program in the country's history. But it did indeed begin to happen. By the time I arrived in Lusikisiki, about eighty thousand people had been put onto treatment at public health facilities throughout South Africa.

MSF's country staff watched the government's rollout proceed, and they were dismayed by what they saw. In district after district, hospitals, rather than clinics, were accredited to administer ARV treatment. Bottlenecks developed almost immediately, and thousands of sick people were put on waiting lists. Thousands of others would never turn up at all. Their local clinics, often within walking distance, remained neglected, understaffed, and without drugs.

For MSF, what they saw only confirmed what they had always believed: that a plague as pervasive as southern Africa's AIDS epidemic would either be fought by nurses and laypeople or not at all.

The South African government was getting it wrong, MSF staff believed, not simply because of its president's and health minister's famous skepticism about ARV medicine. The problem lay much deeper. Ironically, South Africa's health administrators, maniacally vigilant about warding off malignant Western influences, appeared to be trapped in a mentality bequeathed to them by generations of white minority rule.

During the apartheid years, South Africa built a high-technology, hospital-based health system, neglecting preventative medicine. In part, this was symptomatic of a racist indifference to the health of black people. It was also because South Africa was internationally isolated, and developing high-technological competence became a mantra of pride and survival.

When South Africans voted in the country's first democratic election in 1994, they swept the African National Congress (ANC), the previously exiled liberation movement and the party of Nelson Mandela, to power. The new ANC government spoke a great deal about rejuvenating primary health care. It also made some progress. Yet the AIDS epidemic, for Hermann, had shown the limits to its commitment. Faced with a great plague, one that could only be fought beyond the hospitals at the grass roots, the government's feet had gone cold. Despite itself, it could not shake off an old white prejudice: only hospitals, machines, and specialists deliver decent medicine; medicine for the poor is poor medicine.

A battle of ideas was thus in progress. MSF needed to show that in districts where the national government's rollout model was implemented, people died in numbers awaiting treatment; that in Lusikisiki, those who needed ARVs sought them and got them, waiting lists were kept always at zero, and nurses turned nobody away. The question of information, and how to disseminate it, was delicately political. The presentation of success was as important as success itself.

――――――――――――

WHEN HERMANN REUTER came to Lusikisiki, the primary health-care system that he was envisioning would fight a great plague was profoundly unaware of his plans. Of Lusikisiki's twelve clinics, two had reliable electricity supply, one had running water or a phone, and none a fax machine. Few of the medicines on South Africa's essential drug list had ever found their way to the district's clinic shelves, and those that had were there only sporadically. Less than four in ten nursing posts were filled.

Per capita, the district had fourteen times more people per doctor than the national average, and in that sense, Hermann was surely right: either Lusikisiki's battered clinics and overworked staff would fight the epidemic, or no one would.

"During my first week here," Hermann told me, "I went to each clinic. The nurses' first question: 'Are you a doctor?'"

" 'Yes, I am a doctor.'

"Big welcome dance. First time they have seen a doctor coming to the clinic for five years. Lots of excitement. Until I start talking about HIV. They say, no, they don't think HIV is a problem in the community. They don't treat anyone with HIV. Ja, they went to a funeral and someone said the person died of HIV, but we don't know.

"We start testing people in the clinics. Initially, I did most of the tests with the nurses. Positive, positive, positive, one after the other. It was a big eye-opener for the nurses."

I was incredulous. By early 2003, HIV was comfortably the leading cause of death in Lusikisiki. "Are you saying this is how nurses discovered the epidemic?" I ask.

"Yes."

"It's extraordinary that they weren't aware."

"I don't know. Perhaps they were aware. But it wasn't their responsibility. It wasn't for the clinics. Ja, there was home-based care, but it wasn't for nurses, it was the NGOs. Very sick people did not come to clinics. They went to hospital and died there."

Yet even at Saint Elizabeth's, the regional hospital at the northern end of Lusikisiki's town center, there was little talk of AIDS before MSF arrived. I interviewed a staff nurse called Zama, who worked in the hospital's female medical ward in 2003, which by then would probably have hosted at least one AIDS death every single day.

"People were dying of TB, cardiac failure, pneumonia, some of meningitis, some of diabetes," she told me. "We did not differentiate. We did not say, pneumonia is maybe an opportunistic infection of AIDS, and diabetes isn't. It was just: this one died of this, that one died of that."

"When did you first start thinking of these things as opportunistic infections associated with AIDS?" I asked.

"When MSF came and gave a seminar. It changed everything. Suddenly, I was looking at something new. Before then, if you knew that a patient in the ward was HIV-positive you had to keep it a secret; it had to be highly confidential. It was dangerous to ask."

It is an extraordinary tale. In a hospital ward, the leading cause of death among patients is banished from speech and from thought. What was this denial about?

It is perhaps trite to point out that nurses are both medical personnel and people. To what extent did they simply carry into the wards a sense of scandal from the outside? How much of their silence, on the other hand, was the specific silence of nurses? Staffing a hospital ward in the thick of a seemingly incurable epidemic is a grim business. If the people being admitted are destined to waste away and die, and if they keep coming, day in and day out, they become emblems of unspeakable hollowness.

"All over the country," Hermann told me, "AIDS demotivated health workers. Opportunistic infections were treated as acute illnesses; people were quickly discharged to make space for others. Workload increased. Turnover was so quick. Hospital stays got shorter. So much nurse work is admin work. The higher the turnover, the more admin. Patients in hospitals became sicker and sicker, so the workload got even harder. Many patients had neurological problems, confusion: you would get people running out of the wards. There was also lots of diarrhea, lots of soiled linen. And then there was the increased rate of death in the wards. If the person in the bed is just going to die . . ." He allows an elaborate shrug to finish his sentence. "HIV was a nightmare. Health workers hated it."

In some parts of the country, hospital managers would literally police their perimeters to keep the chronically ill out. Hermann has a story about this that remains vivid in my mind. It comes from the early days of MSF's Khayelitsha project, 1999 or 2000, and concerns GF Jooste, the large Cape Town hospital that serves the working-class districts and shack settlements of the Cape Flats. Jooste was critical to the success of MSF's Khayelitsha project. It was the institution to which MSF referred patients who required hospital care; it thus had to have a measure of competence in treating people seriously ill with AIDS.

"I would send people there and they would start crying," Hermann recalls.

"They would say, 'Send me anywhere except there.'

"I say: 'Why?'

"They say, 'People die there.'

"That hospital was overcrowded. It was mainly geared toward surgical patients because of that area. You know, knives and guns and lots of blood. You go to that hospital and you have to go through the security guards. On a Friday night that place smells of alcohol and blood and you need to bleed to be let in there.

"Sometimes I went there on weekends with Treatment Action Campaign people who fell sick, and the guards outside looked at us and said, 'This one is not sick: she can't come in.'

"I said, 'No, she is very sick; she has meningitis.'

"They said, 'What is that? I can see she has HIV. Go home.'

"That was the security guards. I'd tell them I'm a doctor, and that would get me past security. The next line was the nurses. They would say, 'No, this is a chronic patient, take her home.'

"That was the attitude throughout South Africa: we cannot deal with HIV, especially not on a Friday night."

THERE ARE SEVERAL ways to describe what Hermann did when he came to Lusikisiki. I'm not sure which is best. One is to say that he arrived in town clutching the pills themselves, the ARVs, as one clutches a cross or a staff. One can quibble over names and words, but they are to be invested with a force that amounts to magic. For the pills offer nothing less than to halt a deluge of dying. They dare people to drag the disease from its hidden corners, to name it and talk openly of it, and to plan a battle against it, all on the grounds that it need no longer kill.

Hermann came to town promising that in his bag was a force that would confound death. It is the excitement of that promise that conjures out of very little a working health-care system. The pills are billed as the protagonist in a great drama. And so people begin to rally behind the pills. Clinic staff once resigned to the fate that the phone at the Mthatha medicine depot goes unanswered now demand a response. They need the TB drugs, the meningitis drugs, the antifungal drugs on their shelves here and now, because without these drugs, the magic ARV pills cannot fight death. At the local hospital, the wasted patient soiled in her own excrement is no longer a soon-to-be-corpse; she is a project to get right, another piece of the magic, a human being who will one day walk on her own two feet. The management positions in the district that have been vacant for two years are filled because now there is work to do, and if it is not done, the pills will not defeat death.

That the people of Lusikisiki too must join the drama of course goes without saying. The clinic is no longer a place for old women's tired joints and young children's upset stomachs. It is the front line in life's army, the place one seeks refuge from death. With the pills, HIV in the family must no longer be a source of shame. Those who have eluded death must hold their pills up high and celebrate their lives. In every village, those who are alive because of the pills must speak of them, demand that they keep coming, demand that the clinics and the hospitals be working so that the pills can do their work.

It is necessary that all these things happen at once. If the nurses in the clinics are buoyed, but the people stay away and die in their homes, the magic promised by the pills stays dormant. If the people line up outside the clinic in scores, but there is insufficient staff to see them all, they will begin to stay away and die at home. And if there is enough staff, and the people come, but the medicine depot does not deliver the drugs to the shelves, the magic will quickly vanish. Or perhaps the clinics are working well, so well that the sick descend upon them like never before. And so the clinics refer the gravely ill among their patients to the hospital. But the hospital has not enough beds for the influx, and people die at home.

The magic must light up the whole system at once. All is connected. One dark corner can short-circuit the whole.

THERE IS ANOTHER way to describe what Hermann did. Using a mixture of charisma and sheer slog, he built a social movement and stationed its members in the clinics. A cohort of adherence counselors, recruited and trained by Hermann and put on MSF's payroll, did the lion's share of the AIDS work in the clinics. They performed voluntary counseling and testing, prepared patients for treatment, established support groups for antiretroviral users, monitored the adherence of antiretroviral users to their treatment, and collected and collated data. They were as much community activists as health workers, visiting families who had thrown the HIV-positive out of their homes, and staffing the mobile testing units like the one that so unnerved Sizwe in Ithanga.

Hermann recruited six people as pharmacist assistants. Their task was to dispense medicines, monitor low stocks, and place persistent and unrelenting pressure upstream to supply the district's burgeoning need for medicines.

While MSF was planning its Lusikisiki project, Hermann requested that the Treatment Action Campaign open a branch in the town. They did so. Hermann envisioned the branch becoming the central pillar of a popular social movement in Lusikisiki. In the end, it turned out to be a mixture of strong and weak. Around the center of town and in some of the larger villages, TAC members donned their signature HIV-positive t-shirts, giving both the epidemic and its treatment a bold and visible face. TAC activists also worked very effectively among ARV users in the clinic-based support groups, getting users themselves to trace people who had not turned up for their pills, moving into villages where users were being shunned or victimized, and making users literate in the medicines they were taking and in the politics of health care more generally.

But the organization was weaker than Hermann would have liked. Building a lasting social movement in a deep rural setting has never been an easy task. The most talented of the young people Hermann attracted became adherence counselors and pharmacist assistants, thus robbing TAC of the cream of local talent. And so in villages such as Ithanga, few, if anyone, had heard of TAC. Sizwe knew of the adherence counselors from the day they came to test the people, and from the local clinic. Of TAC he knew nothing.

The people Hermann recruited and put on MSF's payroll were young and literate. They lived in a rural town where career prospects were bleak, the course one's adult life might take uncertain. Hermann gave them the prospect of a career, a new discourse with which to understand their lives and their town, and an ambitious project. They took to him and his work with voracious hunger.

It was precisely these people whom Sizwe encountered on that Saturday morning at the school in Ithanga early in 2005. He took them to be members of a new cult, felt his distaste rising, and turned his back. What he had recognized, in his skeptical and fearful way, was the unmistakable fervor of young people speaking a newly learned language, their very sense of themselves invested in a new vision.

A Lusikisiki clinic nurse ensconced in her job in January 2003 was in for an unusual year. Within months, her clinic corridors would host a cohort of busy and animated young people, a new language issuing uncertainly from their tongues. Her waiting room would begin to fill with the victims of a great plague, waiting for her to treat them; and for every one she treated, another three, four, or five would come to the clinic's door.

DID THE MAGIC pills do their work? Any answer ought to be measured and sober.

By mid-2004, a person who entered the waiting room at one of Lusikisiki's twelve clinics could expect to be treated for AIDS: no waiting list, no referral to another institution. Across the country, the number of rural health districts that could make that claim were to be counted on one hand. Given the parlous state of the clinics just a year earlier, the achievement was considerable.

Yet to say that the treatment program had abolished despair, denial, and an accumulation of corpses from Lusikisiki would be a lie. One by one, I interviewed as many nurses and doctors as would speak to me from the medical wards of Saint Elizabeth's Hospital. I never saw any hospital records to corroborate it, but between them they told me that at least one person a day died in their wards from pneumonia, meningitis, TB, or Kaposi's sarcoma. Some had been referred by the clinics, but the vast majority had arrived at the emergency room mortally ill, straight from their homes. This suggested that out in the villages, many people who lived within walking distance of a decent clinic died without setting foot in its waiting room. I knew from my time in Ithanga that soon Jake's brother, and later, Sizwe's niece, might join those ranks.

Also, the mortality rate among those who did start ARV treatment at Lusikisiki clinics was high: one in six died within a year of beginning treatment. After that, the mortality rate dropped nearly to zero, but the beginning was a dangerous time. The primary reason was poor hospital care. Many of those beginning treatment were sick, often critically. And despite Hermann's complaint that the government did not invest enough in its clinics, rural hospitals were also desperately short of staff, expertise, and infrastructure. The wards at Saint Elizabeth's could not manage the scale of the epidemic. Critically ill patients were stabilized and quickly discharged to make way for others.

Nonetheless, in the month I arrived in Lusikisiki, the program celebrated its thousandth ARV user, which meant that more than eight hundred of the souls walking the village footpaths and the town's main street would, if not for the treatment program, be dead or dying.

The program's achievements were always provisional, always a little precarious. The source of this instability was chronic staff shortages, and the effects they might have after Hermann Reuter's and MSF's departure from Lusikisiki in late 2006.

Even at the program's pinnacle, fewer than 60 percent of nursing posts at Lusikisiki clinics were filled. It was a source of great bitterness for Hermann. True, South Africa was suffering from a national shortage of nurses. But it would be hard to argue that the staff deficit in Lusikisiki's clinics was no more than a symptom of national scarcity. The fact is that for the program's duration, the district did not advertise a single clinic nurse vacancy. The problem was one of budgetary starvation, not a skills shortage.

This was one of the symptoms of the philosophical differences between MSF and the South African government. MSF believed that clinics must constitute the front line in the battle against the epidemic, that they were the only health institutions close enough to the ground to reach everyone in need of treatment. Yet the government was rolling out its AIDS treatment program at hospitals, not clinics; across the country, hospitals thus received the lion's share of posts and resources, turning the clinics into neglected stepchildren. MSF's program thus constantly tugged against the logic of national budgetary allocations.

So the dozens of vacancies at Lusikisiki clinics were not advertised. One consequence was that a Lusikisiki clinic nurse looking for a promotion would have to leave the district to get one. The signposts all pointed in one direction—out. It was quite possible that, in the wake of MSF's departure, the cohort of staff it trained in AIDS medicine would gradually disappear.

Even if the district retained its staff, another problem might arise. When MSF began bringing the epidemic's victims to the clinics, nurses' workloads accelerated alarmingly. At the beginning of 2004, a Lusikisiki clinic nurse saw an average of twenty-nine patients a day.

By 2006, the figure had jumped to forty-seven. True, the corpus of energetic, Reuter-trained young laypeople in every clinic alleviated each nurse's burden, making their forty-seven-patient-a-day workload possible. But that is not necessarily how an overworked clinic nurse views matters. The activists and laypeople in her clinic are drawing patients in their numbers, and she begins to resent their presence. In an attempt to regain authority over her clinic, she wages quiet war against the laypeople, and begins to ration her workload by sending patients away.

Even with Hermann still in town, a fault line between nurses and MSF-trained laypeople was evident. Hermann himself wielded immense moral authority in the district health system. A nurse did not ration her workload under his gaze. But when his back was turned, his counselors and pharmacist assistants took flak.

As for the laypeople themselves, they got their inspiration from Hermann. Each had been trained by him. Each had been seduced by his extraordinary dedication, his capacity to work sixteen-hour days, his persistence in inviting them into the world of his esoteric knowledge. There was little question that his departure would depress them. Whether his departure would derail them remained to be seen.

It is quite possible that in his absence, the frenzy in the clinics would give way to a work-to-rule atmosphere. The program would not fall apart at the seams, but it would slow down. Patient intake would decrease, waiting lists emerge and grow.

Soon after I arrived in Lusikisiki, I asked one of the laypeople Hermann trained, to characterize the nurses she works with.

"I'd divide them into two," she replied. "The first is happy that MSF is leaving in a year's time. The second is sad. The ones who are happy believe we give them too much work. They will kick us in the head when MSF leaves. The ones who are sad, they know that they are saving lives now, and that they didn't before, and it brings meaning to their own lives."

I asked her to tell me a story of a nurse who will be happy to see MSF go.

"The other day," she said, "a woman I know came into the clinic. I saw from the marks on her face she had shingles. I was surprised; I did not know she had AIDS. We said hello and talked, and a bit later it was her turn to see the professional nurse.

"When the patient came out, she came to say good-bye. I asked her why she was not lining up at the pharmacy for her medicines. She told me the nurse had said she only had blisters from the sun. She had prescribed paracetamol.

"I was so furious I was almost choking. I grabbed the woman by the hand, took her back to the nurse's room, and said: 'This woman does not have blisters from the sun. She has shingles. There are drugs for this. You must treat her.'

"A few hours later, the nurse came to me and said: 'You must be careful. You must behave yourself here. If you try to be the boss I will chase you away.'"

It would be a little hasty to join the lay worker in condemning the nurses in her first category, the ones pleased that MSF will be leaving, as the villains of the story. From the 1960s to the 1990s, South Africa trained black nurses in the thousands, and herded them into the ground level of its racialized health system. They were subjected to the condescension of the doctors and white nurses above them, and yet were the ones who had to deal directly with the despair of the black patients whom the health system failed. Now, in the context of personnel shortages and workloads unprecedented in their lifetimes, Hermann was asking them to staff the front trenches in a battle against a deadly epidemic.

When I put this to Hermann he nodded his agreement. "The beginning of the program was a huge, huge shock for nurses," he said. "We saw a lot of people die, and the nurses started to see how many deaths were HIV deaths. And now it was their responsibility. For the first time, dying people came to clinic nurses for treatment. It was the nurse's patients dying. Someone comes to the clinic and says: 'Your patient is dead now.'"

To understand the depth of this fear among nurses that they would be held responsible for the deaths of patients, consider their position in comparison to Sizwe's. He was born and bred in Ithanga. Everyone there knows him, his family, where he comes from. He is a local man through and through. What distinguishes him is his modest success. It has courted envy. He worries a great deal about the ill feeling his good life may provoke.

Now consider a nurse, one who lives in a village as poor and remote as Ithanga. She earns a good deal more than Sizwe, lives in a home much fancier than those of her neighbors. With her education, her aspirations, her profession, she stands aloof from the village people around her. She is in all probability an outsider, on contract to work in the village for a time.

She is in so many ways a stranger. And she works on the frontier between life and death. On some days she goes home to her fancy house and a villager who was her patient lies dead in the morgue.

I talked to a nurse at Saint Elizabeth's Hospital who spoke lyrically about the importance of primary health care.

"If it's so important," I asked her, "why are you working at the hospital? Why don't you go to a clinic in a small village?"

"I'm scared to do that," she replied. "I am not from here. People can tell that from my accent. I deal with sick people, with people who might die, and I am an outsider. It is possible they will accuse me of terrible things."

———————

I ARRIVED TO a program celebrating great success, but a little unsure of its future. People were still getting sick with AIDS and dying without ever visiting their local clinic. Whether this was a good or a bad thing remained an open question. If everyone who needed treatment turned up in a clinic waiting room, it was not at all clear that the system would cope.

On the Outer Edge

The first encounter between Sizwe Magadla and Hermann Reuter goes remarkably well. The journalist and his interpreter, who has come to observe the treatment program discreetly to see whether it is suitable for his niece, meet the doctor early on a Monday morning outside the Médecins Sans Frontières offices in the center of town. We are to spend the day at one of the remotest of Lusikisiki's twelve clinics, an hour's drive along a dust road built into the contours of an endless series of valley walls.

Sizwe expresses deference like no one I have seen before. I first witnessed it with his father. He lowers his eyes and watches the floor, and the shape and weight of his entire body demonstrate that he is in somebody else's space. Yet he loses no poise; his own shrunken space is dignified and secure.

And so he is with Hermann on the long journey to the clinic; he is in the doctor's domain: he quietly waits for the doctor's performance to begin.

Hermann is not one to shrink from such an invitation.

"I want to tell you both a story," he says, a few minutes into the drive. "It is a true story about an experience I had in Namibia. I often tell it to Treatment Action Campaign activists when I am giving them a seminar. It is about the chain of events leading to death.

"A child is born in a remote rural area in Namibia. There is bleeding from the umbilical cord. The traditional midwife stops the bleeding using dung."

He lifts his head and searches for Sizwe's face in his rearview mirror. "You know about that?"

"Yes," Sizwe replies. "We do that, too."

"The baby is happy for a while," Hermann continues, "and then after some time she begins to shake. There is something wrong. The child is very sick. Public transport to the hospital comes only once a week. The mother goes to the headman; he is the only one in the village with a car. She asks if he can take them to the hospital. He says no, he is busy. And he goes off to visit his girlfriend."

The telling of the story has transformed Hermann's speech. The adverbs that on other occasions hang so tenaciously on the ends of his sentences have vanished. His words are clipped and purposeful.

"The mother waits two days for the bus to come," he continues. "Finally, she arrives at the hospital at night. The nurse on duty shouts at her: 'If you had come before you gave birth, this would not have happened! I cannot help you!'

"The hospital doctor reports for duty the next morning and he finds the child is dead. This doctor is me. This is a story of mine from Namibia. On the death certificate, he writes that the cause of death is tetanus. Was I correct to write tetanus? Was tetanus the cause of death? Why did the baby die?"

He looks at us both in schoolteacherly fashion and waits for a reply.

"You first," he finally says to me.

"One reason," I say, "is that the midwife had not been educated about tetanus."

"That would have helped," he replies, searching for Sizwe's face again in his rearview mirror.

"Another," Sizwe says, "is that the mother should have gone for her shots while she was pregnant."

Hermann's face lights up. "Why?" he asks. "Why must she be expected to wait for a week for the bus to come, and then maybe have to spend the night in a strange place? Why must it cost her so much money and time? She should have been able to walk to a clinic."

We drive in silence for a while. Sizwe considers a reply, then abandons it.

"The baby was killed by distance from public health care," Hermann says. "She was killed because she was too poor for the government to bother to build her community a clinic. And her community leader was not demanding a clinic because he was a headman with a car who likes to visit his girlfriend.

"I have another story. It is much closer to home. Last summer, I go to the beach at Port Saint Johns. There are lots of school kids on the beach in their school uniforms. They are unsupervised because there is a bar right on the beach, and their teacher is in the bar getting drunk. I hear people shouting, calling for a doctor: there is a girl who is drowning. I say I am a doctor, and the people take me to this obese teenage girl lying on the beach. She is clinically dead. I begin resuscitation. I shout to the people they must call for an ambulance. No ambulance comes. I shout that people must get the teacher. He does not come. He is still getting drunk at the tavern. Still, the ambulance does not come. Somebody finally agrees to take the girl to hospital in a private car. Meanwhile, the girl has vomited; it is a sign of life, even though there is no heartbeat.

"We arrive at the emergency room at the hospital, I tell the nurse who receives us that I am a doctor, and I ask her if she can put pipes down the girl's throat. You see, with drowning victims, you always try to revive the dead; with drowning there is cooling of the brain, which means that brain damage is delayed. So there is always a chance.

"But the nurse on duty says no, it is not the policy at this hospital to work on corpses. I say, please, there is still a chance to save this girl. The nurse says, no, this is a corpse; I will not work on it.

"I am very upset now. I am sitting at the hospital. The girl is dead and all the forms and papers of death are being filled out, and I am very upset. The police offer to give me a lift back to my car. On the way, they try to console me. They say: 'Don't be upset, doctor. It was God's will.' And that is the last straw for me. I start shouting at them. 'Was it God's will that her teacher was drunk in the bar? Was it God's will that the ambulance did not come when it was called?'"

His retelling of the story has released anger. What started as a rote Socratic tale has now been given life by vivid emotion. Sizwe and I are both silent. Hermann's feelings have filled the car and infected us.

"And the nurse," I say eventually. "Was it God's will that she does not work on corpses?"

"No, I left that out." Hermann giggles. He has returned to the present now, the anger of that day back in storage. "Solidarity with my fellow health-care workers."

During the following months, whenever I ask Hermann for his views about a death I have come across—a baby dying of diarrhea, a person whose immunity is still reasonably strong dying of AIDS—he shrugs ostentatiously and his face creases into a picture of ugly sarcasm. "*I* don't know," he says. "Why do people die? It was God's will."

Now, in the car, Sizwe clears his throat and leans forward in the backseat.

"There is no clinic in Ithanga," he says.

"I know," Hermann replies.

"There are no doctors or nurses."

"I know."

"Can you give us some advice. What should we do to get the government to build us a clinic?"

Hermann smiles briefly, leans into the steering wheel with pleasure, and shifts his weight in his seat. One car journey, and the young man from an outlying village is speaking like a nascent activist.

"I'll be honest with you," he says. "Your community applies for a clinic and they will place you on the list behind twenty-three other places that have asked for clinics. They will start building your clinic in three or four years if you are lucky. If you want a clinic sooner, you need to fight. You need to show that there is urgent need for a temporary clinic to be put in until a proper clinic is built. To do that you need the community to start shouting. You do that, you will get your clinic."

Sizwe nods and says nothing.

WE ARRIVE, FINALLY, at the clinic we are to visit. It is too small for its premises: some two acres of bare ground, surrounded by a barbed-wire fence, the clinic a single-story house set in the distance against the back of the property. Hermann parks behind the building, and a dozen or so people spill out of its back door to watch us. We unload the boxes of drugs he has brought with him. Our audience steps back to make a path as we move inside, our arms laden with parcels.

We walk in to a dense body of humanity. Seven or eight long rows of people, each individual on a plastic chair, stretch across the length of the waiting room. There are people sitting on the floor in the narrow spaces between, behind, and in front of the chairs. Others

stand in a tightly packed line against the wall. Given the number of patients it hosts, the waiting room is oddly quiet: just a gentle murmur.
Perhaps people have interrupted their conversations to watch the arrival of the doctor and his entourage.

Hermann is greeted by a counselor. He looks at her quizzically.

"They heard that the doctor was coming," she says blandly.

He takes in the crowd and smiles, but not happily.

"Okaaay," he sighs, largely to himself. "Is there a room I can use?"

Somewhere in his smile there is pleasure: well over a hundred
people have come here at a moment's notice on the strength of a
rumor that he will be visiting. That is a good thing, at least in part.
Even out here, on the outskirts of the ARV program, people come in
numbers because they know that there is treatment to be had. Far
better this bursting room than an empty clinic. Yet this is a nurse-
based system Hermann is building, and the fact that the rare presence
of a doctor has conjured this crowd is not an unmitigated good.

And indeed, once an examination room has been found for Hermann and work is ready to begin, the woman who joins him to assist is
not a nurse in her starched white uniform and maroon epaulettes, but
a lay counselor in civvies.

Hermann frowns. "Where's the nurse?"

"Late," the counselor replies. "She has been on leave with her
family. She had to drive from King Williams Town."

King Williams Town is at least a five-hour car journey from here. It
is nine in the morning. If the nurse managed to leave home at four, she
will be arriving any minute.

Hermann turns to Sizwe and me. We have found two chairs in the
far corner of the room, as close to out of the way as we can get.

"A clinic of this size should have at least two professional nurses
and two staff nurses," he says. "This one has none. So we have one temporary nurse after another. This one, the one who is on her way now,
lives at the other end of the province. She has never practiced ARV
medicine before. And she is doing the work of four people."

I am struck, now, by the import of the didactic tales Hermann told
us in the car. They constituted something of a template over the journey we were traveling. If the people in the waiting room outside had
been born twenty miles from here, on the outskirts of Lusikisiki's town
center, they would have visited a very different clinic. The one in town
has all the facilities of a local metropolis: it has five professional nurses;

its stock of medicines is managed and dispensed by full-time personnel; it is a center of activity for a host of counselors and treatment activists; a doctor visits at least once a week. In this place, there is one temporary nurse who has never practiced ARV medicine. The distance we have traveled this morning suddenly seems immense.

THE FIRST PATIENT to enter the examination room is a beautiful young woman, a most unlikely exemplar of chronic illness. Her thin braids frame a regal, high-boned face, one that exudes health.

Hermann examines the clinical notes in the folder she has handed him. He looks up at her, smiles mischievously, takes another look at the notes, looks at her again, and bursts out laughing.

"You're not sick," he says.

She is shocked and indignant. "I am sick, doctor. It is the glands in my neck."

"They are swollen still?" he asks cheerfully.

"There is no change."

He pushes his chair closer to her, slips his fingers under her braids, and rests them on the sides of her neck. He is still chuckling to himself.

A doctor's visit is too rare to be wasted on patients who are not gravely ill. Usually, the people ushered into Hermann's room have stubborn or complicated opportunistic infections, cases a nurse struggles to diagnose and treat. Whoever is managing the line outside must have slipped up. The young woman in the patient's chair should have been attended to by an assistant.

Sizwe and I have been allowed into the examination room under two conditions. Each patient is to be briefed about our work and given ample opportunity to object to our presence. We are also required to leave the room during physical examinations. Unfortunately, our presence changes the nature of the consultations a little; "a crowded room is seldom an environment conducive to personal talk," Hermann was to tell me later. And so his consultations are perhaps more perfunctory than usual.

Sizwe has described my work to the patient and she hurriedly nodded her consent. She pays us no further attention. Now Hermann hands us her folder. I put it on my lap and we read it together.

She has been on ARVs almost two years; she is one of the earliest patients in the program. Her treatment has been almost trouble-free, the only problem a chronic persistence of mildly swollen glands.

"In nine out of ten cases," Hermann says as he examines her, "the ARVs clear up the glands. This is the tenth. I don't know what to do. I have nothing to offer. There are some things I don't understand."

We read in her folder that she is due to come in for a new batch of ARVs next week. She must have decided to come early when she heard that the doctor would be here.

"Show me her pillbox," Hermann says to the counselor.

"The old patients don't bring them," the counselor replies. "They know their drugs."

The pillbox Hermann refers to consists of fourteen containers, each with its own transparent plastic window and window handle. The containers are arranged into seven rows of two; each row is marked by a day of the week, each individual window by the word *morning* or *evening*.

Hermann looks at the counselor suspiciously.

"She's healthy," he says. "Her CD4 count is high. Her viral load is undetectable. I'm sure she's been taking her pills. But you must not relax with the old patients. It is after two years that they begin to relax. I want you to get all your patients who've been on treatment over eighteen months together and ask them how treatment is going."

He gets up, rummages around in a cupboard, and returns to his chair laden with several bottles of tablets and a fourteen-window pillbox. He puts the pillbox on the table in front of the patient and opens each window. Smiling at her conspiratorially, as if they are playing a game the others in the room will not understand, he opens all the tablet bottles and pours their contents onto the table, mixing everything together. There are small red-and-white capsules, enormous mustard-colored tablets shaped like footballs, and brilliant white, disk-shaped pills. We all watch his performance patiently and in good humor. The counselor is smiling thinly for the first time.

Hermann looks at the patient and nods. "Do your thing."

She responds to the challenge with enthusiasm, sifting through the pile of tablets and slowly filling each of her fourteen windows. She arranges the pills in threes.

"And what are this one's side effects?" Hermann asks, pointing to one of the yellow footballs.

"*Agape*," she replies. Vomiting.

Sizwe's face broadens into a wide smile. He whistles through his teeth. He is impressed. Hermann watches him with evident pleasure and smiles back at him. Once more, the response of the young man from the remote village comes straight out of the textbook of best responses.

The textbook says that a person with Sizwe's life experience will never have witnessed biomedicine as Hermann is practicing it. He will have seen public health campaigns in which people are lined up and vaccinated like cattle; he will have visited inscrutable white or Indian doctors who would never deign to share their diagnoses with him, and who hand down medicines with the imperiousness of a Moses returning from Mount Sinai.

If people are to administer their own lifelong treatment, they must have a lively relationship with their medicines, a relationship at once emotional and cognitive. They must know the name of each pill, its shape, its color, its nickname, all its potential side effects. They are stuck with these tablets for their lives. Their relation to them will at times be hateful and fraught and unhappy. The tablets will perhaps make them sick, fail to stop them from getting sick, change the shape of their bodies. Best to develop a language with which to speak to them.

It is not just the pills, of course. Internal medicine's jargon of measurements—CD4 counts, viral loads—must become instruments through which patients monitor the progression of their health, breaking the seamlessness of a treatment with no end. A viral load is the amount of HIV in the blood. If antiretroviral treatment is working as expected, rendering the virus in her body dormant, the patient's viral load should be undetectable. A CD4 count is a blood test measuring the strength of the body's immunity. A healthy, HIV-negative adult should have a CD4 count of more than 1,000. As the virus attacks the immune system, the CD4 count drops. According to South African protocol, antiretroviral treatment begins when the count drops below 200. When the pills begin to work, the patient's CD4 count begins rising, and stabilizes at levels that rival the strength of her immunity when she was HIV-negative. Consulting her folder, I see that this patient's CD4 count was 181 when she started treatment. It is 512 now.

Her new batch of pills in her bag, she makes her way to the door.

"Was your boyfriend here for Christmas?" Hermann calls after her.

"Yes."

"Condoms?"

"Sometimes."

He turns to the counselor. "Have you explained to her the risks of reinfec—"

"She knows," the counselor snaps.

THE NURSE ARRIVES. Hermann gets up and shakes her hand and makes a great fuss of her.

"Thank you," he says. "Thank you for taking up this temporary post, for helping us out. And thank you for getting up so early this morning."

"Please, doctor," she replies. "This is my job."

The counselor shifts to the far corner of the table to make space for her. The nurse settles in next to Hermann. She is visibly discomfited by the doctor's proximity. She does not know what to do with her hands.

There is a new patient in the room. She is young and very nervous. Hermann settles down in his chair and pages through her clinical notes; she watches him unhappily.

Her case history records that she tested HIV-positive just over a year ago. Her latest CD4 count was taken last month; it is 284. She is, at the very least, several months away from ARV treatment. If things are going as planned, she is attending a support group every other week at the clinic for HIV-positive people. She will soon move on to an ARV support group where she will be prepared for lifelong treatment.

There is an enormous growth on her left thumbnail. Her case history records fungal infection of the fingers, but does not mention any prescribed treatment. Hermann hands the nurse the folder and waits for her to finish reading it. She looks up nervously. He points at the thumbnail.

"What is the correct treatment for that?" he asks.

"I don't know."

He looks down, begins to add notes to the case history, and speaks without looking up.

"I am prescribing griseofulvin, an antifungal medication."

He turns to the patient, begins explaining the treatment, and tells her the fungus will clear up within four months.

The diagnosis and treatment are more than routine. They ought to be second nature.

THE PATIENT SITTING at the examination table is young—late teens, early twenties, perhaps. She is accompanied by her mother. They both wear heavy frowns and grave faces; they are expecting, it seems, to receive news of the young woman's doom.

It is midafternoon. The patients have been streaming in and out of the examination room. By the time we leave, Hermann will have examined some seventy people. The nurse slipped out some time ago to find an examination room of her own; if everyone in this crowd were to see Hermann, we would be here well into the night.

The nervous young woman's last CD4 count was 273. All things being equal, it is not quite time for ARVs. Her clinical notes record that she is in the middle of a course of TB treatment. She and her mother are here because there are sores on her thighs and on her tongue. They do not like the look of them. In the last few weeks, she has also been finding blood in her stool. When they heard that the doctor was on his way, they dropped what they were doing and walked to the clinic.

Hermann takes one look inside her mouth, hurries back to the clinical notes lying on his table, reads for a moment, then slams his pen down in irritation.

"Why is this woman not on ARVs?" he snaps at the counselor.

She shrugs.

"Who was the sister who saw her?"

The counselor picks up the patient's folder and pages through it halfheartedly.

"Was it the sister who was here now? Why is she gone? Does she not like seeing patients with me?"

"She likes," the counselor says, "but she didn't know you needed her."

"I don't need her," Hermann replies curtly. "She needs me."

He gets up and returns to the patient and her mother.

"Has a nurse or a doctor ever spoken to you about the sores in your mouth?"

"No," the patient replies.

"It is Kaposi's sarcoma. We call it KS. It is a cancer that sometimes comes because of AIDS. It is difficult to treat, especially here in Lusiki-siki. The only way to treat it here is through ARVs."

He pauses to wait for questions. Both women are silent.

"ARVs are designed to treat HIV," he continues. "They are not designed to treat KS. It is only a little bit effective."

He turns to the counselor. "Her CD4 count is 273, but she must start ARVs now."

He swivels to face the mother. "Usually, we start treatment when it moves below two hundred. But because of the KS, we must start ARVs now."

He asks the patient to open her mouth and points to the growths. "They will get bigger and bigger without ARVs," he says. "You will not start ARVs today. It is a lifelong treatment. We must first educate you about how to use them properly."

"But if we delay," the mother says, "won't the cancer proceed?"

"It will proceed. But if you don't take ARVs properly it will proceed anyway. If the ARVs are taken the right way, they will strengthen the immune system. Hopefully the immune system will fight the cancer."

Hermann is speaking to the patient's mother, but his words are intended as much for the counselor in the room, who, Hermann tells me later, is among his best. She will be seeing the girl with KS within the next week, perhaps for as long as two hours, to tell her in far greater depth about her cancer and about the treatment she is to receive.

Within minutes, the girl and her mother are gone, their places in the patient's chairs taken by others. The ill come and go with such speed, I struggle to maintain the boundaries between them.

Hermann looks at me and smiles humorlessly.

"What do you think are her chances of survival?" he asks.

"I don't have the knowledge to guess," I say.

"In Lusikisiki, they are maybe fifty-fifty. If she was in Cape Town, they are maybe ninety percent. There she would be hospitalized to test the blood in her stool. She would be put on chemotherapy treatment. Here, the hospital is full and there is only sometimes chemotherapy, usually not. Here we can treat her diarrhea and her TB. We cannot treat her KS. ARVs are not meant for treating KS. Maybe they will strengthen her immune system enough for her to fight the cancer.

Maybe not. Later she will be asked if she has family in Durban." He glances at the counselor to ensure that she is listening. "If she can, she must be treated in a city."

ABOUT FIFTEEN MINUTES later, after another two patients have come and gone, I try to recall the expression on the face of the young woman as Hermann delivered his bad news. I find that I cannot recollect her face at all. I try again and again. Her face will not come to me.

This is my first conscious experience of my own prejudice, the first time I have watched myself write off a life that is still being lived. Now that I am aware of it and begin to look for it, the symptoms will grow both darker and more vivid.

IT IS LATE afternoon. The line outside the door to Hermann's examination room has been whittled away. Five or six solitary souls sit slumped in chairs, waiting to finally see the doctor.

An impossibly large man stoops through the door, straightens himself to full height, and shakes Hermann's hand. He must be six feet five at least. He wears a pair of overalls, unbuttoned to the top of his stomach, no shirt underneath. The pectorals on his bare chest push the flaps of his overalls aside like curtains.

He sits down in the patient's chair. Hermann picks up his folder, begins reading, then drops it. He looks up, his eyes wide, his nostrils flared.

"They nearly killed you last Monday!"

The man slams his hand down on the table. "Yes, doctor! They nearly killed me! They nearly killed me last Monday!"

His baritone is so deep, I look to the table to see if it is still. Sizwe and I glance at one another, wondering whether we too should feel angry.

Hermann is as animated as I have ever seen him. He waves an arm in the air, rallying everyone in the room, the nurse too, who returned with some reluctance about half an hour ago.

"Listen carefully," he says. "Listen to what this man is about to tell us."

He turns to the large man. "What happened on Monday?"

The patient clears his throat loudly and shifts in his chair. He is obviously pleased to be bearing testimony to his ordeal.

"I came Monday to the clinic," he says. "They gave me a bottle of pills. They said I must take the first one now, right here, in the clinic. They fetched me a glass of water. I drank the pill, and then I couldn't breathe. And then I was lying on the floor. I looked at my arms and there were blisters, huge blisters."

"They gave you co-trimoxazole on Monday," Hermann says. "It nearly killed you. You must learn the name of that medicine. Co-trimoxazole. You must never take it again. Also, I am going to write down the names of other medicines which have different names but are the same as co-trimoxazole. You must never take those medicines. I have written it all over your card in big letters."

He turns to the rest of his audience.

"This man has Stevens-Johnson syndrome," he says. "It is an allergic reaction to medicine, a very rare one. He is a gold miner. He went to a clinic on the mines last November. It says here in his notes that he had an allergic reaction to co-trimoxazole. The people here didn't see that in the notes. They gave him co-trimoxazole and nearly killed him."

The big man nods in agreement.

Hermann continues reading for a moment, then looks up at me.

"He was a miner. He got sick. They retrenched him. Sent him back here. Next time you hear the mining houses speaking nice about HIV, remember this story."

"Which mining hou—"

"They all do it," he interrupts. "Even the ones that talk nice."

He turns to the miner. "Why don't you get the union to fight for your job? HIV is treatable now. You can work."

"I don't trust the union," the patient bellows dismissively.

"Why not?"

"They are in it for themselves."

Hermann looks at the nurse. "Do you know what alternative medicine to give him?" he asks.

"No," she replies.

A FEW MINUTES later, in the dying afternoon light, it is just Hermann, Sizwe, and me left in the examination room. My head is down. I am taking notes.

"I don't like what you're writing," Hermann says.

"What am I writing?"

"That it's the nurse's fault that man nearly died."

"Whose fault was it?"

"Whoever treated him at the mine in November. Everybody knows that nurses might struggle to read clinical notes in abbreviations. Doctors understand clinical notes. Other people struggle. My colleague who treated him at the mine knew he was coming to a rural area. If he thought for longer than half a second, he would have known that the clinic in the rural area will give him co-trimoxazole. It is a general prophylactic. Everyone with HIV gets it. My colleague should have educated him. It didn't dawn on my colleague that giving knowledge to the patient might save his life."

"WHAT IS THIS clinic's mortality rate?" I ask Hermann as we make our way to the car. "Is it higher than clinics closer to town?"

"Why do you ask?"

"At Village Clinic in town, you have five experienced nurses. Here you have one temporary nurse who knows nothing about AIDS."

"The workload per nurse is worse at Village than here," he replies. "Everyone goes to Village. It has a strong support group, I am there often, it is a hive of activity, so people go there. Measured in patient numbers it is the most understaffed clinic in Lusikisiki. Here is better."

"Still," I say, "I have seen patients today who might have died if they had been diagnosed by the nurse instead of you."

"It does not take long to train a nurse," he replies. "And besides, poor clinic nursing does not increase mortality rates. If a good nurse sees someone is very sick, she sends the patient to the hospital. If a bad nurse sees someone is too sick, she also sends the patient to the hospital. That is where people die: in the hospital.

"The biggest consequence of having too few nurses is that fewer people start treatment. No nurses, no treatment. That is the problem."

It is Hermann's mantra: Fighting the epidemic is a primary healthcare project. It needs arms and feet, nurses and laypeople, to share the load, and that is all. Their competence will come later; the priority is numbers.

I do not believe him. From the Kaposi patient to the big man with Stevens-Johnson syndrome, I have seen today before my eyes that an AIDS patient who visits this clinic and sees this nurse is far more likely to die than a patient who sees Hermann. And if the Lusikisiki district isn't given the money to advertise its vacant posts, nurses experienced in AIDS medicine will keep leaving, and they will keep being replaced by nurses who know too little, like the one we saw today.

Hermann ought to have answered my question more candidly. Yes, poor nursing can result in mortalities, he might have said, but if ARV treatment is confined to well-trained specialists in hospitals then almost everyone sick with AIDS will die waiting to be treated.

DRIVING HOME IN the sunset, we pass a group of patients walking home. They wave to us.

"Those people are lucky," Sizwe says.

"Why?" I ask.

"Because they live in a place where a doctor, a white doctor, comes to spend the day."

For once, Sizwe's answer does not come out of Hermann's textbook. The doctor does not overhear our conversation. Had he done so, we would have received a mouthful about inherited prejudices against nurses and laypeople.

In the coming months, I will often pause to remember Sizwe's remark. The next time he speaks to me of a white doctor, his words will be far darker and far more complicated.

The Fence
Around AIDS

On the Saturday morning following Sizwe's visit to the clinic, his father, Buyisile, left Ithanga for the weekend. That night, Sizwe went to his mother's place for dinner. He was joined by his sister, Lindiwe, and by his niece, Thandeka, who had a weekend off work and had come to stay. The four Magadlas who broke bread together that evening constituted a full quorum of the bearers of Thandeka's secret. No other Magadla knew of her illness.

What with the old man far away and the four enjoying a simple evening together, somebody plucked Thandeka's illness from its silence and cast it into the discussion. There was an awkward moment in which no one said a word. Then Sizwe asked Thandeka whether she had been sharing her toothbrush. She had: she had left hers at home and had been using Lindiwe's.

Sizwe advised them to stop sharing. Even a healthy person, he pointed out, can break the skin on her gums when she brushes her teeth and leave blood on the toothbrush. Both women apologized. They had not been thinking; one is not accustomed to thinking of these things.

MaMagadla, Sizwe's mother, chipped in for the first time: those who are HIV-positive should also not share towels, she said. They rub it on their private parts when drying themselves, and the AIDS may have given them blisters that split open. And there is also the blood that comes from a woman when she has her period.

Thandeka agreed that she would be careful not to share her towels.

The family fell silent. They soon began speaking of other matters. Nobody had raised the question of what to do. Nor had anyone voiced the uncertainty all four of them felt inside: the question of timing. Next week, next month, next year, or ten years from now, Thandeka would fall sick. It was impossible to say when.

Yet the matter had been broached. Not furtively, in an unseen corner, but over a family meal in the homestead rondavel. Something had been shared, albeit something terribly fleeting and ethereal.

BY THE TIME this family discussion took place I had left Lusikisiki. I next saw Sizwe about a month later. I asked him whether we would go to Mthatha to see the girl who can cure AIDS. He had told me that Thandeka should get medicine from her rather than go to the clinic, for a cure is far preferable to lifelong treatment.

"I don't think so," he replied.

We were in my car once again, driving from Ithanga to town.

"Have you changed your mind about her?" I asked.

"I attended a funeral in Port Saint Johns last Friday." His voice seemed tired and reluctant. "There was a priest there, a priest the people respect. He mentioned the lady from Mthatha. He said she had failed in her promise to cure AIDS. He had watched people go off to see her. They came back and kept getting sicker and died."

He was silent for a long while. I was about to ask him about the priest.

"In any case," he finally continued, "there was a man from another village who has directions to the Mthatha lady's place. I looked for him for two weeks. When he heard I wanted to talk to him he came to Ithanga especially to see me. But the paper with the directions on them was at his home. He hasn't come back since then."

"Do you have another plan for your niece?"

"No. I am sitting without a plan. Maybe I will urge Thandeka to go to the clinic."

"Do you know whether they have taken her CD4 count? It might tell her how far away she is from getting sick."

"I don't think she has had that. I have no plan."

Although more than a month had passed, we had not spoken of our trip to the clinic with Hermann. Aside from his fleeting comment in the car at the end of that day, I did not know what he thought of what he had seen. It was on the tip of my tongue to ask him, but it appeared from his brittleness that now was not a good time.

THERE ARE MANY things about which Sizwe likes to talk to me: his father's life choices, his boyhood memories of herding and hunting, his business plans, his impending marriage. Sometimes, when we go walking together, all I need do is point at something, anything—a circle carved into the hillside by a bolt of lightning, an unusual tree, a hilltop—and a story will flow from him.

About illness he is not comfortable sharing his thoughts. The tension pulls his head into his shoulders and he observes me warily. I am knocking on the door to a universe in which I do not belong—because I am not family, because I am white, because I am a writer, because there are matters about which one does not speak lightly, and others about which one does not speak at all.

But I am here, after all, to write about illness. We are both aware of that: we must either speak of these things or part ways. He has in fact long ago decided to talk to me of the matters about which I want to know. It is a question of how, of the most respectable approach.

I think that the first time was in connection with the twins.

THE MOTHER OF the twins was a schoolgirl, fourteen or fifteen years old, and one of Sizwe's nieces. News of her pregnancy had been greeted with much anger. The girl was sat down and interrogated, and the name that finally passed her lips elicited a frightened silence. Nobody knew the boy, but his name betrayed that he was of the same clan as Sizwe's mother. If the two had indeed had sex, their union had violated a taboo.

Sizwe was instructed to visit the family in question—they lived about twenty-five miles away—to demand compensation. At first he refused.

"It is a very rude thing to say to your mother's family," he told me. "And I did not trust that the girl was telling the truth. These teenagers have sex with many people."

Reluctantly and with some bitterness, he did finally make the journey, and when he returned, it was with good news. The girl had been mistaken: the boy in question was just staying at that place; he belonged to another family and another clan.

"In any case," Sizwe said, "I doubt he was the father. I suspect that the father is from Ithanga. I have been watching. There is a young sangoma who lives near my niece. When she goes into the forest to collect wood, he always follows ten minutes later. Nobody notices because a sangoma does woman's work; he is meant to go to the forest to collect wood."

Sizwe's niece gave birth to twins at about eight o'clock on a January evening. She was attended to by Ithanga's most experienced traditional midwife. The first twin was born healthy, the second gray and unhappy. When I arrived at Sizwe's parents' homestead early the following morning, there was a pallor of heaviness about the place. The second twin had died during the night; the family was preparing to bury her.

Buyisile was in a mood I had not seen before. His face had frozen into a mask of extreme gravity, the corners of his lips pulling his broad mouth into his chin. He moved about relentlessly, first going into his field to untether and retether his goats, then pacing the circumference of his rondavel, then mooning around his workroom, his path trailed by the clattering of tools and implements. He was wearing his igqira's vest, and his powerful, young-man's frame cast a bolder shadow of violence than I had noticed before.

The unexpected death in his family had placed him in a no-man's land. He was, on the one hand, the oldest man in the family, and thus a leader on occasions such as this. Yet he was also an igqira, for whom the rituals of death are contaminating; his role here could at best be no more than peripheral.

After much wandering and muttering under his breath, he chose a burial site at the edge of the family's mealie garden, next to the graves of his three dead children. Sizwe and I and several other men began digging a grave. Within a few minutes, the men had put down their spades and were engaged in heated talk. The oldest among us, Buyisile's younger brother, had remembered that a twin ought not to be buried outside the family homestead. It must be close to where people sit at night. Nobody was certain of the reason. It had something to do with the well-being of the surviving twin.

Buyisile was called. There was a great deal of discussion. He walked off and we followed at a distance. He chose a new spot, this one directly behind his rondavel, and ordered us to dig.

When our work was done, we put down our spades and went to sit on the benches outside the family rondavel. Buyisile watched us closely from some thirty paces away. He was sitting on his haunches outside his workroom crushing herbs with a mallet; the mixture he was preparing protects his medicines from the pollution of death rites.

Without warning, Sizwe's mother appeared holding the corpse out in front of her at eye level; it was bundled in a thin blanket. A procession of seven or eight women followed behind her. She started to sing so softly that her melody periodically disappeared, and the other women cast in their voices and began picking it up. By the time the procession had disappeared around the back of the rondavel, a full chorus of voices mingled with our hushed conversation.

Sizwe's eyes were fixed on a spot in the middle distance. I followed his gaze to find a woodpecker near the top of a tall tree, hammering at its trunk. I smiled at him.

"My friends from Durban would come here for three weeks just to see that bird," he whispered.

After an interval that seemed to last no longer than three or four minutes, the singing ceased. Sizwe's mother reappeared from the back of the rondavel and signaled for us to come. By the time we arrived at the gravesite, the women were gone. We picked up the spades we had used to dig the grave and began filling it in.

Some time later, as I sat on a bench in his rondavel, Buyisile came to sit next to me.

"You have found us on a bad day," he said. "The child of my granddaughter is dead. It is a very dark day for us. When the family is scattered here and there we cannot protect them all. You know that death is coming, but you do not know precisely where. I have been seeing in my sleep for a while now that death is coming, but not once could I tell where it was going to strike."

"What do you see in your sleep that tells you death is coming?" I asked.

He frowned and turned away from me. "When you are here during happier times," he mumbled, "I will explain these things to you. But you are here during sad times, and I can't say more."

He stood up and walked out.

THAT AFTERNOON, I sat with Sizwe and his younger brother Mfundo on a hilltop overlooking their father's homestead. Most of the people who had attended the funeral in the morning were still there. From this height, they looked like charcoal figurines moving in slow motion.

As I recounted my conversation with Buyisile, Sizwe nodded.

"I am also warned when there is going to be a death in the family," he said. "I don't remember any death that did not first come to me in a dream. There are certain visions that mean that death is coming. For instance, a span of oxen plowing a field. Or if it is winter and the land is barren and you dream of a healthy mealie field, that means death is coming. If you dream of shit, of human dung, that is also a sign of death. What else?"

"Cultivated fields," Mfundo added. "Even if it is not winter, a cultivated field could be a sign that death is coming."

"Were you warned of the twin's death?" I asked.

Sizwe and Mfundo exchanged glances. They had clearly discussed this matter in the last few hours, and they were not sure I should hear about it.

"Yesterday," Sizwe said, "I had a terrible headache. It was with me the whole day. It was still with me when I went to bed; I could not sleep. When I finally slept, I dreamt of eating raw chicken, and when I woke up, my stomach was burning, as it always does when I have dreamt of eating raw meat. I thought to myself that a demon must have gotten into my room during the night; they have sent a demon again to feed me raw chicken and attack my stomach.

"Then I heard in the morning that one of my niece's children was dead. I was confused. Maybe the dream was actually about death. Maybe it was not a demon, but my people telling me there had been a death in the family. Except that the visions in the dream were not the visions of death, so I don't know. One does not dream of raw meat when there is a death."

"But either way," I said, "something was in your house last night and came into your sleep."

"Yes. Whether a demon with poison or my people to tell me something, I don't know."

"Who might be trying to poison you?" I asked.

Sizwe looked at me blankly.

"I think it's time to go back and join the others," Mfundo said.

THREE DAYS LATER, I arrived in Ithanga to the news that the second twin had died.

"What happened?" I asked Sizwe. "Was there no one with a car to take the child to the hospital?"

"No, that was not the problem," he replied. "It happened too quickly. The child was healthy and happy when she went to sleep. She woke up in the night very sick. By the morning she was dead."

"Did you dream?" I ask.

"Yes, I dreamt."

He did not say whether it was about raw meat or one of the signs of death. I did not ask.

When I next saw Hermann Reuter, I described the death of the twins to him in all the detail available to me. This was, I imagined, a favorite subject of his: infant death in a village far from medical care.

"From what I have said," I asked, "do you have any sense of why they died?"

He shrugged elaborately. "Who knows? It was God's will."

SOME WEEKS LATER, on a Saturday morning, I walked into a crowded restaurant on Lusikisiki's main street. It is a place where villagers like Sizwe eat their lunch when they are to spend a whole day in town. The patrons assemble at the counter in long lines, choose a piece of raw meat in the glass window under the counter, and then watch it being grilled in front of them. Looking into the sea of faces around the tables I caught Sizwe's eye. We greeted one another silently across the noise. I was surprised to see him; we had arranged to meet in Ithanga in the early afternoon. He made some space on the bench next to him and signaled for me to come.

Seated on his other side was a young woman. She held a tightly bundled infant in her arms. She was a cousin, Sizwe told me. She was passing through, and had spent the night at his place before moving on. After she put him down, her child had fallen ill; he cried without pause until after dawn, dozed briefly, and then awoke crying again. The moment the first taxis of the day began leaving Ithanga, Sizwe brought his two visitors to town to see a doctor. The child had received an injection and some tablets, he told me. They had decided to take a meal before leaving town.

I offered to give them a lift home. Sizwe went to do some shopping. I took the mother and child to my car to wait for him.

Sizwe had been consulting a general practitioner in town for several years. I presumed that is where he had taken his visitors. I asked the young mother what the doctor had said.

"He is not one of your doctors," she replied. "He is an inyanga."

"Do you visit Western doctors?" I asked.

"Yes, often."

"Why not this time? What makes you consult a Western doctor one day and an inyanga the next?"

She laughed evasively and said nothing.

We watched the child together. He started drifting off to sleep and then jolted awake.

"Look," the child's mother said to me. "He is so sensitive."

"To what?"

"To evil spirits. He is responding to something we can't see."

We watched the child. I wanted to ask more questions but felt inhibited by her guardedness.

"He has been sleeping well for two months," she finally said, unsolicited. "Why was he sick last night? The problem is the demons lingering around Sizwe's place."

"Why does his place attract demons?"

"Because there are so many people there all day drinking. They come in and out, lots of people. They go home and sometimes their demons stay behind to make mischief."

By now, Sizwe had joined us. He was listening silently and attentively.

I turned to him. "Why would people who are angry with you set their demons on your visitors?" I asked.

"As my cousin says," he replied cautiously, "demons are mischievous. They have minds of their own. The humans they are attached to go home after drinking, but they themselves linger, just so that they can make some trouble. They often attack my visitors. Last month, my nephew was staying with me and he woke one morning with a razor blade cut above his knee."

"You have not made the long trip to East London for a while," I said, "to get more muthi to protect your place."

"Yes," he replied. "I have been lazy. The other night, two men fought in my place. That is unusual. Usually it is the women customers who fight. It means it is time for more muthi."

"What caused the two men to fight?" I asked.

"Maybe my enemies. Maybe someone sent their demons into these two men, and the demons made them want to come to my place to fight. Maybe my enemy was hoping I would be hurt or killed trying to stop the fight."

"How does your muthi stop them fighting?" I asked.

"It makes them forget. The men come into my shop and they forget that they came to fight. And even after they have left, they never remember that they came to fight. It is foreign muthi from another place. The demons do not see it coming."

He stared at the child.

"Babies are so sensitive. If he looks you in the eye now, tonight he will dream of the things you experienced this morning. If you murdered someone this morning, he will experience it in his dreams later. He will wake up screaming, and we will not be able to make him quiet."

As I DRIFTED off to sleep that night, my thoughts wandered to Sizwe wandering into his own sleep. The idea that falling away from consciousness opens one's body to a medley of visitations unsettled me. I saw a host of souls drift in and out of him through the course of the night.

And then I recalled that some of his visitations were benign, some joyous.

One morning some time after we met, I came to his house early to find him in an ebullient mood. His steps were uncharacteristically light as he moved about his kitchen, his demeanor quietly boisterous. He began to tease me at the slightest provocation.

Over coffee, he told me that Jake had come to him the previous night.

"In my dream, I was sitting in Jake's house," he recounted, "and he walked in. He had come from fishing. He was holding mussels and crayfish and three musselcrackers. His brother was sitting with us. Jake handed him some bait and his brother went fishing.

"He sat down. He spoke. He was very happy. He was smiling and laughing. I was so pleased. He used to visit me before in my sleep, shortly after he died, and he was very sick then, and miserable. Now he was healthy and happy.

"A woman walked into the room, someone from his family. She said to Jake: 'There are always fish when you come from Johannesburg. When you are in Jozi, there are no fish.'

"At the end of the dream, I noticed that there was a fifteen-kilogram bag of King Korn lying on the table. King Korn is used to make *umqombothi*. Jake loved *umqombothi*. I saw this to mean that Jake wants a ritual of beer made for him."

That afternoon, Sizwe paid a visit to Jake's home and told the family about his dream. Yes, they said. He has come to three different people's dreams in the last month. He is asking for stones and a cross over his grave. His grave is unmarked.

"We don't have money for a gravestone," they told Sizwe. "But beer, yes; we will make beer for him."

WE HAD KNOWN each other some three months when Sizwe finally told the overarching story of the place of illness in his life. Until now we had been nibbling around the edges.

We were alone in his bedroom. He closed the door, shutting out both the sun and the ears of eavesdroppers, and told me his tale in the dim light.

Some four or five years back, when Sizwe and his brother were forced to abandon their studies for want of money, Sizwe went out in search of work. The first job he found was temporary, poorly paid, and unpleasant. On a farm some six miles from Ithanga a long-abandoned compound of old metal and wooden structures was to be revived and converted into a chicken coop. Sizwe and about a dozen others were employed to do the work.

After six weeks of daily labor, the men lined up in front of a wooden table and were given a paltry six hundred rand each.

The following day, the proceeds of his first job in his pocket, Sizwe took his parents to town and into the consulting room of the most famous and respected igqira in Lusikisiki. He told the illustrious man that he had been suffering from a burning sensation in his stomach for more than a year, that each night before the burning recurred, something came into his sleep and fed him raw meat.

The igqira asked several sparse questions and then began talking of two figures. One was a man and was short, the other a woman who was tall. They stood at the opposite bank of a river, watching the Magadla family. Immediately, all three Magadlas knew precisely of whom he spoke, a couple with whom the family had a long-standing feud, one that began long before Sizwe's birth.

"He could not have known," Sizwe told me. "He had never been to Ithanga. We had told him nothing about ourselves. And yet we recognized straightaway who he was speaking about."

Sizwe has instructed me to write no more about the identities of these two figures, or the source of the conflict between them and his parents. Suffice it to say that this episode with the igqira is the point to which all of his talk of spirits and illness was leading, the episode he could not possibly omit if he were to tell me the story of his life. The revelations that issued from the igqira are omnipresent; they insinuate themselves into the very trajectory of his and his family's life, explaining why they have become the people they are.

On the day he took his parents to see the sage, Sizwe was a young man from a poor family living through its poorest hour. That he spent his first wages on this expedition suggests that the igqira's words were prefigured, that the sequence of explanations Sizwe was to thread together afterward had been taking shape inside him for a long time.

In the wake of the visit to the sage, a sweeping narrative came together, no less potent for the fact that nobody would ever be sure whether it was true. The Magadla family has its fair share of chronic illness. Aside from Sizwe's recurring stomach problem, he has a sibling who suffers from epilepsy, a source of embarrassment to the family and an illness that it has kept a secret. It is common cause that attacks of epilepsy are triggered by a demon who launches a frenzied attack on its victim from within her own body.

"The demon lives inside you quietly for a long time," Sizwe told me. "Then one day you watch a bird fly past you, and when your neck is turned it gets stuck there, and that is when you fall and begin to shake and foam at the mouth. But what happens with my sibling is not quite the same. In this illness, the sufferers know they are going to be sick and they ask you to hold them. You hold them until their hand starts to shake and you keep holding them until they stop."

Sizwe's younger brother, Mfundo, also has an indefinable nervous disorder. There are times when he wakes in the morning and his right side is numb. He does not know the cause of it.

"It could be from when Sizwe and I were at school," he told me. "Our lives were so tough then. Maybe it is damage that is coming to the surface now."

But then again, Sizwe told me later, the problem began when circumstances brought Mfundo into daily contact with one of the two figures whom the igqira described standing across the river.

It is not just somatic illness. One of Sizwe's sisters is a wanderer. She comes back to Ithanga for a few weeks at a time, then vanishes without saying good-bye, and is not seen or heard of for months. Someone recalled an incident from her childhood. She was preparing to cross a bloated river and took off her clothes; she was being escorted by one of the two figures the sage spoke of. The figure picked up her panties and refused to give them back. The girl came home half-naked and crying.

What was done with her panties? Where are they now? What is the connection between that incident from long ago and her habit of wandering now?

Most important of all is Buyisile. Who kept coming to him in his sleep and calling him to the life of an igqira? Was it indeed his dead grandfather, or was it a spirit disguised as an ancestor? Had the old man been coaxed down a false path that would lead his family to penury? And what of his drifting? His flights from familial responsibility?

As I listened to Sizwe's story, I was struck for the first time by the full weight of what it means to live in a magical world: magical in the strict and narrow sense of a world in which the gap between ill wishes and the means to fulfill them closes. Those who wish to ruin you can do so by little more than wanting it. The trajectory of a family's path through the world, and all the psychological complexity contained within it, can be traced to the envy of others. Buyisile squandering his family's assets, Sizwe and Umfundo's abandonment of school, the chronic illnesses that visit family members: the psychological and the somatic are pulled into one line with a common etiology, an etiology that begins with rottenness within families and among neighbors.

"COULD THANDEKA's HIV have come from the same source?" I asked Sizwe. "From the people across the river?"

"No," he replied. "She got that from sex, probably with her current boyfriend. His previous girlfriend got sick. I think he got it from her and gave it to my niece. Maybe she even got it from earlier. When she left school she went to Durban for a year. We do not know what she was doing there."

He said these things flatly and conclusively, as if there were no more to discuss. But for me it was the very beginning of the story. If witchcraft can explain Buyisile's life choices, the pain in Sizwe's stomach, his sister's propensity to wander, and the numbness in Mfundo's side, why not AIDS?

"When we first met," I said, "you told me of your fear that your enemies had sent their demons to have sex with you while you are sleeping. You—"

"I remember. Sometimes one is not sure. Sometimes, you find yourself wondering about certain things. But I think there is only one way to get HIV."

It is not just Sizwe. I have been confronted by the same response in conversations with at least half a dozen young people in Lusikisiki. We are in the thick of a conversation about illnesses caused by witchcraft. The subject turns to AIDS. My interlocutor declares, by the force of simple fiat, that "there is only one way to get HIV." The discussion can go no further; it is a declaration, and a brittle one at that. A rickety fence is erected around HIV protecting it from witchcraft.

Why? I am not sure. By the time I arrived here, even a place as remote as Ithanga had been saturated by AIDS messaging—on the radio, on billboards, in the town center, on the tongues of people coming from the cities. No other illness has ever been the subject of such sustained publicity. The message that it is sexually transmitted is ubiquitous, universally known, reducible to stock phrases. Perhaps this universal knowledge is used as a shroud to smother, but never to quell, doubt. It stops conversations, but not thoughts.

There is another possibility. The idea that an epidemic of envy is killing the young and the healthy in large numbers is perhaps intolerable. Maybe people separate AIDS from witchcraft in order to protect themselves from the idea that neighbors and family are murdering one another in droves. In the course of this research, I read of a village in Mpumalanga province, more than six hundred miles north of here, where people are no longer prepared to leave their children with neighbors or accept food that was cooked behind closed doors. Perhaps here in Lusikisiki, people are protecting themselves from such a fate. For if AIDS is indeed an epidemic of neighborly hostility, the villages have descended into little more than a state of nature, one in which each soul lives in a cocoon of mutual suspicion. Perhaps it is a need to preserve a modicum of solidarity that pushes AIDS away from witchcraft.

If the fence around AIDS has indeed been erected to keep it from the corrosiveness of witchcraft, it is not a stable fence. I was to watch soon with my own eyes how a shock suffered unexpectedly by a whole village can tear down the fence between witchcraft and AIDS during the course of a single morning.

IF THE INSISTENCE that AIDS is caused by sex rather than witchcraft is born from an attempt to drain the epidemic of social toxicity, it is not at all clear that the attempt succeeds. What are the demons that people speak of: the ones that come to Sizwe in his sleep, feeding him chicken and sex; the ones that made his little nephew sick during the night?

The most commonly spoken of demon in these parts is the *tikoloshe*. He is no more than a foot tall, has an old man's face and a beard to his chest, and a penis so long he carries it over his shoulder. (He can, some say, turn himself into a woman in order to seduce a man.) He is visible to children and to the adults he sleeps with. His favorite habit is to befriend children. Some Ithanga adults have told me that *tikoloshe* lived in their homes when they were young, invisible to their parents.

They were pests, like monkeys, impish and naughty, forever knocking things over and stealing food.

A *tikoloshe* becomes dangerous when his child friends grow up and he proposes love to one of them. In combination with a human sexual partner he is a killer. He murders those his lover envies, and if she envies nobody, he demands that she present him a person to kill. He needs human blood; he is insatiable. The human being who makes a lover of him has entered a deadly pact; she must become a murderer.

The second most common demon is the *impundulu,* or lightning bird. He appears to his human lover as a beautiful young man. In Buyisile's time, he always arrived in Western dress, as if he had just disembarked from the Johannesburg train. He seduces women when they are out alone, collecting firewood or water.

As with the *tikoloshe,* his lover sends him to kill those she hates. And if she hates nobody, the *impundulu* turns on her, and demands the blood of one of her relatives. If she refuses, he kills her. His appetite is never sated. His lover thus becomes a serial killer.

It takes many months before it sinks into my head that those who speak of the shame of the HIV-positive are a hair's breadth from speaking of the shame of witches. Like the witch, the HIV-positive woman has a sexual appetite, and, again like the witch, her sexual appetite is murderous. As much as people try to strip AIDS of evil by giving it a strictly biomedical explanation, it nonetheless remains lodged in an old and poisonous well of fear, of suspicion, and of misogyny.

Kate Marrandi

It was an astoundingly hot January morning. The bodies were jammed into the clinic waiting room so tight I did not know whether the damp on my forearm was my own or someone else's. The soft, soapy smell of hundreds of recently washed bodies mingled with the smell of fresh sweat and the smell of sheer heat, and the line in the corridor outside the consulting rooms had long since vanished into a dense mass of people hemmed in by the walls.

Even here, where the faces were so many they had become interchangeable, she was singular, unmistakable; the promise of death in her face and her body drew you to her like the Hamelin stranger's pipe.

She sat there in her wheelchair amid the crowds, her useless neck dropping her head onto her right shoulder. Her eyes were open wide and unblinking as if she had constantly just a second ago received a terrible fright. Her lips were pulled and drawn, exposing her upper teeth and her gums. She wore a bright pink tracksuit several sizes too big, a sore memory of the space she must have filled before she fell ill.

Two middle-aged women attended to her. The first was using her clinic folder as a fan, flapping it perpetually in front of her dazed face. The second, who wore a wide-brimmed straw hat, had put the woman's head back upright, and was cupping the back of her neck with her hand.

The young man who managed the line had noticed her, too; he took the handles of her wheelchair and shouted in a loud voice for the crowds to clear a path to the consulting room at the end of the passage. He wheeled her chair into the crowd, turning it into a makeshift battering ram, opening space where there had been none before.

I was scheduled to sit in on Hermann Reuter's consultations that morning. I followed the path the wheelchair had made and slipped into Hermann's room after it.

Once the door had closed behind us, the consulting room was disorientingly quiet and empty. In the far corner, a strong fan worked at full throttle. Hermann stood up, walked from behind his desk, found a chair, and sat next to the patient, his eyes level with hers. He put her wrist gently in his hand, and looked at her closely. Then he and the line manager lifted her and put her on the examination bed, holding her neck and her limbs steady; she was so light that one of them could have done the job.

"Which of you is her mother?" Hermann asked.

The woman who had used the case history as a fan walked over to him and watched him as he bent over his patient.

"I am her aunt," she said. "She can't talk. She can't walk. But sometimes she can hear."

The niece was in the middle of a course of TB treatment and had been on ARVs for five months. Her case notes recorded that she had been hospitalized twice since the beginning of December. As Hermann examined her, the appearance of shock left her eyes and she drifted off into sleep. I would not have been surprised if she had died there and then.

Once he was done with the examination, Hermann lifted her off the bed and settled her back in her chair.

"Don't leave her aside," he said. "She must sit with the family. She can hear when you talk. Don't hide her."

"Yes," the aunt replied. As she spoke she held up her niece's neck with firm and gentle hands. "She smiles sometimes when you talk, and when she is feeling her strongest, she can say: 'Hi!'"

At the word "Hi!" her niece rolled her eyes; her mouth broke into a wide smile and a laugh issued from the back of her face.

"Do you understand English?" Hermann asked her.

She grunted affirmatively.

"Did you work?"

She replied with a short medley of grunts, but it was impossible to hear the words.

"She is saying she is a social worker," her aunt said.

Hermann put his hand on the back of her head.

"Your brain has been very, very sick," he said. "The TB got into your brain and made it very, very sick."

"Yesterday, her disability grant started," her aunt said. "The first grant money arrived and she laughed. It was the first time she had laughed. Her granny started laughing and then I did. We were all laughing."

Listening to the story of herself laughing, she laughed again, and we all laughed with her, and she strained for the use of her neck to look up at her aunt. Knowing what she wanted, her aunt bent down into her line of vision.

"You were laughing yesterday," she said, "for the first time."

It is hard to say how a long story gets to be told in a single gesture, but in that moment it was clear that her aunt had poured many years of love and savings into the growth of her niece, and that now she was harnessing that same love to keep her from slipping away.

"Are you also a family member?" Hermann asked the woman in the straw hat.

"No," she replied, "I am a community health worker."

I smiled to myself. Twice in the last two months I had seen this same woman wearing the same hat in Hermann's consulting room. She had sat quietly, as she did now, looking diligent and interested, and had not said a word. On both occasions he had asked her as she was leaving whether she was a family member and both times she had told him she was a community health worker.

I asked her her name.

"I'm Kate Marrandi," she replied, "from Nomvalo village in Taleni locality."

The sick woman had managed to lift her legs and drag her heels to her buttocks. She was preparing for the journey back through the throngs of people outside. Her legs must have been battered on the journey in. Kate Marrandi opened the door, and fragments of noise and heat and smell momentarily joined us.

When they had gone, I asked Hermann whether he thought she would live.

"She got TB meningitis while on ARVs," he said. "Her CD4 count was thirty-nine at the beginning. She was vulnerable to everything."

"She came too late," I said.

"She is being treated with ARVs and TB drugs," he replied. "She will get better than this, but she won't be a social worker again."

SIZWE AND I drove to Nomvalo village a week later. I had taken Kate Marrandi's cell phone number before she left Hermann's consulting room, phoned her, and asked to see her. I was intrigued by her recurring presence in Hermann's room, by her fastidious silence, by the doctor's failure to register her existence.

Her English was not much better than my Xhosa; the directions lying on the dashboard promised to take us somewhere unexpected.

Nomvalo is about forty miles from Ithanga, and the roads between them are slow going; Sizwe and I spent the better part of an hour in the car together. In the silences between conversations I began to think about his niece Thandeka's boyfriend. His previous lover was gravely ill. Thandeka herself had told him that she was HIV-positive. And yet he would not hear of testing. I started thinking aloud. I told Sizwe that I wanted to spend time with him, to get to know him well. I wanted to understand his refusal to test.

"You say you are talking about Thandeka's boyfriend," he said, "but you are also talking about me."

"Perhaps. But you know that your lover is negative. He knows his lover is positive."

"I want to test," Sizwe said. "I think it is finally time."

I nodded and waited for him to continue. It took a while.

"I must get to the bottom of this business in my stomach. You look at me and you think I am well, but I am not well. It has been some five or six years since this problem began. When I wake up in the morning and press my stomach, it is hard and sensitive; it feels like there is some thick liquid inside it. Maybe it is bewitchment, like the sangoma said. But maybe it is HIV. Many HIV-positive people have problems in the stomach. Maybe that is what I have been sitting with. Maybe I am unlucky like Jake."

I concentrated on driving, thought of Sizwe's stomach, and soon felt quite anxious. It was not only the uncertainty concerning the etiology of his complaint, it was also the swaths of territory that lay between symptom and possible cause. The pain in his gut may have been placed there by a terrible anger born more than a generation ago, an anger that had caused an assembly of malicious creatures to inhabit and leave and reinhabit the bodies of his parents and his siblings over a span of decades. Or it may have been sheer chance, as he and Jake blazed a trail of adolescent excitement through the villages of Lusikisiki.

Either way, it struck me that his understanding of the pain in his stomach was crisply social; the somatic was simply an outcropping under which were layers upon layers of family and neighbors and the world at large. I found the idea deeply unsettling. For at the root of this etiology is that one's relation to others exposes one to the prospect of extinction.

"Why now?" I asked. "What has happened recently that has made you ready to test?"

"I am ready. I know that if I have HIV I will die."

"You won't necessarily die."

He turned from me and looked out the window.

"The *umlungus* say that if you take ARVs you will live for as long as you would have if you had never gotten sick. But I know a man who was on ARVs a long time, and he got sick, the very sicknesses you get when you are HIV-positive, and he died."

I do not know what brought on this tightly packed blow of honesty. But he had just knocked down a wall between us. We were somewhere entirely new.

"Why do you think the whites are so keen on ARVs?" I asked.

He responded with an uncomfortable silence. He shifted in his seat, glanced at me briefly, and then stared out the window again.

"I think the *umlungus* want to help people."

There was another silence, this one much briefer.

"Do you think there is a cure for AIDS?" he asked.

"No."

"Some people believe that the whites have developed a cure for AIDS, but that they are holding it back. They are waiting for enough black people to die so that when we all vote in an election the whites will win and F. W. de Klerk will be the president again."

I laughed, and his eyes widened with anger.

"I am not telling you a joke. I am telling you what many people believe," Sizwe said.

He looked down at his chest and cocked his head away from me, as if to erase the entire discussion.

"I have told you a black people's secret. I am sorry I have told you that."

He picked up the map on the dashboard, studied it, and put it back again.

"I think you have missed the turnoff to Nomvalo."

I HAD MISSED the turnoff because one would never have taken it for the entrance to a village. It was an impossibly steep ramp, its gradient perhaps forty degrees, its surface a raw and grainy concrete. From the roadside, it appeared to last only a few dozen yards, leading, perhaps, to a rubbish dump.

And yet we climbed and climbed, and it did not end, and some way up we passed the extraordinary sight of a span of eight oxen harnessed to an enormous bundle of firewood. As the beasts became small in my rearview mirror, the road flattened without warning and we found ourselves in Nomvalo village, a scattered hamlet of round mud huts and square brick houses dispersed across the length and breadth of a broad plateau.

Just as one cannot fathom the presence of a village from the tar road, so one does not get the sense up here that one is at the top of a mountain; from horizon to horizon there is nothing to suggest that the rest of the world is some distance below. It struck me then more forcefully than at any other time that the Transkei is arranged vertically; that unless you recalibrate the sense of dimension coded into your mind you will not find your way about.

As we gathered our bearings, I spotted the distinctive figure of Kate Marrandi in her enormous hat, standing in the middle distance at the side of the road. We pulled up beside her and she got into the backseat and directed us to her house along a rutted and torn-up dirt path. Sizwe introduced himself with his customary warmth and politeness, announcing his first name, his village, his surname, and his clan name. He had not been at the clinic the week before when Hermann examined the young woman in the pink tracksuit.

MaMarrandi's home was that of a poor person. It was made of mud and concrete, and poorly made at that, the far wall of her living room leaning outward, the near wall leaning in, the ceiling slanting toward us. Outside, a few paces from the front door, three piglets guzzled from a trough, their noise filling the room.

MaMarrandi took off her hat to reveal a head of brilliant gray hair. It struck me that she was older than I had imagined back in Hermann's consulting room, sixty at least.

She was not from these parts, she told me; she was Zulu, born in Glencoe in the KwaZulu-Natal midlands. Her father was a devout Jehovah's Witness who read Bible stories to her and her siblings every evening from as early as she could remember, and when she was not yet out of her teens she married a religious man.

In the early 1960s, her church sent her and her husband away to proselytize. They did so with extraordinary diligence, traveling the length of South Africa's eastern seaboard without pause for almost a decade, preaching the word of the Jehovah's Witnesses. Not once did the church pay them for their work. For a living, MaMarrandi found a string of part-time jobs, primarily teaching illiterate adults to read and write.

By the early 1970s the couple had two children. During the course of the next decade they were to have three more.

"We arrived in this area in 1971," MaMarrandi told us, "and we decided to stop here to educate our children. By 2002 the last-born had passed standard ten [twelfth grade]. We had been in this place thirty-one years and the last of our children was educated. The family at home was getting finished. Only the mother of my husband was at home. She needed someone to look after her. So my husband and children went back to my husband's hometown of Matatiele. I was meant to return with them, but I stayed. There was work for me to do here. I had been involved with AIDS, the work was becoming promising for the first time, and I could not leave."

"Please start at the beginning," I said. "Do you remember your first experiences of AIDS here in Nomvalo?"

"Yes, I remember well. The first cases were in 1996. People working in the mines came back seriously ill. We took them to the doctors in the main street and at the hospital. The doctors would say: 'These people are HIV-positive. We cannot help them. You must take them home and treat them with herbs.'

"I remember a girl from Durban. The people in Durban put her on a bus to Nomvalo. When she arrived at Nomvalo station, the people were told they must not touch this girl: she has AIDS. Once you touch someone with AIDS, it is transmitted to you. So they did not touch her. They used blankets to hold her, as if she was a corpse, but she was still alive. They put her in a wheelbarrow and took her home.

"There, she stayed alone. She was in her own hut, and people only came in to give her food. After she died, they dug a grave and they carried her to her grave on her mattress so that they would not have to touch her body. They buried her mattress with her."

She continued without pause: "It was a very difficult time. We believed the disease to be very infectious, and we could not see who was HIV-positive. We could only see once someone was getting sick. Even when the girls gave birth, we didn't have gloves; we helped the girls give birth with our bare hands.

"It was only in 1999 that we started to learn about the disease. Nurses from the hospital came and told us about how the disease only lives in the sexual fluids and in the blood, and not on the skin or in the breath. And people on the radio began explaining. That was also in 1999."

"What were you doing at the time?" I asked. "Were you a community health-care worker yet?"

"I was not working at the time. I was only preaching the Word of God with my husband. But I felt I must get involved. Once the information started coming in, I felt I must go somewhere to get educated about this, and then come back to help."

At about this time, the national government was beginning a policy reversal that was to shape the next era of MaMarrandi's working life. In the 1980s, the South African countryside had been littered with lay health workers trained in a range of fields from midwifery to TB care. When the African National Congress came to power in 1994 the idea of lay health workers fell out of favor. Now, in 1999, as hospitals were getting their first inkling of the horrific burden the great epidemic would place at their door, the idea of lay workers dispersed throughout towns and villages came back into fashion. By late 2003, the national health department would be investing large sums in the recruitment of community health workers across the country, and was soon paying a stipend of five hundred rand per month to some twenty thousand lay workers.

Some criticized it as a measure to keep the sick and the dying invisible and away from the hospitals. Others pointed out that as sickness spread into each village, treatment would be impossible to administer if the health system did not have conveyers of information and knowledge everywhere.

Among the organizations that began training community health-care workers in the late 1990s was the Hospice Association of South Africa. In mid-1999, Marrandi reported to a hospice in Port Shepstone and was recruited into a three-month training course.

"We learned many things there," she said, "including what was happening in the hospitals. When we visited the hospital wards we were not allowed to even whisper the word *AIDS*. The doctors tried to keep it a secret from the nurses because it was feared that if they knew they would not treat the patients. But the nurses knew, and they them-selves were trying to keep it a secret from the patients.

" 'Don't ask in front of the patient what is wrong with her,' one of the nurses told me. 'If she hears it is AIDS, she will die.'

"When we came from our training to the villages we were sent to the hospital. We were given the patients the hospital could not treat. At that time, if you had AIDS the hospital sent you home to be cared for by us.

"And so that was my work. We went to our home villages and we went door-to-door to help the patients to die with the love of their families. We touched the sick person. The family watched. We taught the people how to love the ones who were dying."

"That must have been very difficult," I commented, "this work of changing nightmarish and lonely deaths into peaceful deaths. It must be very difficult to deal with so much death."

"It was difficult for the parents to know that their child was wait-ing for death," she replied. "The parents did not want to know that."

I would soon learn that this was always how Kate Marrandi an-swered a question about her own emotions—by deflecting it onto someone else. I would come to see with time that this ostensible blank-ness was the secret to her work.

"I would arrive one day," she continued, "to find that the patient is not there. She had been taken by her parents to a prophet or an herbal-ist. And so the patient would die far from home among strangers be-cause her people did not want to know that their child was waiting for death.

"But then things changed. Then everything changed. In 2003, Dr. Hermann came. He started to tell us he has got help—ARVs. Nobody believed him. Some said this one has come to kill the people. Even the doctors didn't believe him. People thought he had come to destroy the people with his needle and his blood test. They believed AIDS was caused by politics, by white people."

Sizwe translated these words slowly and carefully, and as he did so, he burrowed his eyes into mine. When he was finished he kept staring at me, and although he said nothing more, he told me plainly with his eyes that what MaMarrandi had said was what he had refrained from saying earlier in the car: that in Ithanga people had wondered aloud whether Hermann Reuter carried the virus in his needle. That is why, when I had mentioned Reuter's name some months earlier, Sizwe jolted as if he had been struck.

"We talked to Dr. Hermann," she continued. "You see, here our nearest clinic is Ntafufu and our hospital is Bambisana. We fall under the Port Saint Johns district, and Dr. Hermann is working in the Lusikisiki district. We are not part of his ARV program.

"We asked him how he can come to us in Ntafufu. He said he could help. We must gather him some volunteers, and he would teach us about the ARVs, and then we could take our patients to Lusikisiki.

"So we stopped working for the hospice and were recruited by another organization that employs community health workers called Bambisanani. We had some workshops with Dr. Hermann about AIDS and ARVs. Me in this village, and others in other villages, we began to take the sick people to the clinic in Lusikisiki. We discovered that after these ARVs have been used by the people, they are not dying a lot now, they are not lying down and dying. But some are still dying: the ones who do not like to listen. If you don't want to stop drinking or smoking you die."

"Tell me," I said, "about the ones who die even though there are ARVs for them. What is it that causes them to die?"

"It is mainly the young people," she replied. "They are living for the present. They don't know about the future. Someone who cares for their life will know that at point x I will be doing this and at point y I will be doing that. The young do not know these things.

"I don't know if you remember, but the first time I met you in Dr. Hermann's room at the clinic in town I was with a young man. He was swollen here." She ran her hands slowly down the sides of her throat. "He was so weak he could not walk. I went to his house and told him he must come with me to the clinic and we carried him to the taxi. At the clinic, I asked Dr. Hermann for ARVs for him. The man was so weak he couldn't go to the support group. I said at the clinic they must give him ARVs. I will teach him at home.

"Then I started to teach him. I told him he must stop drinking beer. He must stop smoking. I told him that his life depended on these ARVs: you are going to be using them for the rest of your life.

"He said, 'Auntie, I was born not smoking and drinking. All of these things I started when I was grown. I can stop.'

"I told him to start with his ARVs, and he lasted two days. On the third day, he sent the little children to buy him cigarettes and beer. I see before my eyes that the young do not know what to do about their lives. I went home for Christmas. I came back on January 3. When I came to his place I saw he was near death. He had gotten so drunk on Christmas Day he did not find his way home. On his clinic card it was written PCP—pneumonia. The following day he died."

"The youth—" I began to say.

"Sometimes I call the youth to the school and meet with them. They need to have sex at fourteen, fifteen. And they will not use condoms. I ask them why not. The boys say sometimes they are just sleeping at their homes and the girls knock on the doors. They hadn't even invited the girls. You do not use condoms in such circumstances. I say, what about AIDS. They say, no, we don't need condoms. I give them advice: be faithful to your partners. They say no. I say, well, then abstain. They say no. I say to them, 'You are a generation of AIDS.'"

"How many people in the village have you taken to be put on ARVs?" I asked.

She rummaged through a rucksack that had been lying in front of her on the table. A pair of reading glasses and a hardcover ledger soon emerged from it. She put the glasses on the end of her nose, opened the ledger and began inspecting it carefully, moistening her fingertips each time she turned a page.

"I cannot say for certain," she pronounced finally. "I think I have about thirty people on ARVs."

"And how many have died?" I asked.

"Only a few. If they listen, they live. Most of them listen."

As I imbibed her stories, it struck me that the position MaMarrandi occupied was quite extraordinary. Nomvalo was located beyond the last outpost of Hermann's treatment program. None of the voluble young activists he had trained was here—no adherence counselors, no pharmacist assistants, no Treatment Action Campaign activists. The local clinic, Ntafufu, did not treat AIDS at all. This entire village's relation to ARVs was mediated through one woman.

An image of Kate Marrandi filled my mind. Her rucksack on her back, her nose keenly tuned to the scent of illness, she knocks on every second or third door in the village. She is invited in, and sits in the family living room speaking softly and paging through her ledger. She coaxes the sick into a taxi to visit Dr. Hermann. It struck me that in Nomvalo what she meant and what the drugs meant must have long become inseparable.

I asked whether we could come back the following month and shadow her, and she agreed. Then I asked if we could visit the very sick young woman in the wheelchair and the pink tracksuit, and she said that when I was back the following month hers would be the first home we would visit.

"How much does the government pay you to be a community health worker?" I asked.

"Five hundred rand per month. So that we can buy soap to be clean when we visit the people."

It was the first hint of irony I had encountered since meeting her, although her face remained so deadpan it was impossible to tell what she thought of her remark.

AIDS Needle

We said nothing to each other as we made our way down the long concrete ramp that connects Nomvalo to the rest of the world. Only after we had rejoined the tar road and were heading for Lusikisiki did either of us speak.

"I am relieved that Kate told you what the people were saying about Dr. Hermann," Sizwe said. "I was worried that it was only Ithanga. When you laughed, I thought, Maybe I am telling Jonny some bullshit that only the people in Ithanga believe. But now we have both discovered that the story is everywhere, even as far away as Nomvalo."

Yet he had not in fact told me the story. Even while betraying the black people's secret on the journey to Nomvalo, he had not been able to say it out loud. MaMarrandi had had to say the actual words— "they thought Dr. Hermann had come to destroy the people with his needle and his blood test." Sizwe had told me with his eyes that this was his story too, that this is what he had been trying to convey to me in the car.

For all our talk on the causes of AIDS, it had taken this trip to Nomvalo to out his strongest suspicion about the origin of the epidemic. It was brewed, not by witches and their demons, but in the vividly imagined laboratories of Western science.

We had known each other four months. Both of us knew that the most significant afternoon of our acquaintance was drawing to a close.

Yet there was strangely very little to say. I considered asking him what he thought of the heart of MaMarrandi's story: for three years she had buried her patients one after the other; now they were getting up and walking. I wanted to ask him to take an imaginative flight with me and wonder what it was like to stand in MaMarrandi's shoes: to know that people you greet in the street every day would probably be dead if you had not come into their lives.

I listened to my internal voice saying these words, and even to me, they sounded relentless and insufferable, and so I said nothing.

Instead, I began to think about Sizwe. It struck me that the trip he had embarked upon with me was radically experimental. Among the things he wanted to discover was whether Hermann Reuter was a villain or a friend.

I believed that Sizwe was entirely open to either possibility, and was gathering empirical evidence. How does one gather such evidence? What is it one is looking out for?

I was thinking of how to formulate the question when he spoke.

"*Ushayela kahle,*" he said. "You are driving well."

I turned to look at him. His face was full of quiet playfulness.

———————

DURING THE FOLLOWING weeks and months, the tale of Hermann's HIV-laced needles began emerging all over the place, always unsolicited. It was usually a Hermann acolyte who told the story.

"Even before Hermann came to our village for the first time, people had heard the rumor that he was bringing AIDS," a young woman called Doli Mapungu, whom Hermann had hired as a pharmacist assistant, told me. "When he arrived, there was a big crowd outside the clinic. Many were not sick; they had come to see Hermann. They said they had heard that here is the doctor who has come to inject AIDS into people. They came to see what he looks like. When he came out, they all stared at him, but no one said anything.

"Then, in the next months, the community saw that dying people took ARVs and they got better. Now, on Tuesdays, the day Hermann comes to the clinic, it is full. If people come on a Tuesday and they find that Hermann did not come today, and only the sister is there, they go home. They want to see Hermann. They love him now. They know him as a healer."

Some weeks later, I interviewed a young man who comes to the clinic in town punctually at eight every morning to manage the lines. He was one of the first in Lusikisiki to begin ARV treatment.

The day he came back from the clinic two years ago to tell his family he had tested positive for HIV, they scolded him.

"They were very angry," he told me. "Not just because I was HIV-positive, but because I had gone to Dr. Hermann.

" 'You have been to the doctor and allowed him to put his needle in you. Do you understand now that you are already dead? Your eyes are open but you are dead.'

"I have not seen my family in a long time," he continued. "Sometimes I want to go to them just so that they can see my healthy body and then remember the words they said to me."

Treatment activists had claimed the AIDS needle story as their own and worked it into a sunny narrative. "The people used to be ignorant, but now everyone knows." Each story they told was a simple variant of this theme.

Yet their narrative was a little too sunny, a little too self-assured. I would soon get to see how much ground they themselves had been forced to give to the idea that Western medical technology embodies malicious intent. Indeed, they had given this ground so thoroughly and so long ago, they were no longer aware of having made the concession.

THE FIRST TIME I asked Hermann about the story of the AIDS in his needle, he gave me a long, sardonic look.

"What do you want to know about it?" he asked coldly.

"Why and how you won that battle. It might have ended very badly."

"Clearly," he replied, "those in favor of treatment prevailed over the others."

He looked at his watch and said he had to go.

Only after this clipped conversation did I discover the ordeal Hermann had experienced. During his early days in Lusikisiki, he had on two occasions arrived to packed clinic waiting rooms; some of the people assembled there had not come to be tested but to ask him to explain what was in his needle. He had had to stand in front of his audience and convince them that he had not come there to kill them.

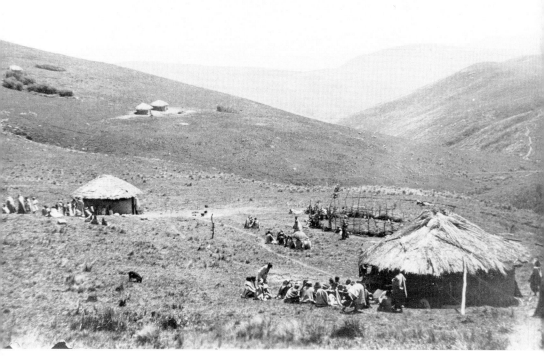

1.

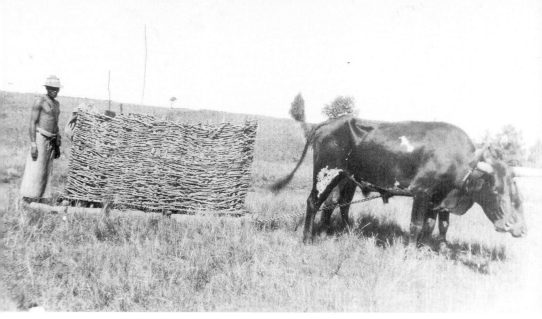

2.

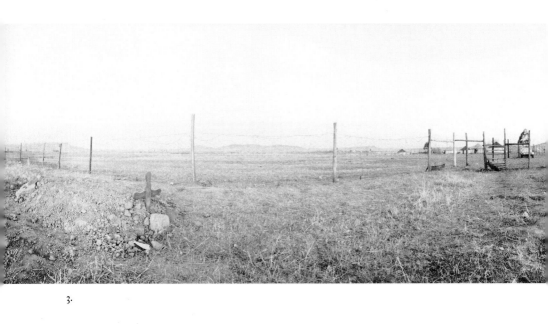

3.

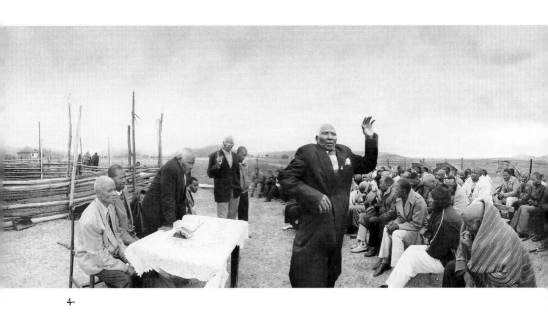

4.

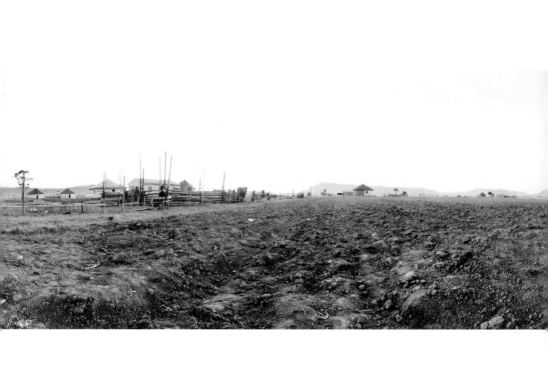
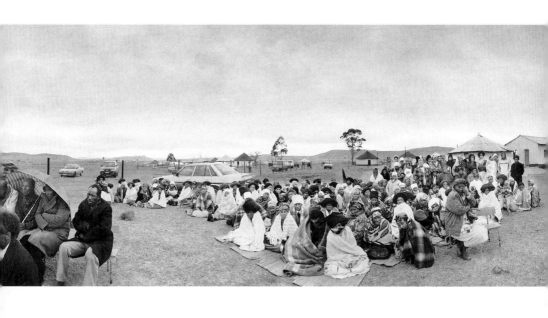

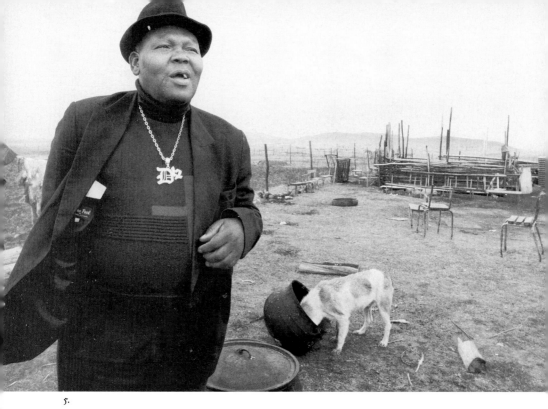

5.

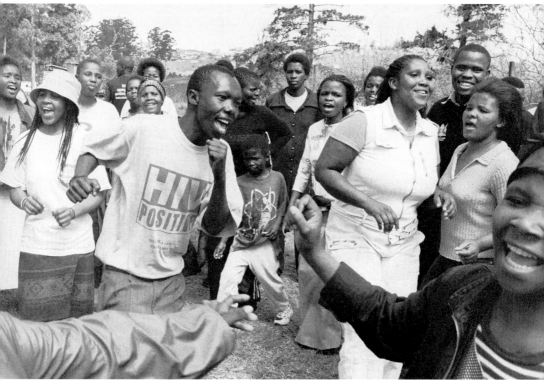

6.

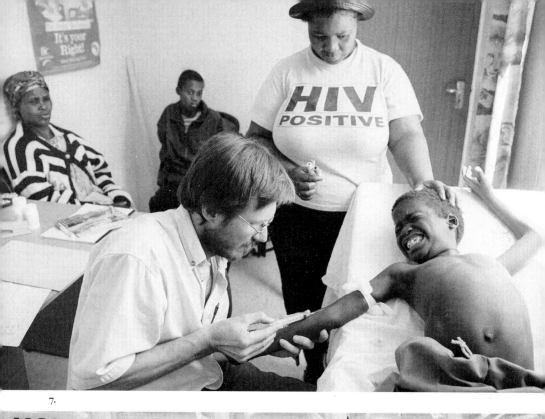

7.

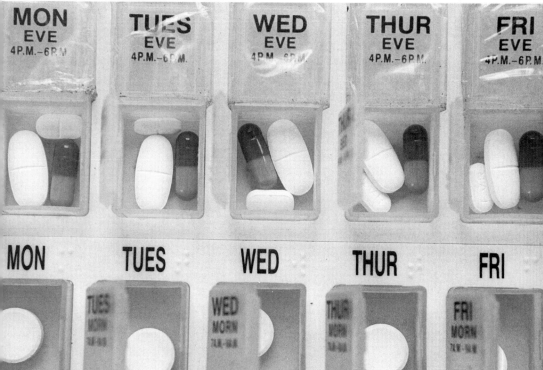

8.

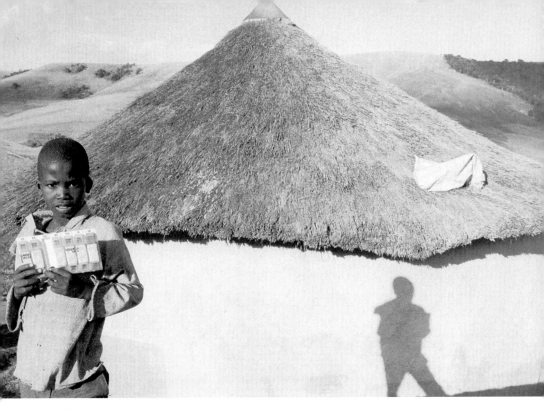

9.

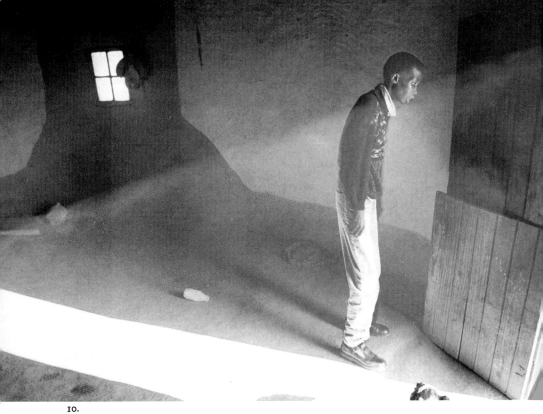

10.

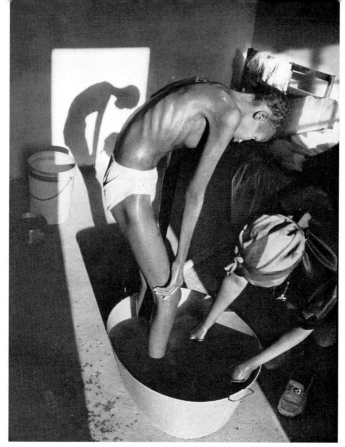

11.

12.

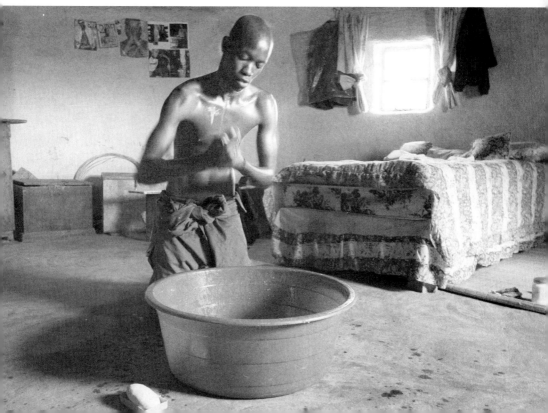

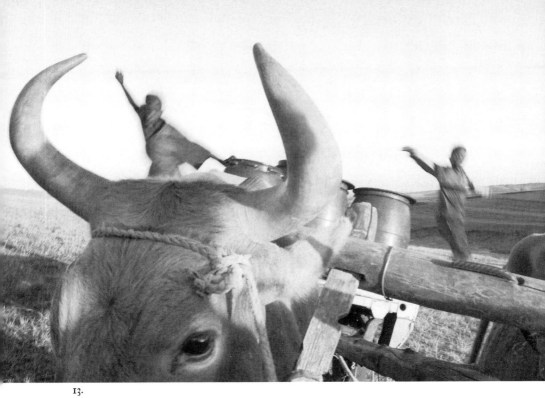

13.

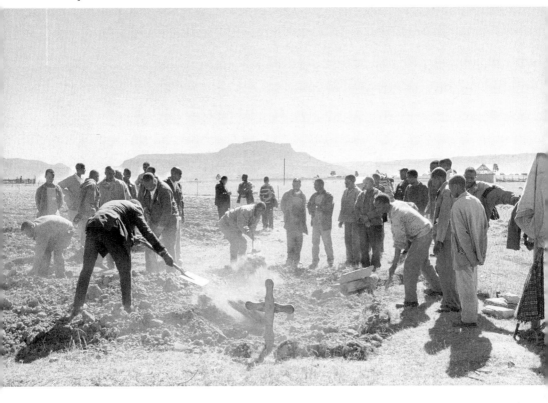

14.

The voices of dissent had grown quiet, and people had come to test for HIV in their thousands. Those involved in the treatment program assumed that the doubts had gone; they spoke of them only in the past tense. In truth, the doubts had retreated into a zone of deep privacy. They were now in the heads and the hushed conversations of people like Sizwe: neutral people, agnostic people, neither in one camp nor another, scouting the landscape for a remedy to bring home to stricken relatives.

AFTER HEARING THE AIDS needle story, I began searching the literature on Pondoland for episodes in its medical history. I was seeking echoes of the fear of Hermann Reuter's needle. I stumbled only upon my own ignorance; the echoes were almost everywhere, spanning the generations.

In the wake of the great flu epidemic of 1918, for instance, of which Sizwe's grandmother still speaks, the flu inoculation kits that public health officials distributed throughout the Transkei and Ciskei territories were greeted with suspicion and hostility. "They often incited whispers that the 'long needle' of the White man [had come] to inject more harm," writes the historian Benedict Carton. The *Christian Express,* for example, a missionary-run Eastern Cape newspaper, "reported in late 1918 that Xhosa-speaking messengers kept one step ahead of vaccination efforts, warning of 'a device of the Europeans to finish off the Native races of South Africa, and as it has not been quite successful, they were sending out men with poison to complete the work of extermination.'"

Once I was looking out for it, the fear of white doctors' needles seemed to crop up in everything I read. In the 1930s, for instance, the anthropologist Ellen Hellman and the psychiatrist Wulf Sachs conducted an extended period of fieldwork in Rooiyard, a shantytown in Doornfontein, Johannesburg. During the time they spent there, rumors swept through the shantytown, which soon proved to be true, that it had been targeted for demolition. Sachs had asked several Rooiyard residents whether he could take their blood and test it for syphilis. He promised to provide medication for those who tested positive.

On a Saturday night in Rooiyard shortly before the place was destroyed, an angry and drunken crowd turned on Hellman and taunted her menacingly. Once she had been pulled away to safety and the crowd had dispersed, an enraged resident blamed Sachs's blood test for the incident.

"The women say [the doctor and the anthropologist] have used our blood against us, the blood they took from us," he admonished. "They say our blood is not good, it shows a bad disease, and so they expel us from the yard."

Indeed, across colonial Africa, medicine was always understood as a vital ingredient in white political power. The needle that penetrates African skin to extract or inject substances into African blood has never been a neutral technology; it is an image that has always been hungry for meaning.

Between the 1920s and the 1940s, for instance, it was widely believed throughout central and eastern Africa that whites and their agents killed Africans in order to steal their blood. The story varied from place to place. In the Kenyan city of Mombasa, it was believed that the fire department captured Africans, extracted their blood, and took it to the medical department for the treatment of Europeans with anemic diseases. At times the belief was a cause for public action. In June 1947, for instance, an angry mob gathered outside the city's fire station to demand that it be searched for a woman whom eyewitnesses claimed had been kidnapped by firemen. And in Tanganyika in the 1950s it was believed that African blood was taken to city hospitals, converted into pills, and fed to whites, who needed them in order to stay alive in Africa.

Indeed, the fear of needles is hardly confined to Africa; it seems to mark every colonial and imperial landscape, every borderline where power is unevenly dispersed and motives are obscure. In Joseph Roth's novel *Job*, set in the early 1910s in a small town somewhere in the Pale of Settlement, smallpox breaks out.

"The authorities ordered vaccination," Roth writes, "and the doctors forced their way into the houses of the Jews . . . About [Dr. Soltysiuk] resounded the lamentations of women and the howls of children who had not been able to hide themselves. The policemen pulled women and children out of deep cellars and down from high attics, out of narrow closets and great straw baskets. The sun brooded, the doctor sweated. He had to vaccinate no less than one hundred and seventy-six Jews; for each who escaped and could not be reached, he thanked God in his heart."

Yet there have also been times when colonial subjects have literally lined up by the thousands for injections. In the Masisi district of Tanzania in the early 1920s, news spread that missionary doctors were successfully treating yaws, a horrific disease that begins with tumid sores all over the body and ends with the sufferer's bones rotting away.

"Thousands flocked to the clinics from all over the southeast," writes the historian Terence Ranger, "until the movement of people took on some of the dimensions of a mass pilgrimage." People spoke of "these wonderful injections" that within four days could have the desperately ill "literally dancing with joy."

IT IS ONE thing to troll the history books for talk of white doctors and needles, and quite another to put episodes in their requisite contexts. In November 1918, when the Spanish Influenza was felling the young and the healthy, and people spoke of the long needle of the white man coming to inject more harm, Pondoland had just commemorated the twenty-fourth anniversary of its formal annexation. Its people were under few illusions that their relationship with colonial power could amount to much more than mutual plunder. There is thus not much mystery in the fact that a little-known white technology was greeted with extreme caution.

The fear of Hermann Reuter's needle came eighty-five years later. He was employed by a nongovernmental organization that had entered a formal partnership with a freshly elected democratic government, one which the people of Pondoland had voted for and identified with en masse. The context could hardly have been more different.

These questions beg: If South Africa's government had felt unequivocal about ARV treatment and had rallied behind it, what would Sizwe have thought of Hermann's needle? Would people have asked in quiet tones whether their government was killing them? Or would Mpondos have pointed out that elements of Western technology have always been benign, that ever since their first encounters with the West, they have picked and chosen among tools ranging from the plow to paracetamol? Would Hermann have been viewed as the agent of a benign, and black, adoption of a helpful technology?

It is unlikely that things would have worked quite so simply. The fears kindled by an epidemic as great as this one cannot be made to vanish entirely by the talk of political leaders. When the young are being decimated, no technology can be stripped of all meaning and made simply benign.

But as things stood, Hermann and his needle came to Pondoland at a time when President Thabo Mbeki had left an air of besiegement across South Africa's body politic. Whether because he could not stomach the notion that he had inherited a country that was sick, or because he believed that those defining the terms and causes of the epidemic were hostile to Africans, Mbeki read calls for universal AIDS treatment as an attack on South Africa's sovereignty and as harmful to its people. While he himself always spoke opaquely about AIDS and antiretroviral medicine, the more vocal of his supporters in provincial ANC centers such as Eastern Cape cloaked ARVs in an ambience of antipatriotic mischief; they had been brought to our shores by people bent on hurting and profiteering from Africans.

In the same week Sizwe and I visited Nomvalo, I had dinner with a local government councilor in Lusikisiki. He was an elderly man, a local ANC veteran, and a fierce Mbeki supporter. It was a warm evening, and we stood in his garden barbecuing steaks, sausages, and mealies, and then ate under the starlight.

We spoke about my work in Lusikisiki.

"I don't trust these ARVs because they are not ours," the old man declared authoritatively toward the end of our meal. He picked up a mealie cob that had been lying on the plate in front of him. "This is ours. If a clever African scientist made an AIDS remedy out of this, I would trust it."

"But mealies are no more African than antiretrovirals," I replied. "Five generations ago, your forebears farmed sorghum. Foreigners brought mealies. You started to use them because they were more productive than sorghum and required less labor to farm. You borrowed something foreign because it was useful, and soon it became yours. It should be the same with ARVs."

"You are just trying to be clever," he snapped, waving the mealie cob dismissively. "What I am saying is that one must be very careful before accepting the offerings of others."

Perhaps I was trying to be clever, but I was momentarily offended by the belligerent nativism of a man who otherwise seemed wise and reasonable. And I was pretty certain that he would not have waved a mealie cob at me if Mbeki had not read the AIDS epidemic as an attack on him and his country's independence. Mbeki did not fabricate the old man's paranoia, but he did draw it to the surface of South Africa's political culture.

About the fear of AIDS needles in Nomvalo and Ithanga I am less certain. The councilor who fed me barbecued mealies was literate, middle class, and immersed in the politics of the provincial elite. Ithanga is only obliquely connected to this world. Without television or newspapers, the village receives its politics third or fourth hand, through this individual and that public service announcement. By the time national debates arrive in such places, they have been translated into a thoroughly local register.

Ithanga's and Nomvalo's forebears had, episodically at any rate, feared the needles of white doctors for at least four generations. That is an inheritance bequeathed to today's villagers. Whether that inheritance was teased back to life by the political choices of an incumbent president I cannot say for sure.

LATE IN MY research, Hermann finally offered me his perspective on the fear of his needle. Scheduled to leave Lusikisiki in a few months, he was slowly working the place out of his system, his thoughts and his emotional investments as much in the future as in the present. His sixteen-hour days had long passed. It was July 2006, World Cup soccer time, and on some evenings he would join his housemates in front of the TV. He had recently discovered the pleasures of roasting fresh Ethiopian coffee beans in a pan on his stove; the beans snapped one after the other like popcorn while he told me his story.

As was his custom, he began by circling my question. He spoke of an episode he had witnessed on an evening some thirteen years earlier. At the time he was working in an emergency room in a large township on Johannesburg's East Rand, a region in Greater Johannesburg that is home to more than two million people. The year was 1993. The ANC had been unbanned three years earlier, negotiations to end apartheid were at a fragile, short-tempered moment, and few South Africans were confident that the protagonists would reach a settlement. On the East Rand, a conflict akin to civil war was in progress. Zulu-speaking residents of the East Rand's migrant worker hostels, aligned to the Zulu nationalist Inkatha Freedom Party, had fought a series of violent battles against ANC-aligned residents in the surrounding townships. Many had lost their lives. The entire country sensed that if the transition to democracy were indeed to fall apart, the unraveling would begin in the East Rand.

At the height of the war, Hermann attended an ANC-aligned meeting in a packed community hall at the very heart of the conflict. Two issues dominated the agenda: the question of armed self-defense, and an ongoing consumer boycott of white-owned businesses.

On the first matter, the meeting was agreed that arms must be distributed to members of civic associations and trade unions so that communities could be defended from attack. The discussion was cogent and sober. It was argued that if weapons were to circulate, they must be put in the hands of workers, who are disciplined and responsible, rather than youth, who are liable to drink and get out of control.

The discussion turned to the consumer boycott. Across the country at that time, consumer boycotts of white-owned businesses in the town centers were enforced by the young. Youths would assemble at township taxi ranks waiting for the taxis that brought commuters home from central business districts and white suburbs. They would search the parcels of each commuter for groceries. Among the more unsettling stories that began to spread at the time were those of young men forcing middle-aged women to drink the cooking oil they had bought in town.

At the meeting Hermann attended, a question was raised about how to dispose of the groceries the youths confiscated.

"One person suggested that the food be given to an old-age home in KwaThema," Hermann told me. "Others said no, it is not safe to do that because the whites may inject this food with poison in order to kill our old people.

"That was for me such a weird logic. If whites can inject this food with poison, why wouldn't they give it to the young people? Why only now during this special crisis, and only for the old people? All the people in that hall who had had such a good discussion about armed self-defense were buying the idea that it was not safe. They used to buy that food at white shops every day and eat it. But now because there is a consumer boycott and they are taking groceries away from people, the enemy will do something malicious to this food to kill the poor old people who will eat it. It was a weird, weird logic for me.

"A few years later, a story circulated in South Africa. You know those oranges that look like they have blood inside, the ones with the red juice? I think they are called blood oranges. The story went round that those oranges have had HIV injected into them and that if you eat them you will get HIV.

"Again, there is a half-truth. It is always when stories mix that they become much more credible. During the time of the international boycott of South African goods in the 1980s, those Outspan oranges were exported to Europe and antiapartheid activists used to pour blood over them in the shops so that people would not buy them. I'm sure that there's a connection between the two stories. Back in the '80s, those oranges were seen as the epitome of apartheid: you had to fight the oranges to fight the regime. And now, a decade later, the story had turned around: these oranges were being used by white people to fight back . . . You know all these things have racial undertones always. It was just amazing for me, these stories.

"So this business when it started happening in Lusikisiki with me was no surprise for me, no surprise at all.

"You must also think of it medically. When I am investigating a patient, for me as a doctor, I know exactly the sequence and what it means to me. I ask questions to gain information. Then I examine the patient, make a diagnosis, and give treatment. That is how I have been trained, that is what I have known my whole life.

"The patient doesn't understand that. For the patient the talking is important. It is not about how to understand the problem. It is counseling. The touching is not examining, it is massaging. For most patients, touch is, you know, from small, when you cough, your mother rubs you. They perceive touching as treating.

"A woman will come to me with an STI [sexually transmitted infection], and I do an internal vaginal examination, and she comes back two weeks later.

"I ask, 'Is the discharge better?'

"And she says, 'Yes doctor, since you cleaned it.'

"I say, 'When did I clean it?'

"She says, 'When you wiped it with your fingers. You wiped it and made it better.'

"So me making the diagnosis, I think the patient is interpreting it in the same way. Actually, the patient is interpreting it in an entirely different way.

"It is the same with an injection. An injection is considered treatment. You prick something. Pricking is introducing, it is not taking out. This idea of taking blood out to test it, it is not easily understood.

"These are difficult concepts. It doesn't surprise me that people see HIV . . . Hermann comes to Lusikisiki. Nobody has HIV. He tells the nurses to prick and suddenly everybody has HIV. Where does the HIV come from? It comes from the pricking. It doesn't surprise me."

"Especially if you are white and no black leaders here are talking about it," I said.

"That probably contributes. I cannot explain to people what I do. I cannot defend myself. And they know I'm doing something against government. There are obviously a lot of questions."

"When did you stop hearing about the HIV in your needle?" I asked.

"It was isolated pockets. Bodweni, some other clinics. It can spread anywhere. Other doctors have been accused."

"I have heard about it all over Lusikisiki."

"It is the story that spreads. It's not happening everywhere. I wasn't challenged about it everywhere."

"What was your response when you were challenged?"

"In Bodweni I showed how the HIV test worked. I pricked myself. I showed them. I tried to explain to them. I gave quite a scientific explanation. I treated the people who tested positive, and people saw I have skills that need to be respected; people who were so sick they had nothing to lose except . . . what is that Marxist word?" He giggles dryly. "Their chains. They were saying, I am going to die anyway: let's trust this doctor."

IN THE END, it was during a conversation with Sizwe that I learned my most memorable lesson about white doctors and black bodies. The conversation was neither about needles nor AIDS; it was about his grandfather's skull.

Driving into Ithanga one morning with Sizwe, I took my eyes off the road for a moment to get a CD out of its case. When I looked up, we were heading for the roadside; I veered straight again.

"Sorry," I said.

"You are going to kill us," he replied calmly. "Maybe the evil spirits are with us. Even this morning in town, there was a taxi that nearly hit us."

"It's just that I was concentrating on the CD," I said.

He cocked his head and peered out at me from between two thick dreadlocks.

"You don't believe in evil spirits."

"No."

"So when we are talking about these spirits, you believe we might be stupid or something?"

The tone of his question was disarmingly earnest; it was as if he had asked me whether I thought it might rain.

"No," I said. "I believe that there is anger and envy, and that they cause people to do terrible things to each other. But I don't think you can use magic to do it. What you say is magic, I say is envy. It is powerful and destructive. It can cause enormous damage. But I don't think you can make someone go mad just because you want them to.

"Do you think *I* am stupid for not believing in magic?" I asked.

"No," he replied. "I don't think you are stupid. Because it is not in your culture. I have never heard of people going to a white person far away to get the right medicines. We know that the Indians are good with medicines. And the Bushmen can use the medicines very well. We know about foreigners from other parts of Africa: they can use medicines. But not the whites."

"Do you not think, then," I asked, "that there is a problem in white culture?"

"No. There is no problem. It is just different."

He said nothing for some time; he appeared to be giving thought to a difficult formulation.

"The problem," he said finally, "is that sometimes we forget that we are different. We do many of your things now, and we are forgetting about a lot of our own things. We believe in the things that are being done by you. We are losing our culture.

"You can see why. My father wanted to keep me at home when I was young because that is how it was in the Mpondo culture. For him, education was not about going to school: it was about teaching the children the culture. But my mom and others saw that our culture was making us poor. She wanted us to learn to read and write. You follow the one who is educated because you see that he is doing so well. And that is good. But maybe you follow too much, or in the wrong way. You follow, you follow, and then you remain with nothing.

"Not so long ago, our ancestors spoke to the sangomas. They warned the family if there was trouble coming; they said you must do this and this to avoid trouble. Today, the sangomas still tell you to do this and this, but the ancestors have not spoken to them."

"The ancestors no longer come because people are losing touch with their culture?"

"Yes. I am thinking of the funeral services, and the things that have changed. In olden times, if a person dies today, tomorrow you go out and tell the relatives from far away. On the second day, the relatives travel to your place. And then on the third day, the person is buried.

"Now, we take the person to the mortuary. He lies there for two weeks, even three weeks. They keep him on ice. He comes back to be buried without his brain or his intestines. They have taken those parts out at the mortuary to stop him from going rotten."

"They take out your brain at the mortuary?" I asked incredulously.

"You don't know this?" He laughed uncomfortably. "We have a belief that if you go there, you come back without your brain, without your intestine, because these things make you rotten, even if you are on ice. In the stomach, for instance, is food, and it takes a long time for the cold of the ice to reach the stomach and make it stiff. So they take them out, and the brain as well."

"What are the implications?"

"We believe the spirit does not come back now. The spirit is left there, with the brain and the intestine."

"They will never become your ancestors?"

"Yes. There are no ancestors now because their spirits are lost."

"And that is because of Western influence?"

"There were no coffins in the old days. In the old days, a rich man was buried in the skin of a cow. He chose the cow himself before he died. He instructed his children to slaughter it and to bury him in the skin. A poor person was buried in a blanket."

During the time I had spent with the Magadlas, they had spoken a great deal about Sizwe's paternal grandfather, Vuyani. I thought of him immediately.

"When your grandfather died," I asked, "did he go to the mortuary?"

"Yes."

"Do you think his spirit is not here?"

"He might be here because he once came to see me. And there are many people who have said he came to them and talked to them."

"When did he come to you?"

"It was quite a few years ago. I had a girlfriend in a village a far distance from Ithanga. I have a cousin in that village. My girlfriend and I always arranged to meet at my cousin's place. I arrived, and she was not there. I was told she had another boyfriend, and she was with him. I waited and waited, and I started getting so furious. I stayed at that place right through the next day, and she came the next night. I was so angry with her. I slept there with her, but it was horrible. We were not talking: the one sleeping facing this way, the other one the other way.

"Then I fell asleep, and I saw my grandfather. And my grandmother, who is still living, was there, too. They were looking for one another. I could see them both, but they couldn't see each other. Eventually, they met, and my dad was with them. They had a talk together. They were not coming to tell me anything. They took no notice of me. They sat down and talked to each other."

"Do you think they were talking about you?" I asked. "Do you think their discussion had something to do with your fight with your girlfriend?"

"Sometimes I think maybe it does not matter what they were talking about," he replied. "Maybe it was not him in my dream, just my own thoughts. You can never say. Maybe if he was really with us, there would not be such strange things happening in my family. Like the fact that we got so poor in order for my father to become a sangoma. If my grandfather's spirit was there in the village, and if he was really watching out for the family, would he really have requested the family to become so poor?"

IT IS TEMPTING to interpret Sizwe's story as an allegory. The Western tools of mutilation lying in the morgue have stolen the spirits of the dead. As allegory, the tale speaks so simply and so vividly of a society dismembered in successive encounters with the outside. Foreign ideas and technologies have been agents of corrosion, and no more.

Yet Sizwe does not mean his story as an allegory. He means what he says: that his grandfather's skull was smashed open, his brain removed with surgical instruments and thrown in the dustbin. He means that a foreign technology has quite literally removed the dead from the living. Once the story is literal, rather than allegorical, it becomes something quite different, something disturbing.

It is disturbing because it conjures an atmosphere of bewildered besiegement, of defensive hostility. That Sizwe is a successful businessman, against all the odds, is a function of his outwardness, his willingness to learn and use things foreign, his awareness that if he does not experiment he is doomed. The story of his grandfather's skull seems to me to come from a dying and reactionary place.

An image of Vuyani in the mortuary sticks in my head and does not leave. Its violence takes expression in sharp smells and plain images: the clinical stench of disinfectant, the wet, meatlike colors of a disemboweled torso on a white sheet. It is not merely a foreign practice that did such violence to the old man, but medical practice: uniquely intimate, uniquely intrusive. It is a dark tale indeed for a man to be telling himself in the midst of a search for treatment to save his niece's life.

―――――――――

WHEN I NEXT see Hermann Reuter, I ask him if he has heard of the business of the removal of the brains and the gutting of the stomachs.

He has not. But it does not take him long to begin imagining.

"You've never seen a postmortem?" he asks.

"No, I have not."

"A postmortem isn't complete until you have cracked that skull and taken out the brain. You cut it into slices to see if there's any hemorrhage or bleedings or blood stoppages or abscesses.

"It's quite a procedure to get through the skull. If somebody has seen that once, it's a very, very strong picture. People work in these morgues who don't always understand what is done and why. It is they who do it. The doctor doesn't saw through the skull. It is a proletarian job, done by people who go back to their villages and describe what they have seen and done. They must crack it open and then the doctor looks at the skull and sends part of it away to the laboratory. And the story spreads."

"And intestines?" I ask.

"Intestines I'm not sure. I mean, internal organs do get sent away for pathology tests. I don't know if sometimes intestines blow up and they just throw them away. Close up the body to make it look pretty. I'm sure sometimes they don't stuff the intestines back. People are lazy. Doctors are lazy. Postmortem people are lazy. They just throw it away and incinerate it somewhere. These stories probably spread.

"Very few people actually get postmortemed. But when it does happen, it happens at the morgue. So it happens to one or two people and the story spreads, and soon it's common knowledge that it happens to everyone at the morgue."

VUYANI'S GRAVE LIES among the ruins of what was once his Great Home, about halfway up one of Ithanga's steepest hills. The family moved from there many years ago; it was high above the nearest source of fresh water, and the trip home from the river was too arduous for all but the youngest and strongest women. If Sizwe had not pointed out the grave, I would not have seen it: a gentle, unmarked mound, covered in long grass.

We leave the gravesite, and on the journey down the hill, we begin talking about Graeme, one of the bird-watchers who established Sizwe in his business. Graeme is a lawyer. The discussion turns to his education, and then to my education, and together Sizwe and I calculate that between us Graeme and I spent a cumulative seventeen years studying at university.

"Do you think," Sizwe asks, "that if a black person reads too much he can go mad?" He speaks with an uncertain voice, as if he is risking embarrassment.

"Why?" I ask.

"Because many black people who go away to study go mad. But maybe it is because people who are jealous of their success bewitch them. Maybe it is not that they have read too much."

"But say it was because they read too much—"

"I want to ask you something else," he interrupts. "Do you think that if we sent the *umlungus* back to Europe and kept their wealth here, the wealth would eventually run out?"

"You want to send us away?"

"No. I'm just asking. Do you think the money would run out and we would be in trouble?"

"Where would I go?" I ask. "My grandmother is from a tiny country called Latvia. I have never been there and I don't speak a word of the language."

"I am teaching you Xhosa nice," he says. "You will find someone like me from your grandmother's country. But in any case, I am just asking: do you think the wealth would all run out?"

We walk for a while. He is irritated that I have not answered his question.

"Even a small tribe like the Mpondos," I say at last, "even you, we in South Africa need you. If you were chased into the sea we would be in big trouble."

By now we are walking on a wet forest path surrounded by trees and undergrowth. Suddenly, he throws his arm across my chest.

"Mamba!" he shouts.

I have already begun to launch myself off the path, the adrenaline coursing through my legs, when it comes to me dimly that he has tricked me. By the time I have recovered my senses and regained control over my body, I am three yards back from where we came.

He is beaming at me and laughing his head off; it is a flat, boyish laugh, triumphant and satisfied.

Voting Day

The day after Sizwe wondered aloud what might happen if I and my kind were sent back to Europe was March 1, 2006. In Ithanga and across South Africa, it was municipal government elections day.

When I arrived at Sizwe's place early that morning, he looked at me skeptically.

"Where are you going to vote?" he asked.

"I can't," I said. "My ward is in Johannesburg and I am in Lusikisiki."

He took this in and nodded, his disapproval entirely private and barely detectable. He went to stand in the doorway, looked out, and remarked, somewhat absently, that by midday Ithanga would be unbearably hot.

"I don't want to talk about the weather," I said. "I want to talk about the fact that I am not voting. You disapprove. I saw it in your face."

"No," he replied. "It is just something I have noted. And now we move on."

He said this with such finality that it seemed rude to push the point.

We put on our hats and began walking slowly across Ithanga toward the school, where Sizwe was to vote. Already, about a half mile away, we could make out a stumpy snake of voters protruding from the school's front entrance.

We met Sizwe's mother on the way, and she asked me where I would vote, and then we were joined by an uncle of Sizwe's, who also looked at me askance and wondered aloud where I was going to vote.

By the time we arrived at the school, I had the sense that my relationship with this entire village had been recalibrated. I was no longer just the one who hangs out at Sizwe's place, or the one who asks the Zionist Christians about their belief that their prophets can cure illness. My difference was now also marked by my relation to the political order. That I was white and not voting, and they black and en route to the school to cast their ballots, reestablished the meaning of who I was. I felt the presence of "black people's secrets," as Sizwe once put it, darting between the polite and masked faces around me.

In the line, Sizwe greeted an elderly man with his broadest and most generous smile.

"*Molweni Zizi,*" he beamed.

The old man clearly enjoyed the appellation, and soon the two were chatting happily. Once he had left us and made his way to the voting booth, Sizwe turned to me.

"Do you know what is *Zizi*?"

"It is the name you use to address a member of the Dlamini clan."

"Yes," he said. "That is exactly what it is. And do you know who else is Zizi?"

"Thabo Mbeki."

He took out his broad grin once more.

"You are so right, my man, you are so right. We have Zizis here in this village, and Zizis there in the government in Pretoria."

I marveled at Sizwe, at the invisible strand that linked him to the president via the old man, at the bond that had wrapped itself around everybody standing in the line. Democracy had not treated this village especially well. When the adults of Ithanga converged on the school to vote for the first time in April 1994, they had been told, on radio, and on election platforms, that their vote would bring them running water, electricity, proper roads, perhaps a clinic. More than a decade later, there isn't a soul here who has forgotten that every one of these promises was broken.

Nor is anybody especially naïve about the character of local politics. When I asked Sizwe whether he knew the ANC ward councilor for whom he was about to cast his vote, he spoke of a well-off man who lived in a smart, brick-and-mortar house about twelve miles away, in a village with electricity and running water.

"Will he be good for Ithanga?" I asked.

"He is not smart enough to be good for Ithanga," Sizwe replied. "If anything is going to happen in Ithanga, it must be negotiated with the chief and two or three other men who are close to the chief. And they will not let anything happen that is not good for them. They will run circles around this ward councilor. It will be too difficult for him in Ithanga."

And yet these acidic observations cannot burn the thread that binds the Zizis in Ithanga to the Zizis in the Union Buildings in Pretoria. If there is anyone in this village who did not go down to the school on March 1 to cast her vote, I doubt she would have shamed herself by saying it out loud. It is axiomatic: to be black, here and now, in the early years of the twenty-first century, is to vote. And to vote is to vote ANC.

DRIVING AWAY FROM Ithanga through the dusk on an evening in early March, I listened on the radio to a postelections talk show. A political analyst was accounting for why more people had voted ANC than in previous local government elections, despite the fact that ill-tempered protests about housing shortages and poor services had preceded polling in several towns. "What many analysts don't understand," the analyst said, "is that voting is neither a calculus nor a trip down the aisle at the supermarket. Party loyalties are an extension of one's identity."

I had just seen precisely that firsthand in Ithanga. But I had also seen something else. If party loyalties are an extension of identity, there is a flip side: during the few seconds that it takes to cast a vote, many components of one's identity are suppressed. At some point during the day, Simlindile, who may or may not want to ruin Sizwe and his business, joined the line to vote; and so did the two figures on the other side of the river, who may or may not have been trying to destroy the Magadlas for a generation; and so too did Charlie, who watched his nephew die of AIDS, and then snatched his estate from under the widow's nose.

Yet the moment they joined the line they were none of these

things. They were shorn of all detail. The particularities that constituted the community of Ithanga dissolved. In the line, everyone was
cleanly and simply a black person in early-twenty-first-century South
Africa. Thus everyone voted, and voted ANC.

What is the content of this clean, shorn identity? What is it that ef-
faces the differences between people and draws them to the school to
vote? Were I to ask Sizwe, I am not sure how, precisely, I would phrase
the question. Yet I think I have already learned some of the answer. I
suspect it takes the form of a grand narrative, one that begins with the
annexation of Pondoland in 1894, and encompasses the crushing of
the great peasant uprising of 1960. It culminates in Mandela's release,
in Oliver Tambo's homecoming to Pondoland, in voting day on April
27, 1994, when political independence returned after a century-long
absence.

I suspect, too, that the fear of the white doctor's needle, and the
tools of excision that lie in the morgue, are markers in the same narrative. To be black is to have been robbed and violated, and to vote is an
act of retrieval.

It is an immense power and is thus extremely beguiling: a nationalism of such force that on an appointed day it can suspend enmity
and reconfigure a community into the shape of a simple line. And yet
if this is what binds, if this is what gives a village an image of itself, it
cannot be all good. For it seems to me that the empowerment of standing in the line and voting is fused with the disempowerment of suspecting the doctor's needle as an instrument of genocide. They seem
two sides of the same identity, two faces of the same defeat.

And indeed, it is hard not to recall that just a year earlier this same
school was the stage of another public drama. Then, too, many Ithanga
villagers lined up outside the school door. They were waiting to be
tested for HIV. And if today's ritual constituted an act of unity, the previous year's event fingered individual people and separated them out.
Those who stayed in the school too long emerged bearing stigmata of
shame.

Nomvalo

A month after our first trip to Nomvalo, we visited Kate Marrandi again. She had been waiting for us. The moment we entered her front door, she hoisted her rucksack onto her back and handed each of us a banana. Sustenance for our day's work, she explained. We were to visit six patients, as she called them, a carefully chosen cross-section: the well, the ill, those adhering cheerfully to their treatment, and those struggling against it.

On the way out, Sizwe and I both admired a guava tree standing in an orchard opposite MaMarrandi's house. Against our protestations, she opened the orchard gate, made her way to the tree, and shook it with a degree of strength that surprised us both. She returned with two guavas for each of us. We added one to our respective bananas and ate the other on the spot. They were floury inside and tasteless, and when we grimaced MaMarrandi laughed at us and shook her head. Then we followed her across Nomvalo's maze of pedestrian paths. She quickened her pace as the journey proceeded, and it was not long before we two fit young men were struggling to keep up with her.

"She is like an ox," Sizwe remarked, once we had lagged behind far enough to be out of earshot. "You look at her and you think she is fat and old, but she could carry one of us under each arm and she would not get tired."

I do not know what our presence meant to MaMarrandi, only that she was clearly very pleased to have us shadow her. And I knew better than to ask, since it was already plain that she did not speak about herself. In any event, the spirit with which she received us radiated a warmth that seemed strangely infectious. As we struggled to keep up with her and spoke behind her back, Sizwe and I were both possessed by light-headed cheerfulness.

Our first stop, MaMarrandi informed us after some twenty minutes of walking, was to be the home of a patient who had died. She wanted to introduce us to the dead girl's aunt and grandmother.

We entered a good, large home, one with many ornaments, thick carpets, and a tidy lounge suite. A woman walked across the room to greet us. Before I had a chance to introduce myself, a picture on a side table caught my eye. It was a framed studio photograph of a young woman.

The moment of recognition came like a sharp slap across the cheek. Looking out from the healthy face in the photograph were the eyes of the skeletal being in the pink tracksuit I had seen in the clinic waiting room a month earlier. I swiveled and stared at the one who had welcomed us, and she was indeed the woman who had made her sickly niece laugh in Hermann's consulting room.

She greeted us warmly and then turned her back to summon her mother, leaving us alone in this cluttered and ornamented room with her dead niece. The poised and carefully arranged face in the photograph lent every object in this place a terrible heaviness.

MaMarrandi had settled on a bench adjacent to the lounge suite and was staring blankly ahead of her.

"How long has she been dead?" I asked.

"Tomorrow will be three weeks. It has been ten days since we buried her."

The girl's grandmother appeared leaning heavily on a stick. She was ancient and bent over, her torso veering over her legs, and she breathed as if a jumbled collection of instruments and tools was rattling around in her lungs. She walked up to Sizwe and me in turn, grasped our hands, told us to sit, and sat down carefully opposite us, her stick clattering to the floor, the flurry of activity lifting the volume and intensity of her wheezing.

MaMarrandi smiled at her and laughed.

"Tell them when you were born, *Gogo*," she said.

"I am told that by the time of the *umbathalala* I was walking," she replied in a surprisingly strong voice. "My mother was pregnant with my younger brother. The *umbathalala* was taking the pregnant women, and everyone was concerned for my mother."

The *umbathalala*—the great disaster—is the 1918 flu epidemic. She was about ninety years old now.

Once she was settled and breathing more easily she began to talk in a continuous stream.

"The sadness in this household is carried in my chest," she said. "The night after my granddaughter died my TB deteriorated immediately and the medicine no longer worked. Every day since her death it is more difficult to breathe."

She turned to MaMarrandi: "You will be coming tonight? You will come here after your work is finished and we will read?"

"Of course I am coming, *Gogo*," MaMarrandi replied. "What else do you think I would be doing tonight?"

The old lady beamed and nodded, and her chest rattled.

"It is not just her lungs," MaMarrandi said to us. "The girl passed away three weeks ago, and since then there is very little sleep in this house. On the third night I came here and I read to *Gogo* from the Bible for one hour, then another hour, and her breathing went quieter and she went to sleep. I went home, it was late, I got into bed, and then there was a pounding on my door.

"'*Gogo* has woken up, and she wants you again,' they shouted.

"I went back in the middle of the night. And that is how it is here every night. I come and read with *Gogo* and we go to sleep together. Early in the morning I go home to wash.

"Both of them can't sleep," Kate continued, "they both of them see Zukiswa standing in the doorway late at night." It was the first time that day I had heard someone utter the dead girl's name. "Zukiswa says nothing, and they don't know what she is thinking. It is only when I come and read that she disappears."

Throughout our conversation Zukiswa's aunt sat a little apart from us and stared out the window.

"We are grateful to MaMarrandi," she said finally. "She is *Gogo*'s medicine to sleep."

And then she began talking about Zukiswa. One after the other, she chronicled the ailments from which her niece had suffered since she was a small child. And in this long, scrupulously detailed list, she kept returning to a chronic condition that had first visited her at the age of fourteen: disabling headaches that kept her in bed for weeks on end.

Although she did not once draw an explicit connection between these childhood illnesses and her death, I understood her to be inferring that the origins of the ailment that killed Zukiswa were to be found long ago, when she was not yet a young woman, but rather a virgin girl. I understood her to be saying that this death had nothing to do with sex. She was, I thought, attempting to grab her niece from the clutches of a nameless shame.

ONCE WE WERE on the road again, I asked MaMarrandi if she had known Zukiswa well.

"She was born in '74," she replied. "The same year as my daughter. They attended school together."

"Why did she die?" I asked.

She repeated the story of the fourteen-year-old's chronic headaches. "They were so bad that she had to drop out of school in standard eight [tenth grade]. The doctors could not find the cause of her headaches, and many people believed she was sick because the ancestors had called her to heal. But she did not train to be a diviner. The headaches backed off a bit. She would start with a temporary job, then the headaches would come again and she would stay home for a while."

"I thought she was a social worker."

MaMarrandi smiled. "In her last job she worked for social workers. She would photocopy the people's IDs and do work around the office. During this last job, she started getting terrible headaches again. The people did not think it might be HIV. Everyone thought it was the old problem.

"She used to come to my place often because she liked to eat my guavas. I counseled her. I tried to get her to test. She resisted. I told her she was getting very sick. Eventually, when she conceded and we went to test her blood, her CD4 count was thirty-nine."

Perhaps, then, all the talk about the history of headaches was not about retrieving Zukiswa from a shameful death. What was at stake, perhaps, was the guilt of those still alive: they had mistaken AIDS symptoms for an old illness, and so they had not coaxed her to a clinic to test until it was too late.

WE VISITED MAMARRANDI'S six patients back-to-back during the course of the day.

The first was not at home. We left a message with a neighbor and were about to leave when MaMarrandi caught sight of her making her way up the path from the river, an indistinct figure carrying a large bucket of water on her head. As she drew closer, and the contours of her body took shape, it became plain that she was sick. Her thinness was the unmistakable thinness of the chronically ill; the curves of her body had been flattened into rigid lines, her breasts small against her chest: a young woman transformed into a lanky and undernourished prepubescent. Her face was marked with the raw outcroppings of a skin disease, and the sweat of her labor had run from her temples down her cheeks and into the crevices and ruts between her scars.

She put down her bucket and invited us into her room, a square, mud structure with a single bed, an older dresser, and no more.

"How are you feeling, Nosiviwe?" MaMarrandi asked.

"I get dizzy when I work," she replied. "And my stomach runs every day. And I feel like I have a blister on my ankle."

"Did you follow my advice? Did you go to Saint Elizabeth's?"

In a sullen tone and with bowed head she told MaMarrandi that she had visited the HIV unit at Saint Elizabeth's many times, and had attended the support group for people beginning ARV treatment three weeks in a row. Each time she had been sent home empty-handed because she had nobody to sign for her pills.

"They will not give you pills," MaMarrandi told her in a quiet voice, "until they have trained a member of your family to help you take them. And to know the side effects. The family must know the side effects."

"I myself know," the young woman said. "Three-TC causes dizziness and headache. Nevirapine burns your liver. E-five-rands [Efivarenz] gives you dreams."

"Why do you not take your sister with you?" MaMarrandi asked.

"She is pregnant. She gets very short-tempered."

"Who will you take, then?"

"I will ask my mother."

"Will she go with you? Do you want me to talk to her?"

"No. She will come."

ONCE WE HAD left, I asked MaMarrandi why she thought the young woman was struggling to get her family to support her.

"I don't know," she replied. "I would have to sit down with them."

"What do you think her chances are?" I asked.

"It is good that she tested when her CD4 count is still high," MaMarrandi replied. "It is 201. The problem is that she drinks. I am not confident that she will give up drinking."

"Why?" I asked. "Does she have problems with her family? With men?"

The three of us were walking in single file along a narrow path. All I could see of MaMarrandi was the back of her straw hat and her rucksack.

"The whole family drinks," she said neutrally. "They've been all of them drinking since they were children."

PATIENT NUMBER TWO was out for the day, and after a brief chat with her mother, we departed. Number three was a middle-aged man called Vuli. He lived alone in a three-room house. When I asked him about the history of his illness, he stiffened his back ramrod straight and began speaking in clipped, staccato sentences, as if giving a set of instructions to a large gathering.

He contracted TB in 2003, he said. It did not go away. In 2004 he tested HIV-positive. His CD4 count now was 337, so he was not ready to start with ARVs. But he was sure he still had TB because he felt sick all day, every day, and he had very little energy when he woke in the morning and none at all when he went to sleep at night. He was going to the clinic for a sputum test the following day, and he was sure he would test positive.

While he was speaking, MaMarrandi rummaged through her

rucksack and pulled out her reading glasses, her black exercise book, and a number of glossy leaflets. Now she had a leaflet in front of her, a pen in her hand, and her glasses on the end of her nose. So poised, she began:

"I am advising you to go to the support group at the hospital in Lusikisiki," she told Vuli in Xhosa. Sizwe translated quietly in my ear. "I know it is taxi fare and half a day away from home, but it is very important to go there. You will get lots of knowledge. You will learn from other HIV-positive people there. And you will learn the importance of having a decent breakfast every day. You will be taught to eat coffee and porridge and bread with peanut butter. These things will give you strength for the day. The food will also be a reminder for you to take your pills. At the support group, they will also tell you to have a good lunch: beans and soup with pieces of meat.

"You will be advised to play, to exercise. I know it is difficult for an old person. But you must go to neighbors and talk and not be lonely, because company is also like exercise. Also, you must go and knock on the doors of others in this village who are HIV-positive. You must talk to them."

"Where will I find them?" he asked dismissively. "They are hiding themselves."

"Whenever you are feeling uncomfortable," MaMarrandi continued, ignoring his rhetorical question, "you must go to the doctor. Because HIV-positive people can get sick suddenly, and it is important that you are treated."

She took off her glasses, put them carefully on her lap, and looked at him squarely.

"Now I'm going to talk about a difficult thing. You must reduce your smoking, and then slowly stop it. The TB tablets will not work if you smoke. And after you are on ARVs, they will also not work. And the other difficult thing is drink. You need to stop drinking so that the TB medicine will work well in your body. And in any case, if you get drunk at night, you will forget to take your tablets in the morning.

"But all these things become easier with support. You have raised the point, and I know it is true, that it is difficult to meet people here who are HIV-positive because they are shy. We are in the process of convening a support group in the very near future, there in the community hall. It will happen soon."

He laughed humorlessly. "Your support group will fail. Everyone is running away. Everyone is hiding. The only people I have met who are HIV-positive are the people at the clinic in town. They are from other villages. I just greet them, and then we go our own ways."

"Some people get confused when they discover their HIV status," MaMarrandi continued doggedly. "They want to kill themselves. At support group, they meet people who have already started up. The other people say: 'I was also like this. I wanted to kill myself. Then I went to the support group and it has changed my life.'"

He nodded impatiently, cupped his chin in his hand, and waited for MaMarrandi to announce that we were leaving.

OUT ON THE village paths, MaMarrandi began speaking about him unsolicited.

"I am scared of what will happen with that Vuli," she said. "A man whose immunity is dropping like that cannot be alone talking to no one, eating dry bread, not cooking. He is stubborn. His stepmother lives very near him. He could go there for meals and for company. He will not."

"What are your plans for him?" I asked.

"I could go there every day and cook for him and eat with him. I could give him food and company. But I cannot do that. My husband is not here. I am a woman alone. He is a man alone. I cannot go to his house every day and close the door. I need to start this support group. I cannot help that man alone."

For the first time, I was struck by the delicacy of Kate Marrandi's position. Her presence in this village had maneuvered talk about AIDS out of the depths of secrecy, but not yet into the light. She had taken it only as far as an awkward twilight zone, one that was no longer private but not yet public. The sick discussed their illnesses with her, behind closed doors, but seldom with one another. One woman, traveling from home to home, substituted for a public forum.

We had found MaMarrandi during a transitional phase. So late in the history of the epidemic, she was attempting to turn AIDS into the subject of formal public discourse, an issue that people would meet to discuss in Nomvalo's public spaces. The circumstances under which she was doing so were very trying indeed. Had she lived in a village within the Lusikisiki district, she would have had a clinic, nurses, two or three adherence counselors, and a doctor's weekly visit to help her bring AIDS into the light. She would have taken her place as a worker in the movement Hermann Reuter's charisma had inspired. Here in Nomvalo, the nearest clinic did not treat AIDS, nor did its nurses want to talk about it. She was working almost entirely alone.

I AM NOT sure whether MaMarrandi deliberately chose to visit her more troubling patients first—as if the course of our day together should serve as a metaphor for the progression of her work—but at the remaining homes we visited she was greeted like a hero.

From Vuli's place we walked through the middle of the village and back along the path on which we had started the day's journey. We were still some fifty paces from the home we had come to visit when we saw a young girl standing at the fence and pointing at us. "*MaMarrandi ukhona!*" she shouted. "MaMarrandi is here!" By the time we came to the gate a family of five had put down their tools and assembled to greet us—there was a man, a woman, and three children.

"Go and call your uncle Leonard," the woman said to the young girl who had announced our arrival. "He will never forgive us if he does not see MaMarrandi."

Mats and chairs were brought out, and we sat together in a circle waiting for Leonard to come. There was no question of anyone getting on with their chores while MaMarrandi was here.

Leonard, it turned out, was MaMarrandi's patient, and the father of two of the three children. He was not from Nomvalo: until recently, he and his family lived in a village about sixty miles away. Illness had brought them here.

The previous year, he and his wife had both become sick with AIDS. She had died very quickly, less than a month after she had first taken to her bed. The two children were packed off to live with an aunt at the other end of the province, and Leonard had been brought here, to his brother's home, to die. MaMarrandi had learned that there was a sick man in the house, had visited him, and taken him to Hermann. That was a little over a year ago. He was now reasonably healthy and building a house with his own two hands some five hundred yards from his brother's place. His children had been called from their aunt's village to join their father at his new home. Having been scattered by illness and death, Leonard and his children were settling into Nom-valo.

He crossed the lawn in front of us wearing overalls covered in plaster and paint. He shook MaMarrandi's hand vigorously, then Sizwe's, and then mine. Sizwe explained who we were and what we were doing here. He listened carefully, and when Sizwe was finished he took off his cap and began speaking with great formality.

"My name is Leonard Noxaka," he said. "My place is just across there. I live in Nomvalo because I was very ill and was taken here to the house of my older brother. It was expected that I would die. I am HIV-positive. Through MaMarrandi I began to take ARVs last year. One by one the sicknesses lifted until this day I am left only with one problem."

He pulled up his shirt to reveal a display of shingles welts running down his side.

"The skin itches," he continued, "and sometimes the itching goes below the skin and into the body. It is not nice."

He dropped his shirt back into place and put his arms at his side.

"I am united with my children. A year ago, they thought they were orphans and were living with a woman who may have been their blood relative but was a stranger to them."

He sat down and turned to MaMarrandi and in a long, steady stream began describing the state of his body, beginning with his head and ending with his feet. As he spoke, it became clear that there was nothing in particular to report to her: he was well stocked with drugs, reasonably healthy, and in good spirits. And yet MaMarrandi's visit had been absolutely vital—of sufficient importance to bring this household to a standstill—in and of itself. It was as if describing the state of his body to her were as much a part of the treatment as the drugs themselves.

As I sat listening to Leonard, an occurrence in my own life from more than a decade ago, one I had not thought of in a long time, came to me quite vividly. I was living in the southeast of England at the time and had resolved to give up smoking. Somebody told me of a doctor named Andrew Rutland who helped people quit smoking. I made an appointment with him and found a quiet, sullen man who dispensed almost no advice at all.

"Give up on Monday morning," he said. "And come back to me in a week."

I gave up that Monday, and the agony of the first few days was gnawing and torturous and utterly unrelenting: by Friday I thought I might go insane. I hung in there. I clung bitterly to the renunciation, and to the feeling that the renunciation was good for me, and the feeling took the form of an image of the silent Dr. Rutland planted in the front of my mind.

I went to see him a week later and told him I had not smoked.

"Good," he said quietly. "Let's make another appointment for three weeks' time."

During the following months, the sensation of clean air moving through my lungs became ineluctably attached to the idea of Dr. Rutland. At times he seemed to have lost his corporeal form and taken his place in my very breath.

MaMarrandi grabbed my wrist and spoke to me, interrupting my thoughts.

"I am so pleased with this one," she said. "He follows all the instructions. It's a pleasure dealing with someone who follows all the rules."

I had not been mortally ill when I visited Dr. Rutland. Nor had the question of my children's future been at stake. My experience was a far cry from Leonard's. Nonetheless, as the day progressed, Dr. Rutland's presence in my mind grew larger and larger, such that I could not think of MaMarrandi's work without thinking of him. Perhaps this is a little too speculative, based as it is on one fleeting observation of Leonard and MaMarrandi together, but it seemed that she stood in the space between him and his pills and gave them their meaning. It was almost as if she took the pills first, chewed them thoroughly, spat them out, and then gave them to him. By the time he had swallowed them, which bit was antiretroviral and which bit MaMarrandi had become indistinguishable. She was the affirmation of the idea that there is a daily regimen that keeps one alive, keeps one's children from becoming orphans.

And if this was so, what accounted for the difference between Vuli and Leonard? The one, surly and lonely and stubbornly entrenched in his loneliness, could not wait to eject MaMarrandi from his house. The other, surrounded by the children he had almost lost, and a brother and sister-in-law who had witnessed his resurrection from his deathbed, embraced MaMarrandi with all the force of his desire to remain alive.

Perhaps it is as simple as that. In desiring to remain alive, one sur-
renders to the fact of one's dependency on others: on one's children to
be a father, on one's brother to be a sibling, on one's pills, and the one
who has brought the pills, to remain all of these things. Perhaps
Leonard's attachment to MaMarrandi was no more than an expression
of his will to live.

Which makes the glimpse we saw of Vuli's bunkered-down life an
unpleasant portent.

———

WITH THESE THOUGHTS fresh and incoherent in my mind, we arrived
in the midafternoon at our final appointment for the day, a large
compound of several mud rondavels and square brick structures. They
formed one long line stretching across the length of the property, leaving
me with the incongruous feeling that we had entered the grounds of a
school. MaMarrandi told us that a famous chief once lived here, and
that the person we were coming to see was his granddaughter.

"Who was the chief?" Sizwe asked.

"Konkhotha."

Sizwe raised his eyebrows. "He was very famous. He was one of
those chiefs the other chiefs came to when it was not clear how to settle
a matter. In my grandfather's time, people in Ithanga would walk two
days to come and see him. Even my grandfather came to see him once.
Maybe he stayed in one of these rooms."

The old chief's granddaughter came out to greet us. She introduced herself as Thobeka and shook our hands firmly. She was in her
early thirties, I guessed, and like the first person we had visited in the
morning, her face was marked with the raw scars of a skin disease. She
brought out a broad mat from one of the rondavels and we sat under
the shade of an old pin oak, a strange tree to find in these parts, since it
is doubtful that a white family has ever lived in Nomvalo.

Thobeka reminded me that we had met in Hermann's consulting
room some months earlier. She had come with her brother. Both siblings had contracted TB some time earlier, Thobeka while living in
Durban, her brother here. MaMarrandi had knocked on the door of
the two sick siblings, and had taken them to Hermann. Both discovered that they were HIV-positive. Thobeka's CD4 count was 120. Her
brother's was next to nothing.

"My brother passed away," Thobeka said quietly.

As she said this, I noticed for the first time that the grand compound in which we sat was hushed and almost entirely empty. Whether it was the backdrop against which she spoke or merely the fright in her voice, it seemed, as she mentioned her dead brother, that she was expressing more than mourning and grief; her tone seemed to express a terrible vulnerability that had to do with the emptiness of this place.

In cue with my thoughts, a very old woman emerged from one of the houses and made her way toward us. She was perhaps as old as Zukiswa's grandmother, her hips quite stiff, her progress across the lawn a long, slow shuffle.

Thobeka introduced her as her grandmother.

"It seems God is not with me," she announced sharply by way of a greeting. "He is taking my children and leaving me alone."

"*Makhulu* [Grandmother] has been sick," Thobeka said. "Since my brother died she has been getting a headache so bad that when it attacks her she can't get out of bed."

"And he is not the first to leave me," the old woman added. "He is not the first."

Her eyes moved between me and Sizwe.

"Did you bring some beer?" she asked curtly.

Sizwe said we had not. She brushed her hand at us irritably, as if she had just dismissed us from her home.

"Since when does a person come here without beer?" she mumbled as she turned to leave.

Sizwe chuckled to himself. "She thinks it is still the days of the big chief," he said.

"Sorry, *Makhulu*," he shouted after her. "Next time we will bring."

Thobeka smiled thinly and watched her grandmother disappear into her house. She began speaking at length, and her talk soon took the shape of a broad commentary on MaMarrandi's work.

"I was sick," she said. "I knew nothing of HIV, nothing of ARVs. I was lucky I came back here from Durban. The one who convinced me was Kate. She was the one who took me to the doctor. I asked Kate to write down everything the doctor said: what I must use, what I must not use.

"It has been five weeks with the ARVs. I have a few side effects, as Dr. Hermann said I would. I have a rash. I have a pain in the side of my body. These things will go away. I have my instructions from which I live: to eat healthy, to take my pills at the right time. To not smoke. To not drink."

These strictures—do not smoke, do not drink—had punctuated the course of our day. They drew the line between the compliant and the recalcitrant, between those who embraced MaMarrandi and those who resented her. In MaMarrandi's understanding of medicine, they also drew the line between those who would live and those who would die.

I wondered about them. To drink heavily while on medication for chronic illness is undoubtedly unadvisable. A person who is habitually drunk forgets to take his pills, does not eat well, drifts into a state of absence, and increases viral replication in the body: the chronically ill must maintain a vigilant relation to their bodies that alcohol erodes. So if a person is dependent on alcohol and about to start antiretroviral treatment, he should quit drinking completely since he cannot drink in moderation. But there is no sound medical motivation to prohibit all ARV users from drinking, still less from smoking. It does not hinder people from taking their pills, nor does it impede the drugs' work in the body, nor aggravate their side effects. AIDS doctors like Hermann do not tell patients that the success of their treatment requires them to stop smoking.

And yet the chorus of laypeople who staff the ARV treatment movement at its grassroots do. Community health workers such as MaMarrandi, adherence counselors, support group chairpersons, and even nurses—I have met scores of people who state as an article of faith that those who smoke or drink while taking ARVs will die. It is an injunction that seems to have arisen organically from the front lines of the campaign.

When I asked Eric Goemaere, the head of Médecins Sans Frontières in South Africa, about the origin of the injunction against smoking and drinking, he expressed irritation.

"I'm a little annoyed," he said. "I'm definitely not a puritan. I am not a religious person, either. I don't want to re-create a church around ARVs. What I definitely don't like is that it excludes some people."

We were sitting in his office in Khayelitsha. He nodded to the busy street outside his window.

"Men in Khayelitsha go through a tough time before they get on the ARV program. People say to them, how many of you can say you don't drink? There is a prejudice against drinkers, and it extends to men. Men are unemployed here, so they drink. So I tell our counselors they are going too far. Let them have the occasional drink. And for God's sake, let them smoke."

He mused quietly for a while.

"Look at that picture behind you," he said. It was an enormous photograph, the frame filled with singing faces. "It was taken when a thousand people in Khayelitsha got onto treatment. They are all there in their t-shirts. It is important for people to believe they are part of a club, perhaps even a church. It is a sense of *ubuntu*. If you want to create a club, you must create rules. Because otherwise everyone is in, which means nobody is in. It is amazing: they set up artificially a number of rules; it was never pushed by us. And they give challenges to each other."

Artificial, perhaps, inasmuch as the rules do not make medical sense, but not arbitrary: one surely cannot use any old set of rules to define the boundary of one's club. What is the significance of these particular rules?

Those who begin treatment must make a public renunciation. Watched and judged by an audience, they must deny themselves alcohol and nicotine. In Nomvalo, that audience is Kate Marrandi. Closer to the center of the treatment program, it is a support group of peers. In either case, one must submit one's powers of discipline and restraint to a public test.

I took these thoughts to Judge Edwin Cameron, among the most vocal, and probably also among the most self-reflective South Africans on ARV treatment. Cameron is a judge at South Africa's Supreme Court of Appeal. In early 1999, he became the first South African in high public office to disclose to the nation that he was HIV-positive. He is now a leading figure in South Africa's treatment movement. We sat in a bay window in his house in Brixton, Johannesburg, and I told him of the prohibitions on smoking and drinking I had encountered in Lusikisiki. At first, he found my story perplexing: he had not come across these prohibitions before. But as we talked, so he began thinking out loud.

"I knew my status for eleven years before I started treatment," he said. "During that time, I did not realize that this virus inside me represented an enormous contamination, a sense of self-rejection. I only began to understand these things when I realized that the drugs were working. Once the viral activity had been stopped in my body, I stopped feeling contaminated. I'm aware of having viral reservoirs, but

I don't feel contaminated, not in relation to you, or friends or people I meet, or sexual partners. There's a liberation from a sense of self-disentitlement which successful treatment brings.

"It's a redemption of sorts. And like a spiritual redemption, you've got to cleanse everything. The more I think about it, the less surprised I am that it takes the form of a physical cleansing—cleansing your contaminated body of smoke and drink."

If this is right, Kate's patients, who must stop drinking and smoking and must swallow their pills, are cleansing themselves of a judgment, a reproach, that is at once physiological and moral. What is this reproach that has gotten into the blood and taken the form of a virus? Cameron suggests that his self-rejection was for being gay. Is it, for Kate's people, that the idea of the virus is attached to that of licentious lives, that to renounce smoking and drinking is also to renounce sexual adventure?

There is, it should be said, something menacing in these renunciations. I recall that on the day we first went to see her, MaMarrandi spoke with sharp accusation of those who smoked and drank and died. It is as if the living were pointing an accusing finger at the dead, announcing that they had died by contamination. Perhaps it is hard to cleanse and to heal in the absence of an enemy or a scapegoat. One can hear it in Thobeka's harsh tone when she talks of those who shun or fear ARVs: she draws a divide between friend and foe in bold and angry strokes.

"There is a problem here in Nomvalo," she said. "There are those who are saying the ARVs kill the people. And they say it because they do not want to stop smoking and drinking. They hear that before you go on ARVs, you go to a support group and you are told that smoking and drinking makes the virus strong. And then they say, 'No. These ARVs are dangerous. They will kill us.'"

"Yes," Kate said. "When they start ARVs they are told to stop. They agree. They stop for three months, and then they smoke hard, they drink hard, and they die. People then see they have used ARVs and died, and so they blame the ARVs."

SIZWE AND I had barely spoken to each other during the course of the day. He had translated and I had listened, but we had not been alone since morning.

Now, in the late afternoon, as we tailed the brisk-paced MaMarrandi back to her home, three young men, wearing vests and baggy
pants and looking like they belonged on an urban street rather than a
village path, greeted MaMarrandi warmly.

She stopped and waited for us to catch up with her.

"All three of those boys are on medication," she said. "One for
mental problems. The second one for TB. The third one for HIV." She
laughed heartily. "I took all of them to the clinic."

Sizwe stopped, turned around, and stared at them.

"Such healthy-looking boys," he said. "They are strong and
healthy."

We walked on side by side.

"Today has shocked me," he said. "Everywhere we go we meet
people who look healthy but are on medication. This one for his blood,
that one for his lungs, all the rest for their HIV. If there was a Kate in
Ithanga, would we all be on medicines, too? Do we just walk around ill
without doing anything about it? Everyone here is on some drug.
Maybe I would be, too, but I'm too scared to test."

Testing Day

In early March 2006, the organization that employed Kate Marrandi, Bambisanani, told her that it was time to bring HIV into the open in Nomvalo. A professional nurse who worked for Bambisanani, Sister Sicwebu, would come to the village on a Saturday in April with a mobile testing unit to test anyone who cared to volunteer, for HIV. In the meantime, Kate was to prepare the ground; she was to begin training several of the people she had shepherded onto antiretrovirals as voluntary testing counselors.

The idea was this: On one morning in April, dozens of Nomvalo's residents would test for HIV. Several were bound to test positive. They would be drawn into post-test counseling with a fellow villager, and invited by their counselor to join the village's newly constituted HIV support group. Nomvalo's ARV takers were thus to become activists after a fashion, the pioneers of something akin to a village movement. They would draw the asymptomatic carriers of the virus out of the danger zones of invisibility and ignorance; they would use themselves as testimony to what a future on lifelong treatment looks like. Perhaps they and their forum would come to constitute an authority in the village, one that would settle once and for all the question of what AIDS means in Nomvalo and how one goes about living with it.

In preparation, MaMarrandi went to the chief, discussed her plans with him, and asked for permission to have voluntary HIV testing conducted in Nomvalo. He responded with enthusiasm, and insisted on calling a public meeting to urge villagers to test. She also asked to speak at the services of Nomvalo's Zionist and Apostolic churches, and urged the congregants to test.

By the time Sister Sicwebu arrived on an early Saturday morning in mid-April, every soul in Nomvalo knew she was coming. The public discussions that preceded testing day had elicited a great many opinions, some irritable, some cautious, others dark. At the public meeting the chief convened, he had called on people to test, and the words and phrases he used had elicited some disgruntlement.

"The government does not need its people lying down and getting sick," the chief reportedly said at the meeting. "You have an obligation to go and test."

MaMarrandi had been sitting in the audience during the chief's speech. From behind her, she heard a man's mocking whisper.

"What does that mean? That the government is forcing us to be tested? Do my veins belong to me or the government?"

To that she heard another voice, this one much louder than a whisper, reply: "We are like cattle that must be dipped."

And then another voice: "The chief is the government's herdboy."

And then muffled laughter.

The day before the tests, MaMarrandi went to Nomvalo's central spaza shop to buy potatoes and tomatoes. Outside the shop, she joined a group of middle-aged men.

"We are not going to test," one of them said to her. "It is a waste of time."

"Why is it a waste?" she asked. "What if you are sick?"

"So what if we are sick?" another replied. And they told MaMarrandi that they would never test for this virus, because it was put in one's body by witches and their demons, and antiretrovirals were useless in the face of witchcraft.

Despite these murmurings of fear and doubt and resentment, a great many people turned out to test, so many, indeed, that Sister Sicwebu had to return the following day to finish her work. Some who came were young and still at school, others grandmothers and mothers with grown children. Almost all were women. Men confined themselves to watching and talking.

Nomvalo is small enough for everyone to know everyone else. And, whether as participants or observers, everyone was interested in testing day. Things probably unfolded just as they had the previous year in Ithanga, when the nurses came to test and the counselors to counsel, and Sizwe had noted who went in, and how long it took them to come out.

By the end of the day, about a dozen Nomvalo women had tested positive for HIV. I cannot say for certain, but given that they were counseled by fellow villagers, and that a great many pairs of eyes must have watched them on their way to and from the testing unit, it would be surprising if their status was still confidential by the following morning.

For MaMarrandi, it was a moment of achievement. By our joint and, admittedly, rough calculations, about one in five Nomvalo women between the ages of fifteen and forty-five had now tested positive for HIV under MaMarrandi's direction during the last three years. Few of them would have tested in her absence.

Yet it was also a delicate time for MaMarrandi. The virus and the question of treatment were out in the open like never before. Several Nomvalo women were to wake up on Sunday morning vulnerable and exposed. They had to be scooped up very quickly into a forum of their peers, one where they would feel the presence of collective sympathy and the absence of ill-feeling; where they would hear a confident and simple account of what to expect and what to do over the coming weeks, months, and years.

———

ON A MORNING some two weeks after testing day, Sizwe and I sat on a bench in the corner of MaMarrandi's living room. Opposite us sat five women. All had been on antiretroviral treatment for various lengths of time. Among them was Nosiviwe, the woman we had met carrying water from the river, with flaming sores on her face and nobody to accompany her to the clinic. Now her face was clear and smooth, her body once more that of a woman. The sight of her was truly startling. We had last seen her only five weeks ago.

"You look wonderful," Sizwe said, beaming with amazement and with pleasure. "You look so healthy I can hardly believe it is you."

She smiled and played with her hands.

"I am feeling okay," she mumbled with embarrassment.

"Who did you find to accompany you to the clinic?"

"My neighbor. I have been on the pills four weeks."

This morning she was to take her place as MaMarrandi's most precious asset. For we were here to attend the first support group meeting, where those who had just tested positive would talk to those on treatment, and if there was ever proof that MaMarrandi's pills could raise the dying it was Nosiviwe. She was one of those fortunate patients for whom the pills work almost immediately with neither side effects nor any of the infections triggered by the rebuilding of the immune system.

We sat and chatted and looked at our watches. The meeting was meant to have begun at nine and it was now after ten-thirty. Every woman who had tested HIV-positive two weeks earlier had been invited, but none had showed up.

"It is the weather," MaMarrandi said impassively, staring out of her open front door. "When it looks like it is going to rain, people stay in bed until lunchtime."

It was not the weather. It was something else, something far more substantial. Where the story begins depends on to whom one speaks. I like to think it starts with the two girls who attend one of Nomvalo's Zionist churches.

MaMarrandi had told us the story earlier.

"The first of these girls," she began, "went to test on the day the nurse came. She tested positive. She was shocked. She was very upset. She went straight to the house of her best friend and told her what had happened. So this second girl, she also went to test, and she also tested positive.

"Here were these two girls now, both very shaken, thinking about what they must do. They came to me. They said: 'Ma, you brought this test here, and we have tested positive, so tell us now what to do.'

"Now, Sister Sicwebu only had the means to test for HIV. She could not test people's CD4 count. But we had checked with Ntafufu, the nearest clinic, and they confirmed they were able to take blood for the CD4 count. So I advised the girls to go to Ntafufu clinic and ask the nurses there to take their blood. 'And then we will take it from there,' I told them, 'because that count will tell us how to plan.'

"The following day, they came back to me, and they said, 'Ma, the nurse at Ntafufu sent us away. She said she does not deal with AIDS. She said we must go to Lusikisiki because they deal with AIDS there.'

"I was angry with the Ntafufu people because they had gone back

on their word. I was forced now to send these two girls to Saint Elizabeth's Hospital in Lusikisiki. But I made a mistake. I gave instructions
in English. I said 'CD4 count,' whereas I should have told them in
Xhosa. I should have said '*bala amajoni*'—'count your body's sol-
diers.'

"They went to the hospital and by the time they got there they had
forgotten these words 'CD4 count,' so all they said to the nurses was,
'We tested HIV-positive in Nomvalo; the community health worker
there said we must come here.' And the nurse said to them, 'You must
go home and not come back until you get sick.'

"So now the two girls came back from the hospital empty-handed.
They were very confused. They went to their church to share with their
prophet what had happened to them. And at the church they were told
that if they pray they will get better. God will make them better, not
pills. That was when they began to deny that they were HIV-positive.
They started to visit this one"—she pointed to Nosiviwe—"and told
her that she must stop taking ARVs and come and pray."

Nosiviwe looked up from her hands for the first time. "I told them
that if they want to pray they must pray," she said quietly. "But my pills
are helping me."

The woman next to her thumped her fist on the table. "They say
Jesus Christ is the one who will help you," she shouted. Her voice was
like a battering ram crushing the very idea of the poor Zionist girls.
"You must tell them to go to their Jesus and leave us with our pills, because we are going well on them."

When I told Hermann what had happened to the two Zionist girls
he smiled at me laconically.

"Do you understand that this is a classic symptom of understaff-
ing?" he asked. "It's a variant of a very old story. Ntafufu clinic is, I
don't know, maybe 60 percent understaffed. They've just made available a new service, CD4 counts. When an understaffed clinic has a new
service, they get scared. They worry about overwork. And so when
people ask for the new service, they say no, go to Lusikisiki. And at Lusikisiki, maybe they were unfortunate enough to find a nurse who was
also too overworked and thought no, I am tired of attending to patients from the Port Saint Johns area. They must go to their own hospital.

"Once people have visited a health-care institution and have been
turned away, they don't come back. The local institution that was best

staffed and most receptive to Kate's two girls was the Zionist church, so that's where they stayed."

He is right: Kate had been forced to send her new and vulnerable charges into the health-care system like messages in a bottle tossed into the ocean.

Whether precipitated by the two Zionist girls I am not sure, but shortly after they began to voice dissent, others who had tested positive in mid-April started to register protests of their own. Rumors that had circulated through Lusikisiki's villages at the start of the treatment program now came to Nomvalo.

"Some of them are now claiming that the drugs are very dangerous," a woman who had not spoken previously said. "They say that the big oval pill, the one that is shaped like a rugby ball and is hard to swallow, that one will make you give birth to a deformed baby. The baby will come out the same shape as the pill, without arms or legs. And they say that the pill that is a little red-and-white capsule with the powder inside, that one will make you mad. And the third pill, I forget now which one, they say it gives you epilepsy."

The inversion is cruel. In the ARV support groups, each pill is handled and named and nicknamed, the side effects associated with it learned by heart. The coupling of detailed knowledge with familiarity is meant to strip the veils of mystery off the drugs, giving their users a measure of mastery over them. Here, the idea of individuating the pills is mimicked, but only to underscore their treachery.

"What exactly do people say?" I asked the woman who had spoken. "Many people believe that epilepsy and madness and deformed babies are caused by demons. Do they believe there are demons in the pills?"

"They do not put it like that," she replied. "They are scared. Some people have bad dreams when they start with ARVs and people hear that. Other people have such a low CD4 count that they die soon after they start ARVs. People see that. They are scared."

"But you are right to talk about demons," the last woman who had yet to speak finally said. "Because some of these girls who tested positive last month do not believe us. They believe we are mixing our ARVs with traditional medicines. They do not believe that ARVs can stand alone and make you survive."

"What does that have to do with witchcraft?" I asked.

"They are saying that there are two ways to get AIDS. One is through sex. The other is through people, people who hate you. They say that with this much AIDS, it can't just be sex. They say that if it was sex, so many people would not have tested positive last month. They say that people have learned to make AIDS."

"How do they give it you?"

"While you are sleeping, their demons come holding a syringe and they inject you. You are sleeping deeply. You do not even know that it has happened."

"And why do they think you would lie? Why would you hide that you are taking traditional medicines?" I asked.

"I don't know. But there is medication that is being advertised on the radio. It is called Magwagota. You can buy it from the chemist for 245 rand. People say that can cure both kinds of AIDS: AIDS from sex, and AIDS from the demon's injection."

"As well as AIDS from the *makwerekwere*," added the woman with the battering-ram voice.

"What is that?" I asked with exasperation.

"A few months ago," MaMarrandi said, "a nurse from the hospital was caught stealing a baby. When they interrogated her, she admitted that she was selling the baby to a *makwerekwere* sangoma. They say he was using parts of the baby, its arm, maybe parts of its face, to make AIDS."

"Where did you hear about the nurse stealing the baby?" I asked.

It was Sizwe who answered. "Everyone has heard it," he said. "Even in Ithanga we have heard it."

"Do you believe that the foreign sangoma is making AIDS?" I asked MaMarrandi.

"I don't believe they can make AIDS," she replied. "I believe they can do the things they advertise on their pamphlets. They can help you find things you have lost, they can help you be successful with money, to make your case go well at court. But not AIDS."

I was reminded of my conversation with Sizwe some months earlier about the witchcraft that had beset his family. It could explain his father's waywardness, his sister's nomadic drifting, and it could account for his stomach ulcer: but not AIDS. A line had to be drawn. The meaning of an epidemic that killed the young had to be narrowed.

And so it was now with MaMarrandi. Testing day, it seems, had detonated an explosion in the center of Nomvalo. Never before had the virus been so public, so very much on the surface of the world, so clearly attached to so many villagers. In the wake of this shock, the meaning of AIDS had shattered in all directions like shrapnel from a blast. Every fear that had ever been whispered came out onto the village paths. Demons with their injections, ARVs and their toxins, foreign sangomas and their dead babies: each splinter scratched out its own tale, but all bore the same warning—evil intention. Whether neighbors or foreigners or the invisible manufacturers of drugs, the intention was to kill. It was as if, in the wake of testing day, Nomvalo had awoken to an epidemic of murder.

MaMarrandi's task was to gather together the splinters, to clean up the surplus of thoughts and fears, to restore to the virus a simple and coherent meaning. Yet the meaning she gives to AIDS cannot take the form of a well-told story or a crisp definition: it comes alive only through a medical process. A clinic whose nurses accept patients who come to get their blood tested; a doctor who visits weekly; two full-time adherence counselors who shepherd the ill onto treatment—these are the tools that carve out MaMarrandi's definition of AIDS. A long twenty miles separated her from these things. She was trying to stand in for an institution.

"It was these crazy muthis that killed Vuli," the loud-voiced woman barked. "That crazy prophet and her muthis."

"Vuli is dead?"

"When you met him he was waiting for his results," MaMarrandi said calmly. "He got them two days after you saw him. His CD4 count was 230."

"Why did he die with a count of 230?" I asked. "He did not look very sick when we saw him."

"He was staying alone. I was always advising him to go to his stepmother's family and stay with them. He was stubborn. He said no, he would cook for himself. He didn't eat well. And as a man, he was drinking very heavily."

She sighed, got up from her chair, and reached for her straw hat, which was hanging from a nail on the wall.

"Perhaps we should go to the church people," she said. I had suggested earlier that we visit the leaders of the church who had told the two Zionist girls to pray.

"How did you feel when Vuli died?" I asked, once we were out on the paths. "Angry? Depressed? Responsible?"

"I feel sorry. Above all, I feel sorry. I went to his stepmother to tell the family to convince him to stay with them. He was stubborn. He wanted to stay alone. I went as often as I could to help him, but like I told you last time, I am a woman and it is difficult to help a man living alone. People will call me names. I needed a woman to assist me.

"Now one of the prophets in this village came and gave him some special water to inject inside him with an enema. His stomach swelled. People put him in a wheelbarrow and took him to his stepmother. When he arrived there, his stomach started running terribly. He died that same day."

———————

WE COULD NOT find the Zionist church people. I asked to see the two girls who had told Nosiviwe to forget her pills and pray, and we could not find them, either. I arranged to come back the following day. Still, they were not available; the church people had gone to another village for a meeting, the girls were in town. Could we visit one of the others, one of those who had spoken about the pills deforming babies? We looked but could not find them.

I thought of coming back another day and finding them myself, without MaMarrandi. I hesitated. It would constitute a betrayal. She did not want us to speak to those who scorned her work. It would seem like talking about her behind her back.

———————

I WONDER HOW things will go in Nomvalo over the coming months and years. For now, those whose HIV-positive status is public knowledge are divided into two groups. The first have AIDS and are on ARV treatment. The second are asymptomatic, and most have, for the moment, denounced ARV treatment. As for the rest of the village, they are not sure. They will watch both groups keenly. They will observe who lives and who falls ill and dies. The outed are the unfortunate subjects of an empirical experiment.

If this is so, if an uncertain village is watching closely in order to learn, what will it see? I don't think the answer is all that simple. On the one hand, there is Nosiviwe. Five weeks earlier she had carried her looming death in the shape of her hips and on the surface of her skin. Her body had reclaimed its health so fast its progress could be observed by the day. But is Nosiviwe representative of the aggregate evidence? The ones who tested in mid-April are asymptomatic. Many will not fall ill for years to come. The ones on ARVs have AIDS. They are on a long and fitful journey of recovery. Sometimes their drugs will make them ill. Sometimes their drugs will fail to prevent them from getting TB and pneumonia. They are far more likely to get sick in the next year or two than the ones who tested positive in mid-April. The village will be watching for evidence, but the evidence will probably lie.

I wonder, also, how much that matters. It is one thing taking a position on AIDS when watching others from a distance; the gallery has never been a thoughtful or generous place. Falling ill oneself is another matter entirely; there is nothing like the emergency of one's own failing health to expel dogma and invite openness. MaMarrandi will still be there looking out for the sick. She will knock on their doors, and sit in their living rooms with her reading glasses on the end of her nose and her hard-backed ledger on her lap. And she will offer to accompany them to the clinic. How many will say no? Those who are uncertain are prone to experiment. Many will go with her, no matter what they are saying now. They will be examined by nurses, their opportunistic infections will be treated, and they will be invited into a forum of HIV-positive people.

Perhaps AIDS in Nomvalo will remain in its current twilight, neither public nor private, many people on drugs, their relation to their treatment mediated through one woman.

WE VISITED KATE Marrandi again in July to discover that her support group had struck upon another problem. At around the time she had been preparing for testing day, she recruited a Nomvalo woman to help with her community health work. Her name was Vuyokazi. She was in her early forties. She had lived in Nomvalo her entire life.

A few minutes after Vuyokazi walked into her first support group meeting, which consisted of the five people we had met in MaMarrandi's house on our previous visit, a woman put up her hand and objected to the new health worker's presence. A second woman endorsed her sentiments, and then a third.

"The problem," MaMarrandi explained, "is that they are sick and Vuyokazi isn't. She grew up in this community and she used to chase the same men as these women. They don't trust her with such a sensitive thing as AIDS. They are worried that she will use her knowledge of their illness as a weapon against them. They think maybe she will go around disgracing them."

I thought immediately of the time, some while back now, when Sizwe had shared with me his fears of Simlindile, of the many pairs of eyes that watched him prosper, of what might become of his business if it were known in Ithanga that he was HIV-positive. To those who have it, the virus, it seems, places a magic flute in the mouth of its victim, drawing all the people in his past who have ever resented him.

I thought also of MaMarrandi herself: she is able to play the role that she does because she has emptied herself of meaning. She is elderly and unimplicated and did not come of age in this village. She has envied no one, competed with no one: she arrived here fully formed. To do her work, she must guard her blankness with vigilance. She must never, for instance, close the door behind her in the home of a man who lives alone.

———————

MAMARRANDI TOOK US to a patient we had not met before, a teenage girl who lives with her mother and infant child in a hut at the summit of a steep hill.

She fell pregnant last year and reported to a clinic, where she tested HIV-positive. She was ill with TB and put straight onto treatment. Her son, who is three or four months old, tested negative.

"Do you still see the father of the child?" MaMarrandi asked.

Sizwe sat next to me and translated quietly.

"Yes, I do. But we do not have sex."

"Did he test?"

"Yes. He is negative."

MaMarrandi raised her eyebrows and looked at her patient skeptically.

"Your white blood cells are protected by the ARVs," she said. "If you have sex with someone positive, their infection is maybe a little different from your infection and it will come and attack your cells. When it comes time to test your viral load, the nurses will find that the virus is there and they will say you have not been taking your ARVs. It will be because of what happens to your body when you have sex with your boyfriend. It will be difficult for you to survive.

"My advice: either your boyfriend must wear a condom every single time, or you must forget about sex for the meanwhile. Rather do something else: do something that will amaze you. You left school when you fell pregnant. Go back to school. Get your matric [high school diploma]. Your mother can look after your child in the mornings. Do something for yourself."

"You are right," the girl said. "I have stopped and started school too many times."

Her tone is bland and unsuggestive. It is difficult to know whether her agreement is just an acknowledgment of MaMarrandi's authority, or something more substantial.

MaMarrandi turned to Sizwe and me. "Do you have any questions for the patient?"

"Do people in Nomvalo know your status?" I asked.

"People on this side of the village know."

"How does that feel?"

She pointed to the door as she answered, a gesture to the world outside.

"I don't feel bad. I tell them myself. When they ask what is wrong I say *amagama mathathu.*" "Three letters"—H-I-V.

"Some people are ashamed for others to know. You are not."

She shook her head earnestly, almost stubbornly.

"No, I am not. Because those who believe they are negative, how many of them have tested? They know in themselves that maybe the only difference between us is that I have tested."

"Some people in Nomvalo say that there is more than one way of getting AIDS. There is sex, and there are traditional ways."

"Yes," she replied. "Some say they get it from bewitchment. Others say sex."

"Do you believe it is possible to get it both ways?"

She glanced furtively at MaMarrandi.

"I do not agree with the way of the wizards. It is from sex." She paused, and when she began speaking again it was MaMarrandi she addressed. "What's difficult for me is that even old ladies are HIV-positive. I don't know why."

MaMarrandi took off her reading glasses, folded them carefully, and put them in her breast pocket.

"Maybe I should explain," she said. "The pensioners, the men, after pension day, when they have money in their pockets, they sleep with young girls. They give them money and then they sleep with them. They come back to their wives with the disease. Also, there is a way the old women get the virus themselves. You have, just for example, an old lady with a shebeen [unlicensed tavern]. When the young boys come and drink, she watches for the one with a lot of money. He calls her *magriza*. She doesn't like that. She does not like being seen as a granny. She will propose love to him to show she is not a *magriza* and she will get the disease from him."

The girl persisted. "But there are other cases that are even more difficult to explain," she said. "I know a child who is five years old and HIV-positive, but the mother is negative. What happened? Even the mother asked the nurses at the hospital how it could be that her child had the three letters."

"Yes," MaMarrandi said. "There are children as young as five or six who have sex. The little one maybe had sex with someone who is HIV-positive. There is a story about my own granddaughter. Her mother was heating some water to bathe her. She was eighteen months old. Two little ones came: a boy of three, a girl of seven. They came and took my granddaughter. When the water was ready for her bath, they brought her back. She was crying terribly. I checked the child. There was something wrong with her private parts. They were damaged. I called the little boy. I offered him food. We talked nicely.

" 'Who did it?' I asked him.

"He said the girl did it. She put a stick in my granddaughter's vagina. The girl denied it. We took the baby to a doctor. He shouted at us. 'Why do you not care for your own kids?'

"Kids are naughty when they are alone."

"That's strange," the young woman replied. "At the hospital they said maybe a healer used an old blade to cut the child, a blade used on an HIV-positive person. Or they said maybe a careless nurse used an old needle."

WE LEFT THE young woman and her child, and on the village paths I caught up with MaMarrandi and walked in stride with her. I listened to the sound of her steady footfalls, and of the cotton on her arms brushing the cotton at her sides. Occasionally I glanced sideways at her impassive face, covered now in a thin film of sweat.

In all the hours I had watched her working with the ill, she had betrayed nothing. She appeared to have emptied herself of all save for a silent and limitless compassion. She had answered all my questions about herself so frugally that I soon gave up. It was as if she had decided long ago that to do this job in this village she must become a blank unit of care.

Back in the hut with the teenaged girl she had revealed a sliver of her vantage point for the first time. It seemed to be that of an exasperated woman, of conservative Christian morality, who believed the world to have become unhinged: the very old sleeping with the very young, the children running amok as soon as the adults turn their backs, an orgiastic anarchy spreading this epidemic into every second home.

"When you were growing up," I asked her, "was there much less sex than now?"

Her face remained impassive and her gait steady, but she began to speak and did not stop for a long time.

"You can't compare that time with this time," she began. "They do not listen today. When we were growing, we grew up in groups—young adult girls, middle girls, and young girls. The oldest group had their boyfriends who were about to ask them to get married. They looked out for each other, and they cared for the middle group: they made sure that the middle group does not do wrong things. The young adult girls would watch the girls in the middle group closely and when they noticed that one of them is maturing to a certain stage they would approach her and tell her it is time for her to have a boyfriend. They would sit her down and tell her what to do. They explain that you must not have sexual intercourse. The boys as well, they had adult boys teaching them how to behave. When they reached the point they got married, they knew it is time now to have intercourse in order to give birth.

"Today, they are not listening. There is something called freedom that is confusing them. If you tell them it should not be like this, it should be like that, they tell you that you are abusing them. And so we have a generation of AIDS."

We walked in silence for a long time. Her soliloquy was so thick with irony it muted me. She is the one in this village on the side of reason and simplicity. She is the one whose work is to drag the virus from the mire of treachery it inspires, to wash off the resentment and the envy and the bile, to wrap the afflicted in a plain garment of medicine and empathy. Yet her own moral imagination had suspended some of the medical knowledge she has learned. She is as aware as anyone that children neither ejaculate semen nor secrete vaginal fluid. So what is it that passes between them? How do they infect one another with AIDS? It is surely the sex itself, the surfeit of sex that has spilled over the boundaries of orderly categories. As if corrupt human practices are quite literally diseased.

It struck me that what I had been thinking of as her limitless compassion is in fact something else, something more admirable, perhaps. It is forgiveness. For the epidemic she has given over her life to fighting is an epidemic of excess and perversity.

I wracked my brain for its thin and rusty knowledge of the New Testament. "What do you think of the Book of Luke?" I asked her. "Did you know it well when you were a child? Was it among your father's favorites when he read to you?"

She laughed. It was more a query than an expression of amusement. "Why do you ask me that?"

"I am thinking of Jesus on the cross. When he says, 'For they know not what they do.'"

"That is not a passage I think of often," she replied. "Actually, when I was a child, my favorite story was from the Old Testament: the story of Samson. It made me feel very strong when I heard it. It shows that even when you think you have nothing, you actually have all the strength you need to accomplish your task. Whatever that task may be."

We were approaching the car. She asked for a lift to Lusikisiki.

"I have to deposit money for my son," she explained. "His college fees are due today."

"How do you manage to pay for your son's college?" I asked. "You live in a house built from mud and trees. You earn five hundred rand a month. Your husband has also done Christian work his whole life . . ."

By now, MaMarrandi was laughing heartily. "Jonny! Jonny! Jonny!" she exclaimed between bouts of laughter. Sizwe began to laugh, and then I did, too, reflexively, because there was no choice.

"It is easy," she said. "It is so easy. Five hundred rand a month? A person can live from a fifth of that, from one hundred, and still be fat and healthy."

Support Group

Kate Marrandi's difficulties, as Hermann Reuter pointed out, are the symptom of an unlucky geography. Nomvalo is close enough to decent AIDS medicine to sniff it, but no more. The village institution most responsive to the anguish of the HIV-positive is not the local clinic but the Zionist church.

How would the story of Kate's work have been told had Nomvalo been uprooted and put down within walking distance of a Lusikisiki clinic?

Finding out is, of course, a simple matter. Over the course of a three-month period in mid-2006, I sit in on several HIV support group meetings at Lusikisiki clinics. Sometimes Sizwe accompanies me. Sometimes I go with activists from the Treatment Action Campaign and watch them work.

By mid-2006, the youngest of the clinic support groups is more than two years old. In theory, each of the twelve clinics has two support groups: one for HIV-positive people, another for those on, or about to initiate, ARV treatment. Some are chaired by Médecins Sans Frontières adherence counselors, others by Treatment Action Campaign activists, still others by long-standing support group members. Each is held in the outdoors on clinic grounds, under a tree or against a clinic wall, the bum of every member on government-issue plastic chairs that were borrowed from the packed clinic waiting rooms. That they are conducted out in the open, in full view of passersby, is both their signature and an emblem of their most urgent aspiration: to take the virus and those it afflicts from their secret places of shame.

The most eccentric feature of the support groups is their cosmopolitanism. An odd observation, perhaps, in the context of a rural town in the depths of the old Transkei; but Lusikisiki is about as unequal and diverse a place as you will find in any countryside anywhere in the world. Around the town center are tiny suburbs of four- or five-room houses with satellite dishes, a complete range of household appliances, and a good car or two in the driveway. Twenty miles away is MaMagadla, Sizwe's mother, who fetches water from the river and firewood from the forest, has never seen a working television or attended a day of school, or traveled any farther than the one-horse town of Kokstad.

The support groups assembled on their plastic chairs under the trees make for an unlikely sight: a cross-section of Lusikisiki, right through, from one side to the other. There are the adherence counselors and the Treatment Action Campaign activists, young, clever, testing the limits of a new identity and a new confidence. Some wear jeans and TAC t-shirts, others crisply pressed, button-down shirts and chinos. Among them are women in baggy trousers, cropped haircuts, and cloth caps, who carry in their body language and their faces the universal signature of an out-of-the-closet dyke; the TAC has been the catalyst for the unlikely emergence of a lesbian subculture in Lusikisiki.

Alongside the dykes are middle-aged, buxom women from the villages in their starched skirts, their hair wrapped in brightly-colored cloth, the accoutrements of their excursions to town in supermarket bags at their sides. Next to them, middle-aged gold miners returned to their home villages when they fell ill; young, unemployed men living on their grandparents' pensions; men and women cast out of their homes because of their illness and living in a tin shack settlement to the north of town.

From this motley jigsaw of Lusikisiki's people comes the most remarkable talk. Men and women who, under other circumstances, would have come no closer than to brush against one another on the town's main street, here exchange views on clitoral orgasms, and semen, and anal sex; proper conduct in matters of love, marriage, parenthood and nutrition; and, of course, drugs. There has surely been nothing remotely like this in Pondoland's history.

When a batch of people who have freshly tested positive join the support group, the discussion explodes into shards that disperse across every aspect of life.

A shy, middle-aged man in a red-and-black checked shirt clears his throat, tentatively tests his voice, and begins to speak: "If I stay with my child," he asks, "is my baby safe? Can we still live in the same house?"

A hefty woman, her head wrapped in bright orange cloth, stands up and replies: "That depends. Is this baby your girlfriend or your off-spring? Because some men refer to their girlfriends as their babies, and I need some clarity on exactly what you're talking about before I can give you useful information."

"I'm talking about my son," he says with indignation. "He is four-teen months old."

A TAC activist named Akona joins the discussion: "The virus lives inside your body," she says, "mainly in your semen and in your blood. You cannot infect your child. You can cook for him and bathe him and do everything a parent does."

"But when I cook for him, can I taste the food before I give it to him? And what happens, for instance, if I put his dummy in my mouth, and then he sucks it again straight afterward?"

"There is some of the virus in your spit," Akona replies, "but very, very little. The medical scientists say you need gallons of spit to infect someone, much more spit than is in your mouth. You can taste your child's food. You can do everything normal. You will not infect him."

Another man stands up to ask a question. At the beginning of the meeting, he had announced that he tested HIV-positive two months ago, that when his CD4-count results came back they measured 316.

"My girlfriend doesn't know her status," he says. "I told her I was positive the day I got the results, but she refuses to test. And she says she would rather die than use condoms. But I have learned here that I must use condoms for my own health. I suspect she is HIV-positive, and that she has a plan. She wants to go to the police to tell them she got HIV from me. I do not understand her behavior. I do not trust her."

"You must not jump to conclusions," a man responds. "Denial is a very strong force. After I tested positive I went to the mother of my children and told her. She refused to believe me. It took three months before she went to test."

"That's all very well," the aggrieved man replies. "But every time we have sex she could be infecting me with another strain."

"You are right to worry about that," Akona says. "But you are probably wrong to suddenly treat your girlfriend as a stranger with criminal intentions. I do not know her, but I would be surprised if she is trying to harm you. Probably, she cannot come to terms with the fact that she might be positive. She is not ready to face that. You must try to help her."

ON A MORNING in early spring, I sit in on a support group at the clinic that has Ithanga in its catchment area. It is a tough walk from Sizwe's home: two and a half hours at a brisk pace, up a series of tall hills and down the other side.

I find an empty chair and cast my eye over the assembled people. Among them is a face so familiar and yet so out of place that at first I fail to recognize it. We make eye contact, and in that brief moment of mutual recognition his eyes bulge with fear. He springs from his chair like a jack-in-the-box, turns his back, and flees to the shelter of a tree some twenty steps away. He stops and swivels, takes in the scene he has just fled, breathes deeply and watches furtively, calming himself, deciding on a course of action.

His name is Vukani, and he is a regular drinker at Sizwe's spaza shop; I must have sat with him at least a dozen times.

I watch his eyes until they meet mine. I smile and nod a silent greeting, and I try to tell him with my face that I will not inform Sizwe or anyone else that I have seen him here today. He looks back at me with strained and studied nonchalance, as if I am making a fuss over nothing, as if his moment of panic and flight were a figment of my imagination. The chairperson opens the meeting and Vukani listens to proceedings from his place under the tree. After some time, he makes his way back to his chair and sits down.

The support group is an old and solid one, and much of the discussion is taken up with the management of various associations that its members have formed. There is a group that grows vegetables together in a nearby village; it is almost time for planting, and they request that the support group assist them in buying seed, and in acquiring wire for a protective fence. There is also a knitting group; its members want the support group to subsidize the purchase of wool.

A middle-aged woman speaks. She is clearly a long-standing figure here; the chairperson refers to her as MaDlamini. She says she wants to report a problem in her village. "The question of stigma is not resolved at my place," she says. "There is an HIV-positive woman not far from me, and when I go to visit her I am badgered. They tell me she is infected and I must not go and visit a person like that."

"Clearly," the chairperson says, "we must ask the TAC to go door-to-door in that area and talk to people. There is clearly not enough work being done there."

"The TAC has been twice to my village," the woman replies. "It seems that it does not help."

Yet precisely what she has said and what she wants remain ambiguous. Is she in fact the woman in her village whom people are discouraged from visiting? And if so, why has she conjured another person from her stigmatized self? Or does she mean what she implies: that her own status is not known in her village, that she watches the victimized woman in guilty silence, protected by the shelter of her secret? Perhaps what she is asking is for the TAC to saturate her village while she takes cover and watches from the privacy of her own home. Perhaps she hopes that by the time they have done their work she can come out into a world in which she will not be shamed.

This is, ironically, something the support groups do for their members in powerful fashion after they have died. At Lusikisiki's clinics, one in six people die within the first year of beginning ARV treatment. The support groups thus know death well. When a member dies, the group makes contact with the grieving family and asks permission to attend the funeral wearing their slogan-emblazoned t-shirts. If the family says no, they stay away. If it says yes, they arrive in large numbers, "HIV-positive" or "viral load undetectable" in bold purple letters across their backs and their chests. They assemble under the funeral tent and they sing old freedom songs, the lyrics no longer about guerrillas and machine guns, but about blood tests, CD4 counts, ARVs, and viral loads. The voices and t-shirts of the singers become the ceremony's emblem; it is now an AIDS funeral, the one being mourned has died of AIDS: visibly, audibly, undeniably.

The discussion turns to the clinic itself. A woman complains that there has been no co-trimoxazole on the pharmacy's shelves for several weeks. Co-trimoxazole is a general prophylactic for people with diminished immunity. It is required by a broad spectrum of patients, particularly those preparing to begin ARV treatment. Another woman reminds the group that the new clinic doctor did not pitch on his appointed day last week, that three people who were meant to begin ARV treatment were left waiting, and are still waiting now.

I am attending the meeting with Akona, the TAC activist who, in a previous meeting at another clinic, had assured a young father that he could taste his son's food. "What do you plan to do about this problem?" she asks.

"We will report it to the TAC's clinics organizer," someone says.

"But he is not here. And the clinic is here. Is there not a better course of action?"

"We should appoint a delegation to approach the sister in charge of this clinic," says a young woman. "She is sitting just over there."

"I think that is better," Akona adds. "But let us choose some of the quiet ones to the delegation. Let everyone get some practice at speaking."

Among those who have not said a word is Vukani. He and four others are appointed to approach the sister in charge. He listens attentively as the meeting briefs the delegation on what to say. He speaks for the first time: he asks the minute taker to ensure that her notes are accurate; he does not want to forget what it is he must take to the nurse.

To appreciate the meaning of this discussion under the trees, it is necessary to plot it on a timeline. Three years ago, doctors did not visit Lusikisiki clinics and there was no co-trimoxazole on the shelves. Three years ago, it was an unusual Transkei patient who knew the name of the drug she had been prescribed, let alone possessed a layperson's account of what it does in one's body. The very idea of taking action to put a drug on a shelf was nonsensical, for it was in the nature of things that drug supplies were erratic, a fact as immutable as the hills that lie between Ithanga and the clinic.

It is necessary to go back further in time. From the early 1960s to the early 1990s, the Transkei was run by a Bantustan government with a tinpot brutality bordering on madness: the sort of government that could arrest a person in his own home and lock him in jail without trial or fathomable reason. The idea of demanding that a drug be put on a shelf, or that a doctor arrive at his appointed time, is without precedent. The social movement to which AIDS medicine has given birth is utterly novel in this part of the world, the relationship between its members and state institutions previously unheard of.

Yet if it is a novel movement, an aspect of its novelty is surely its uneasiness and its ambivalence, for the identities of some of its members are exquisitely opaque. As I watch Vukani listening to and memorizing his brief, I am struck by the slipperiness of his place in the world. This afternoon, he will take part in the most innovative social action of his times: a patient demanding from the head of his clinic the drugs and doctors necessary to tackle a great epidemic. When that is done, he will undertake the long walk back to Ithanga; by the time he arrives home the things he has done and the person he has been during the course of the day will vanish into the invisibility of his interior. He will get drunk at Sizwe's place and play the clown.

By strange coincidence, on the very day I see Vukani at the clinic, I am reading a book about other places and other people that nonetheless speaks directly to the things I have seen. *Love in a Dark Time*, by the gay Irish writer Colm Tóibín, is a collection of essays about gay lives before the advent of gay politics. One after the other, the characters who fill its pages live masked, double lives, their very beings animated by the fear of who they are and the scandal of their possible discovery.

"The gay past is not pure (as the Irish past can often seem too pure)," Tóibín writes. "It is duplicitous and slippery, and it requires a great deal of sympathy and understanding."

I do not know Vukani well enough to see inside his heart. But I suspect the doubleness that has come to constitute his life since he tested HIV-positive reaches as deep inside him as would a forbidden love of men. It takes a great deal of shame, a great fear of one's self, to have to scale a series of hills and walk two and a half hours every Thursday morning, in order to embrace one's identity as a man with a virus.

I wonder, though, just how solid is the wall between his two lives. In the support group, his HIV-positive status is public, but not public. Back in his life, his status is secret, but not really secret, surely. I can hardly have been the first person he knows to spot him sitting under the trees in the support group meeting. And in a village as small as Ithanga, it cannot have gone unremarked that he disappears into the hills in the direction of the clinic every Thursday morning.

His health status is secret but not secret. People don't know, but they do. He lives his life in a twilight where everything is and isn't.

IN APRIL, I attend a support group meeting at Village Clinic in the center of Lusikisiki. It is the oldest, largest, and most cosmopolitan of all the support groups. Sizwe is with me. He places his chair against mine and translates the Xhosa proceedings in a quiet murmur. He is a natural: he listens and translates at the same time, his English unbroken and lively, his intonations performing each speaker's character.

It is clear from early on that there is going to be trouble. The meeting is chaired by a woman called Thembisa. I do not know whether she is from MSF or TAC, or just a long-standing member of the group, but she has about her the demeanor of an activist, of one who must guide the discussion without bulldozing it. There are two women in the group who have signaled from the start that they are going to challenge her authority. One has bright yellow cloth spun around her head. The other is strikingly obese. They whisper to each other while Thembisa is talking, and cluck their tongues loudly to show their displeasure.

Somebody has placed the question of condoms on the agenda. Thembisa leads the discussion.

"They are something that can make a hypocrite out of you," she says. "Today I tell people to condomize; tomorrow I come to you with a big, pregnant stomach."

"It is hard," a middle-aged woman in the group responds. "For twenty-five years my husband and I have had sex without a condom. He is not used to it. He doesn't like it."

"Your husband is one thing," Thembisa says. "He knows your status. But if you sleep with a man who doesn't . . . Yo! If he is negative, and you make him sick, he can take you to court and you can get ten years. You must disclose your status."

The woman with the bright yellow headdress is shaking her head in disagreeement. "It is hard to tell someone you are positive," she says sharply. "If a man proposes love to me, I cannot tell him my status. Even at home it is difficult to disclose. How much more difficult with a stranger?"

Thembisa frowns irritably. "You don't just jump into bed with someone. It goes slowly. When you are in bed with him, you ask him to use a condom. If he refuses, you suggest that you go and test together. If you walk out of here and sleep with someone flesh-to-flesh, I will blame you for killing him."

The fat woman speaks for the first time. "Maybe you see a man," she says, "and you really want to sleep with him." She slams the back of her hand into the palm of the other. "It is urgent. You want him. You must have him."

A few people giggle shyly. Thembisa brushes off the challenge with a dismissive wave of the hand. "There is no such situation," she says.

"Yes there is. You can love a man immediately and propose love to him."

"Please," Thembisa says. "If you love him and he loves you, you must know each other's status. Otherwise how can you even talk of love?"

A TAC activist has appeared from nowhere and joined the discussion. Her name is Nomasamaria.

"There is no debate here," she says. "Since you know your status, you must use condoms. It is simple."

"I am not saying no condoms," the fat woman says. "I am saying you can meet someone today and sleep with him today if you love him. And in that situation, you cannot disclose your status."

"In any case," Thembisa says uncomfortably, suddenly changing the subject, "people still need to be taught how to use a condom. It is no use using them if they are not going to work."

She marches off in the direction of the clinic, leaving Nomasamaria to chair the meeting, and returns a moment later carrying a large wooden penis, a pair of surgical gloves, and a box of condoms. She stands on a chair in the middle of the meeting, tucks the penis under her arm, and puts on the surgical gloves. Some people giggle. Two very dour-looking women in long, starched shirts stare expressionlessly. Another takes out a scrap of paper and a pen and watches carefully, preparing to take notes.

A man who has been silent until now swaggers over to Thembisa and tries to grab the penis from her.

"You will embarrass yourself," she says, lifting it high in the air, beyond his reach. "You are *isishumane*. You do not know how to do this. You have no experience."

"Why the gloves?" he asks. "Are you afraid to handle meat?"

"Go away. You are making a fool of yourself." She stands on her toes and lifts the penis higher.

Thus, Sizwe and I look on as a mottled patchwork of Lusikisiki's citizenry gather around a young woman who stands on a chair and holds aloft a large wooden penis like a pagan idol.

I chuckle out loud. "Is this what Moses saw when he came down the mountain with the Ten Commandments?" I ask Sizwe.

"I don't think Moses saw anything like this," he says quietly.

A woman who has not spoken before puts up her hand.

"Is it true," she asks, "that if you put hot water in a condom, you will see fly larvae?"

"I have heard that, too," another woman comments. "I have heard that the slippery substance on the condom is HIV. Is that true?"

"It was true of the old condoms," someone replies. "The ones that used to come from America. Today they get the condoms from other poor countries, made by black people and Indian people. They are safe."

"Indian people? Why should the ones made by the Indian people be safe?"

Thembisa is distracted by the gloves and the penis. Nomasamaria says nothing. The explanation goes unchallenged.

Excitement about the wooden penis ebbs; Thembisa gets off her chair; the discussion drifts toward the last item on the agenda. The support group is organizing a party, a beach *braai*. It will take place next Saturday. Most of the discussion is taken up with the question of expenses.

"Does anyone's boyfriend drive a bus?" a woman asks. "If we can save on taxi fare, we will be okay."

"Doesn't your boyfriend work in a butchery?" another asks. "Can he supply the meat?"

"If everyone brings their boyfriend," the woman with the yellow headdress says, "there will be no problem with expenses."

"But this is not a party for boyfriends. It is for the group."

"Then the group must find a way to pay."

THE MEMBERS OF the support group vanish in pairs and in threes into the thick crowds of Lusikisiki's market street, leaving Sizwe and me alone in the clinic's garden. Thembisa had held a penis aloft, but I wonder whether the meeting's proper object of contemplation should not have been a vagina. The discussion, it seems to me, had been nothing less than a tour through its many meanings: a source of pleasure and exuberance, a path to money and subsistence, a site of risk and selfishness, an occasion for restraint and responsibility to others.

I once arrived at Hermann Reuter's house on a Sunday morning to find him absorbed in anthropologist B. A. Pauw's classic study of Transkei churches, *Christianity and Xhosa Tradition*. "All these women's groups in the churches," Hermann had said excitedly, "all these forums generations ago where the women had space to talk. TAC has re-created them with the support groups. It is one of their biggest achievements."

I am relishing talking to Sizwe now, for the meeting has delivered a veritable feast for discussion: the men largely silent, those who did speak curiously inarticulate or meek, the women boisterous and ob-streperous and free with their mouths, the discussion proudly and un-ashamedly taken over by the question of female desire.

"Let's go," he says, before I can say anything. "This place has made me so anxious."

I look at him properly for the first time in a while. All morning I have been listening to his voice without taking in his mood. He is gray and troubled. He fidgets with his hands.

"About what?"

"Everyone here today looked healthy. And yet everyone here was sick. I looked from one face to the next one and wondered whether it was possible that they were all sick. And if it is true, if they are all sick, it is possible that everyone in Ithanga is sick. The whole village. Everyone. Me. My mother, my father, the people who drink in my shop. Everyone."

Ithanga's Kate

A few days after we attended the support group meeting at Village Clinic, Sizwe knocked on the door of Jake's brother, Xolela. The previous year, Xolela had gone to a distant clinic where nobody knew him and had tested positive for HIV. Sizwe had silently watched his health decline over the months and knew that Xolela was going to die; "Jake's mother is going to lose another son," he had told me sullenly. I had responded with an outburst: I had told him that there was medicine for Xolela a few miles away, that he was choosing to allow Jake's mother to lose another son.

Now, Sizwe knocked on Xolela's door and told him that he wanted to take him to Village Clinic to test all over again.

"I am unemployed," Xolela said. "I cannot afford the taxi fare."

"I will pay for you," Sizwe replied. "I will take a day off work and we will do the whole thing together."

I cannot say for certain what precisely passed between the two men, but it appears that Sizwe laid great stress on the disability grant of 790 rand per month Xolela would receive were it found that his CD4 count was less than 200. You are poor, Sizwe told him. The money will not hurt. And I will be with you: from the moment you get in the taxi until you get your results, I will be there.

They boarded a taxi early the following morning, arrived in the town center shortly after nine, and took their place in Village Clinic's crowded waiting room. On its route to town, their taxi had passed within a couple of miles of the clinic where I had encountered Vukani, and two others besides. I am not sure why they chose Village over their local clinic: perhaps because Sizwe had accompanied Hermann and me there, and believed that Xolela might see a doctor rather than a nurse; perhaps for the sake of anonymity. If it was indeed the latter, then that overpopulated waiting room became yet another arena of the epidemic's twilight, for it is certain that Ithanga people, or people who know Ithanga people, would see them, and would remark on the fact that they had been there. And why else would two young Ithanga men spend the morning in Village Clinic's waiting room unless one or both of them suspected that he had the three letters?

It was almost lunchtime before they were ushered into a small office for Xolela's pretest counseling. When the counselor asked Xolela whether he'd tested before he said no.

"I got angry when he said that," Sizwe told me when we next saw each other, about three weeks later. "But my anger passed quickly. He was not accepting. I thought to myself, That's okay. I understand that he is not accepting."

Ten minutes later, they were back in the counselor's room; she showed Xolela the bars on the test kit into which his blood had vanished: he was HIV-positive, she said. They listened politely to her posttest counseling, but when it was over they insisted on seeing a nurse.

"It was long after lunch when the nurse could finally see us," Sizwe told me. "The clinic was already half empty. She explained like Kate, but not nearly as well. She just said very quickly you must do this and this and this. Don't smoke. Don't drink. Luckily, he has already stopped smoking, and he hardly drinks."

The nurse also told him that she would not take his CD4 count, that he must go to his local clinic for that. From now on, she told him, every aspect of the management of his illness, from support group to the initiation of treatment, must take place at his local clinic. She was abiding by one of the fundamental principles of the MSF program: the closer your site of treatment to your home, the more likely you are to adhere to your treatment.

The following day, Sizwe gave Xolela money for another taxi ride, this one to the local clinic, to have blood taken for a CD4 count. On his way home, Xolela stopped by Sizwe's shop, asked to speak with him privately, and told him in all the detail he could remember what had happened at the clinic, from the precise words the nurse had used, to the counselors he had met and their names and the things they had said, to a description of the needle that had found his vein.

Sizwe has become Kate, I thought to myself. Or Xolela's private Kate in any event. He is the one who mediates between Xolela and his treatment. When time comes for Xolela to take his pills, Sizwe will be the one to chew on them first, spit them out, and hand them over.

Xolela returned to the clinic the following week to get the results of his CD4 count. He got back to Ithanga just before dusk and went straight to Sizwe's spaza shop. He stopped at the front door, looked over the heads of the drinkers, and found Sizwe's eyes behind the counter. Sizwe nodded and stepped outside.

"He said that his CD4 count was 107," Sizwe told me, "and I was so shocked I could say nothing for a long time. Okay, Xolela has been sick, but he is a strong man, much stronger than me. How can a man be so strong, and yet so close to dying? It made me worry about my niece, Thandeka. How long has she had the virus? What is her count? She looks healthy, but maybe she is nearly dead, too."

"What did they tell Xolela at the clinic?" I asked.

"They told him he must go onto ARVs, but not yet. He must first attend the support group to learn about the drugs."

"How's he doing?" I asked.

"He is okay. He needs to talk a lot. Almost every day, he comes here to my place in the late afternoon, and we go somewhere quiet to talk. He needs to tell me everything that's happening."

———

XOLELA IS NOT the only one to whom Sizwe had decided to become a Kate Marrandi. A few days later, he told me another story, of a relative called Vuyiso, a man I had not met, from a village some distance away.

"It started with a skin disease," he told me. "His skin went very dark, almost black. That cleared, but then he started getting a running stomach. He has had it over three weeks now. It seems it is permanent. He came to me a while ago. He wanted to talk about money. There was going to be a big ceremony for his daughter. We call it the bucket ceremony. When a daughter of the family is getting married, she is given many, many things that are put in a bucket, and she takes the bucket with her to her new home. Vuyiso asked me if he could borrow three thousand rand for the bucket ceremony. I gave him two thousand rand. The ceremony was last weekend. I arrived and Vuyiso was not there, at his daughter's own ceremony, for which he had humbled himself to raise money. He was too sick to attend."

"How do you know it is AIDS?" I asked.

"It is clearly AIDS," he said cautiously. "The skin, the running stomach. All he has done is get medicine from the chemist. I said to him openly when he came to see me, 'Maybe you must go and test for the virus.' He said, 'What can you do if you have AIDS? I don't want to know.'

"Next week, I am going to take a day off and make a trip to his village. I will sit him down and urge him to test."

"What will you tell him?"

"That having AIDS does not mean you are going to die. That you must go to test. It is like asthma. It is something you are sick with for a long time, but it is not death. You never get completely well. You are not quite right. But you do not die. You can live and you can work."

"WHAT HAPPENED THAT made you change your views?" I asked.

"About what?"

From the tone of his voice it was clear that he knew what I had asked. He had taken my question as a criticism, as a call on his inconsistency.

We had come from visiting a relative of his in a district that was new to me. I had parked the car on a tall, narrow ridge, and we were leaning against the hood. The scene before us was unlike anything I had seen in the Transkei. In all directions, the land rolled away for miles. To the south, there were wide grasslands and forests and a blurred hint of the sea. To the north, a series of valleys disappeared over the horizon, lending the scene a hyperbolic sense of depth. Stand on almost any piece of ground in the Lusikisiki district and you feel that much of the world around you is hidden. Here, it seemed you could see everything.

"About AIDS," I said, "when we met—"

"I know. When we met I was against even testing. And I did not believe that ARVs worked. You are right, I have changed my mind. It is for two reasons. First, I have seen four, maybe five people at Ithanga get very sick, and then get nearly better on ARVs. Also, the trips I have done with you—to Kate, with Dr. Hermann, with the nurses—I have seen the work the nurses do. But mainly it is the girls from Ithanga, the very sick girls who went onto ARVs and are well now."

And yet the girls of whom Sizwe spoke went onto ARVs and started getting better some time before he and I met. They were among those who tested one Saturday morning when the counselors and the nurses came to the school at Ithanga, the day the entire community watched to see who went in, and who took a long time coming out. When Sizwe and I met, this day stood out in his mind as a warning against testing for HIV.

"So what changed? Did you speak to these girls about their ARVs?"

"No. They do not say they are on ARVs. But you see them getting into the taxis to go to the clinic, and you watch their health and you see that they are getting better. And people talk and you hear the rumors that they are on ARVs. You do not talk to them about it. You watch and you hear."

I began to say something, but he interrupted me and began speaking of something else. He did not want to talk about why his views had changed.

I did not think it was the Ithanga girls who made him change his mind. I thought his views on the Ithanga girls changed because of the things he and I had seen together. That this was a source of discomfort for him troubled me. To my mind, the reasons for his shift were both obvious and unembarrassing. It came directly from an experience he and I shared.

The first thing I believed we grew to share was a bond between ourselves and the ill; it was something we brought back from our time with Kate Marrandi. She lifted our spirits, mine and Sizwe's alike. At the end of each day that we were with her, we drove back to Ithanga feeling light and serene and nourished. We watched the sick ones surrender themselves to her care—the care of a faithful mother, plodding the footpaths in a calm and ceaseless search for the ill, never a judgment on her tongue. I think there were times both of us identified with her patients; I think we took part, vicariously, in their surrender to her. In those moments, the epidemic disentangled itself from the jeers and the whispers, and was enveloped in a gentle solidarity.

We also experienced something else together, something connected to the feelings we imbibed from Kate, but different.

Together we saw that the epidemic has no boundaries, that those who were ill were interchangeable with ourselves. Before our trip, the epidemic was contained: it resided in Jake, who was dead; in Sizwe's niece, for whom he would one day surely find a healer with a cure; and in the girls who had been foolish enough to have their blood taken before the curious gaze of their community.

Indeed, the outing of the foolish girls had been a convenient foible, an illusory means to contain the virus. They allowed for the epidemic to be named and placed and pushed to one side. As they went about their business, silently watched but never openly confronted, the girls who had tested positive became the members of a parade to be jeered and pilloried. The audience, by virtue of being the ones who jeered, were freed from the epidemic.

And that, indeed, is the heart of the poisonous work done by the virus's strange twilight. These souls whom everyone knows but does not know are ill, gather the virus into one cage: a high fence is erected and the healthy affirm their health by staring in from the outside.

On our journeys, we saw too much for this illusion to hold. Wherever we went, the virus was in the healthy and the sick, in those who coughed and those who breathed freely, in those with the scars of a fungus on their faces and those with clear skins. That was precisely what Sizwe had been telling me throughout our journey: that the epidemic had lost its boundaries, that there was no caging it any longer.

Why was he so reticent to acknowledge that this experience had caused him to take stock? Why was his change of heart a cause for estrangement between us?

———————————

THE FOLLOWING DAY he offered an answer, albeit obliquely and cautiously.

"One of the things I have changed my mind about since my trips with you," he said, "is the question of shingles. I thought this is something you should know, since clearly you are very interested in what changed my views.

"Previously, I did not think that shingles was a symptom of HIV. We used to associate HIV only with diarrhea, and with weight loss. Shingles we thought was witchcraft. It is caused by the *ichanti* or the *umrulo*. These are snakes sent to you by demons. They crawl on you in your sleep, and where they touch your skin you are left with shingles. I saw lots of people getting shingles. I think they all tested HIV-positive, and were too ashamed to tell people. So they let it be believed that they were bewitched. They would go to the inyangas, and the inyangas would say, 'Yes, you have been bewitched. I can treat you.' The inyangas treated them, and then they died.

"When I was traveling with you, I saw people with shingles. The nurses said this is a symptom of HIV. And I saw that some people with shingles did not die. They got better."

I immediately remembered the first of Kate Marrandi's patients we met, Nosiviwe, the water carrier with heavy marks on her skin. I remembered vividly how, on our second trip to Nomvalo, when we saw that she had gained weight and that her skin had cleared up, Sizwe had beamed at her and remarked on her skin. I recalled his joy well, but had no idea until now precisely what was at stake.

Throughout our journey he had been conducting these empirical tests in private. I wondered about the line that divided the things he shared easily with me and the things he kept to himself. About those who envy him and will see him destroyed, he was eager to confess and to share. But about the silent experiments he had been conducting on AIDS and its treatment, he was deeply reluctant.

I recalled that twice during our acquaintance, I had said things that he interpreted as a judgment on both himself and the entire milieu that had shaped him. The first was when I asked why falling ill with AIDS was a disgrace. "Is it not a disgrace where you come from?" he had asked with surprise and embarrassment. The second time was when I laughed at his account of the white conspiracy to win back political power by decimating blacks. "I am relieved that Kate told you what the people were saying about Dr. Hermann," he had said. "I was worried that it was only Ithanga. When you laughed, I thought, Maybe I am telling Jonny some bullshit that only the people in Ithanga believe."

At question in these encounters was the integrity of the local knowledge that had been bequeathed to him. The matter at stake was one of pride and humiliation. He knew that twentieth-century South Africa had gutted his world, leaving it without roads or lights or clinics, or decent jobs. Perhaps he also wondered whether it had left his world without wisdom.

I thought that the same was at stake when he compared inyangas and nurses on the question of shingles, and more broadly, when he decided to shepherd ill people to the clinics. That he had changed his mind on this question perhaps signaled a cultural defeat, a belittlement of his world. And thus an elevation of my world and a victory for me. It was a deeply unpleasant victory, one that was thrown in my lap while I was looking elsewhere.

Mabalane

On a Saturday in mid-July we attend a funeral some distance from Ithanga. I will only come to understand much later that the journey Sizwe maps for us today is intended to take back the victory I have won over him, that he is to put a wager on the superiority of Mpondo wisdom.

Sizwe never met the one who has died: she is of his clan, and the funeral tent is filled with clansmen and -women whom he knows only from rituals and ceremonies. The dead woman's parents are Zionists, and the members of their congregation have assembled in the tent in their numbers. The women are in thickly starched red-and-white uniforms, while the men wear spectacular crimson robes on their bodies and expressions of austere religiosity on their faces. Each carries a chest-high staff. One of them wears a high, gold-embossed bishop's hat and clutches a crucifix some seven or eight feet in length. They form a wide crescent around the coffin, the crucifix rising with some drama from their left flank. They sing and preach in turn, without interruption, for the duration of the morning. There is nothing mournful in their singing: it is frenzied and urgent, and it mobilizes in its members a blistering energy.

Sizwe gets up to leave the tent and invites me to join him. I shake my head and stay. This gaudy yet spare theater, lavishly camp but powerfully earnest, has me feeling both melancholy and mesmerized: the thought of getting up and walking out makes my legs feel heavy.

It is with this, I think to myself, that the support groups must compete when they descend on a funeral. Freedom songs and t-shirts versus bishop's hats and staffs and a thunderous singing that evokes an ancient god. There is no mention this morning of the cause of the woman's death. She was thirty-two and had been ill. That is all.

I remain in the tent for an hour or so, and then leave and look for Sizwe. I bump into him almost immediately.

"I was coming to call you," he says. "There is someone you must meet."

He leads me around the back of the tent. A number of young men are sitting in the sun on a long bench. Sizwe introduces me to one of them.

"This is a cousin of mine," he says. "His name is Mabalane."

He is perhaps thirty at most. He is dressed in creased blue overalls and he is very shy. He smiles at me nervously and looks away.

"He is an inyanga," Sizwe says. "And he has been telling me about a cure he has developed for AIDS. He says he has cured many people."

The young man glances at me quickly and nods, then bows his head and fiddles with a button on his overalls.

I look at Sizwe closely: there is urgency in his face, but I cannot read its source. Has he donned the role of the diligent research assistant, searching for interesting subject matter on my behalf? Or does he hope that he has found a cure for his niece Thandeka's virus, that this business of spiriting the ill to and from the clinics for their blood tests and their drugs and their endless support group meetings can finally come to a close?

Of his thoughts about Thandeka's illness and his plans to deal with it I have stopped questioning him long ago. It is not something he chooses to talk about. On the day he agreed to accompany me to the clinics as my interpreter, he said his primary motivation was to see whether ARVs might be for her. Since then, he has answered my questions about his quest in monosyllables. Talking of Thandeka, I guess, would mean talking of the private empirical tests he has been conducting for himself on the efficacy of ARVs; that is something he will only share with reluctance.

"I would like to see his place and his medicines," Sizwe says. "It is not far from here. We can take your car."

IT IS A ten- or fifteen-minute journey, much of it on overgrown pathways more suited to carrying pedestrians than cars. At times we move no faster than we would have had we gotten out and pushed.

I turn on my Dictaphone and we begin to ask Mabalane about his work.

"The ancestors started calling me when I was very young," he says. "It was the 1980s. I was a small boy. There was big fighting at that time. The young men's associations were fighting wars against one another. And then there were other people who were struggling against the government. The ancestors came in my dreams and told me to do this and this and this. I went as far as Natal to get muthi for people to stop the bullets entering them."

"What are the diseases you have learned to cure?" I ask.

"Any disease. If someone comes with an illness I cannot heal, I tell him to go. As soon as I go to sleep, all the ancestors come, even the ones I have not seen before." He nods in Sizwe's direction. "This one's grandfather, whom I never met in life, my grandfather introduced him to me in my dream."

"How do you recognize AIDS?"

"I need a card from the clinic. The patients must go to the clinic and come with the card saying they are HIV-positive. Then I give them two liters of medicines: they are herbs I have been told to fetch in my dreams. When the two liters are finished I tell them to go back and test again. The test will be negative. I don't reduce the AIDS like the doctors. I kill the disease." He pauses a moment, and then adds: "I charge two hundred rand for the two liters. But if the person doesn't have the money, I give the muthi anyway, to save their life."

"So many people have died from AIDS," I say. "If the ancestors know how to cure it, why have they let so many people die?"

"The people only trust the doctors," he says sorrowfully. "They don't want traditional herbs. They trust Western doctors and they die."

My thoughts turn immediately to Hermann Reuter and what he would say about this rival. I have tried to draw him out several times on the question of traditional healers. Always, he greets my inquiry with a long silence, then shrugs and begins speaking of something else.

MABALANE'S HOME IS that of a very poor man. A flat, barren square of ground enclosed by a waist-high fence, two stocky, one-room structures at each end. One is his house, he tells us, the other his workshop. We are not in a village, but on empty land along a busy district road. The sparseness and the sound of the traffic lend the place a feeling of forlornness.

Mabalane's wife is sitting on her doorstep and nods at us silently. I smile at her momentarily, but am distracted by the presence of two dogs. One is a very young pup, perhaps six weeks old. She is tethered to a post outside the workshop; she strains at the end of her rope in an attempt to join us. The other is skeletal, and barely conscious, and lies on his side breathing heavily. As we get closer it is apparent that his head is desperately swollen, as if a tennis ball has been inserted under the skin on his forehead.

He opens an eye at the sound of our footfalls: he is blind, his iris hidden somewhere behind his eye socket, his cornea a milky white.

"He was shot some weeks back," Mabalane says, crouching over his animal. "He is going to die any day from now."

He turns his back on the dog, searches the ground, and picks three herbs. He hands one to each of us, and asks us to chew it and then spit it out. An herbalist's working space must not be polluted by the presence of people who have come from a funeral; the herb cleanses us of the recently dead.

The workshop we enter is dark and windowless. On the floor in the center of the room, several dozen bottles are piled haphazardly: half-pints, one-liter cold drink bottles, beer bottles. Some are filled to the brim with herbs, others are almost empty. Herbs are scattered all over the floor, from one corner of the room to the other. Among the bottles is a well-polished turtle shell.

"This man should be a sangoma," Sizwe murmurs quietly. "This is a sangoma's place."

The remains of two creatures hang from the ceiling on low hooks. One is the coat of a genet. The other is an owl, its broad wings stretched wide, its torso a rotting and mutilated cavern.

"That owl," I say, "why do you keep it there?"

"If I kept it on the floor the rats would eat it," he replies.

"Yes," I say, "but what is its function here?"

"When somebody wants to bewitch this place," he replies, "they send an owl. I make a fire in which a piece of this owl is burnt. The owl that has been sent to bewitch me smells the fire and knows not to come here."

He gets down on his haunches, chooses three bottles, pours out a generous portion of herbs from each, mixes them together, and empties the cocktail into a supermarket bag. He rolls the bag up tightly and throws it across the room into Sizwe's lap. Sizwe reaches for his wallet in his front pocket, finds two hundred-rand notes, and puts them down next to him on the floor.

"I notice that you use three herbs for AIDS," I say. "It is just like the doctors. ARV therapy uses three kinds of drugs."

"Yes," he says. "One herb is for TB, another is for diarrhea, and the third is for headaches. When you mix them together it cures AIDS."

"Do you have to travel far into the forest for these herbs?" I ask.

"No. They grow right here in my yard."

We leave the workshop and he accompanies us to our car.

"A man from East London came here a while ago," Mabalane tells us unsolicited as we are leaving. "His name is Mr. Simgo. He took a sample of my medicine to test in a laboratory in Bisho. I am not sure when he is coming back. But I am not worried about his test. Whatever the results, I know that my medicine cures AIDS."

WE RETURN TO the funeral, pick up Sizwe's mother and two other people who are going to Ithanga, and drive home. By the time we are alone together again, it is almost dark. We are standing outside Sizwe's shop.

"What do you think of these herbs?" I ask.

He stares at the ground and does not reply for some time. "I'm not sure," he says finally. "If it does cure AIDS, why do more people not know of it? Even at the funeral, where the people know Mabalane well, nobody had heard of it. But who knows? And what is there to lose?"

"The herbs are for Thandeka?"

"The main problem is her boyfriend," he says. "Maybe these herbs will cure her and she will be reinfected by him. And then we will not know whether it has worked. Maybe what I must do is, I must visit the boyfriend and instruct him to go to Mabalane to buy two liters of medicine. Then I will sit Thandeka down, give her these herbs, and tell her not to have sex with her boyfriend for two weeks. Then I will take her to the clinic to test again."

"The discussion with the boyfriend will be difficult," I say. "He does not want to know about AIDS."

"I have had some practice with people like that recently," he says dryly. "And anyway, enough is enough. He is a sick man."

He pats his pockets, checks his jacket, then looks up and smiles sheepishly.

"I have left the herbs in your car."

I COUNT TWO weeks from the afternoon Sizwe bought the herbs from Mabalane, and mark the day in my diary. It comes and goes. Eight or nine days later, I get a call from Sizwe. I am at home in Johannesburg. He says he has phoned to say hello and to see if I am well.

He is awful on the telephone: stiff and proper and awkward. But I am too curious to wait another week until I see him.

"Did Thandeka and her boyfriend take the herbalist's medicine?" I ask.

"They both took it." A long pause. "When the two weeks were over, they went to the hospital. Both tested positive. They had their CD4 counts taken. Hers was 435. His was 402. They were told to come back in three months to have their blood taken again. And if either of them gets sick before the three months is up, then they must come back immediately."

He relates these things to me blandly and without emotion. But I know that a heavy burden has lifted from his shoulders—to know that Thandeka's CD4 count is 435, that there is still plenty of time, that she is not at death's door, that there is now a protocol to follow.

"Mabalane did a very good job," Sizwe says. "I am happy with him."

"How so?"

"If it were not for the herbs, Thandeka's boyfriend would never have gone to test. Perhaps even Thandeka herself would have done nothing until she was ill or dead. I am very happy with Mabalane. I must make a special trip to thank him."

MUCH LATER, PERHAPS as long as nine months, Sizwe and I find ourselves driving past Mabalane's place. Neither of us has spoken of him in a long time. I nod in the direction of his house.

"Have you seen your cousin lately?" I ask.

He laughs. Puzzled, I laugh back.

"What's funny about Mabalane?" he asks.

"I was responding to your laughter," I say. "It was you who laughed at the mention of him."

A long pause. "When you wrote about Mabalane in your book," he says, "why did you say that the fence around his property was knee-high?"

"I don't remember. Did I say it was knee-high? Is it knee-high?"

"It is about the height of the stomach. You exaggerated. You wanted to show that the man's place was fucked up. What fool wastes his time and money building a knee-high fence? Anything can get over it, even a small dog."

He had said nothing of this when he first read the chapter about Mabalane. That was some six weeks ago. It was one of those thoughts, I guess, that one holds back. Now he is telling me he has seen his world through my eyes, and what he saw was people with useless fences around their gardens and useless bottles of herbs in their rooms.

"Where else have I exaggerated to show that things are fucked up?" I ask.

He shrugs. "I'd have to go back and look."

I recall his defensiveness on the phone when I asked him whether Mabalane's cure had worked, and I think I see what he is protesting against when he shields his cousin from me. He is protesting against a collective humiliation. Black people have gotten sick in droves and line up outside the clinic to get the medicine the white doctor has brought. It is humiliating. Before the gaze of their community they are outed as the bearers of a disgraceful disease; they must sit in support groups run by fiery young women and for the rest of their lives they must swallow ghastly pills that serve only to remind them that they are sick and that each cough or bout of diarrhea could lead to death.

He wants very much for an end to this, and for the end to be delivered by a dose of Mpondo medicine; a gift from the ancestors that heals one now and forever and puts an end to the lines outside the clinic and the counselors in the school hall.

I have rubbed his face in it. I went to Mabalane's place, and what I saw was a knee-high fence.

Nombulelo

The person Sizwe has approached to become Ithanga's Kate Marrandi is a single woman in her mid-fifties named Nombulelo. He chose her because she was once trained as a field-worker by an orphan support organization that is now defunct.

"The work is not very different," he says. "Maybe it will not take the clinic so long to retrain her, and she can start work immediately."

We visit the nurse in charge of the local clinic, and she agrees that Ithanga does indeed desperately require its own dedicated community health worker. If she is embarrassed that it has taken this long to attend to a village in her jurisdiction, she does not show it; with easy authority, she tells us to send Nombulelo to her.

Nombulelo's home stands at the very bottom of Ithanga's narrow valley basin, and the path from Sizwe's place to hers is so steep and slippery that I spend much of the journey walking crablike, digging the sides of my shoes into the mud.

"How well do you know Nombulelo?" I ask. "Will she be as good as Kate?"

"She can read and write as well as Kate," he replies. "So she will be good. The thing that can make her not so effective as Kate is that she grew up in Ithanga. Her whole life she has competed over men in this village. It will make her work very difficult."

"Is she married?"

"She used to be married. She separated from her husband many years ago. Over the years she has been the girlfriend to several men in this village."

"How has she supported herself?"

"She has a big homestead like a man. She has made money selling oysters and crayfish to the hotels on the sea. She is a very clever woman. She has learned how to save money. Much cleverer than most of the men of her generation: they throw their money at women and at beer and they and their families die poor. Her son, he has gone off to study. Me, I couldn't finish matric because . . ."

His sentence trails off, and he shouts a greeting to a man a hundred yards below us.

Described by Sizwe's tongue, she is a giddy combination: an unattached woman who builds a home as a man ought to. He is surely right: she must be both the best and the worst person to be drawing the epidemic into the open. If Sizwe's spaza shop courts such envy, then what of a woman who invented her own business and has slept with husbands of her fellow villagers to boot? I imagine she must marshal admiration and resentment in equal measure, that the idea of her conjures both promise and scandal.

She is waiting for us. She sees us from some distance away, locks her front door, and joins us on the path. She is small-boned and thin. She greets me quietly, puts her head down, and does not speak. She is shy. Throughout the walk out of Ithanga, I do not get a proper look at her face.

In the car on the way to the clinic, I ask her how she will begin her work, and she says her first task will be to start a support group in Ithanga.

"What is your strategy?" I ask. "People are so scared here for their neighbors to know they are positive. How will you get them to come together in broad daylight and sit together in a group?"

"I will attend every funeral every weekend, and I will speak to every mourner," she says. "I am not HIV-positive, but I will tell people that I am. That will give them the confidence to come to me. They will trust me if they think I am HIV-positive."

"You are sure that's wise?"

"My work will fail if they think I am negative," she says authoritatively. "People are too disgraced to confide in people who are negative. The people who are negative talk about them at funerals and at functions. They whisper about them. How will they confide in me if I am someone who might whisper about them?"

"Would your position not be much stronger," I ask, "if you could show them both that you are HIV-negative and that you embrace them? Isn't an important task to break the divide between the positive and the negative?"

"It will not work," she says. "They need to have trust in me."

Listening to Nombulelo, I wonder where the epidemic's peculiar twilight ends. For Sizwe is here in the car, a fellow villager who knows everyone she knows; might he not one day, in the course of casual conversation, tell drinkers at his spaza shop that the rich, single woman in the valley is only pretending to be HIV-positive? Among the things stored in the village's stock of common knowledge—the same stock in which the ARV girls' regular taxi trips to the clinic are stored—will be the notion that Nombulelo pretends to be positive in order to tend to those who pretend to be negative.

"You are not married," I say. "Does that affect the way you do your work?"

"A married woman could not do this work," she replies crisply. "She would not have the freedom. Her husband wants her to cook, to do this and that, to wash his clothes. Doing this job properly means being called out at any time. You must have love and commitment, and you must be unmarried."

WE PARK OUTSIDE the clinic. Nombulelo disappears into the gloom of the building's interior to her appointment with the nurse in charge; Sizwe and I settle under a tree a few paces from our car.

"What do you think of the fact that she is going to lie about her status?" I ask him.

He looks away, a cold, disinterested expression on his face.

"All the counselors do that," he says. "Even the ones who came to Ithanga that day last year to test the people at the school. They tell you they are HIV-positive and on drugs and alive and well, in order to charm you into saying you are HIV-positive."

"How do you know they are lying?" I ask.

He laughs hollowly and says nothing.

"Seriously," I say. "How do you know?"

"Some are HIV-positive. Some are not. The ones who lie, what they are doing is wrong."

Several recent events lie in the background to our discussion, shaping its meaning. Hermann Reuter's four-year stay in Lusikisiki is to end soon; Médecins Sans Frontières will be handing the treatment program over to the Eastern Cape Department of Health. There is a great deal of apprehensiveness among the counselors, pharmacists, and community health workers Hermann trained. They worry about the future of treatment in Lusikisiki in the absence of its pioneer.

"These ones who charm the people by saying they are HIV-positive," Sizwe says, "if they are worried about Dr. Hermann leaving it is because they are worried about their jobs. But I think their jobs will be okay. The people have been shouting at Thabo Mbeki, for letting the people die. So, maybe, if they shout loud enough, the government will now employ these ones from MSF to stop the people from dying."

Had I closed my eyes while he was talking, I would have sworn that his comments were soaked in sarcasm. But the expression on his face suggests that what he means is unclear. Both to me, and to him. Perhaps the movement Hermann built here consists merely of people in search of salaries and positions; they beguile the ill into humiliating themselves in order to feather their own nests. Perhaps they are nonetheless saving from death the people they have tricked. Perhaps both of these things are true. Perhaps neither is true.

When he chose to accompany me to the clinics he was utterly uncertain about ARV medicine. His journey was experimental. Now that our travels are almost over, he has made decisions of much consequence: he has taken Jake's surviving brother to get antiretroviral treatment, he has coaxed Thandeka and her boyfriend into getting their CD4 counts taken, and he has found a Kate Marrandi for his village. And yet all these decisions are provisional. If he wakes up tomorrow morning to discover that he was wrong—that the drugs will leave with Hermann Reuter, that people quickly develop resistance to them and die, that those who brought them to Lusikisiki always knew this to be a ruse—he will not be surprised.

"These are not easy times," he says. "In my parents' and my grandparents' day, they got lots of sexually transmitted infections, but they did not die. Those diseases were made by people and AIDS is made by people, but in those days, sexual diseases did not kill."

"You know that AIDS is made by people?"

"Look over there," he says, pointing over my shoulder. I turn around. The front of a wide forest faces us from the middle distance. It climbs a hill and disappears into a valley. From somewhere beyond the horizon, a scrawny trail of smoke twists into the air.

"We have a saying in Xhosa," he continues. "When you see smoke like that in the air, it means there is someone underneath, at the bottom. Some people have been lighting a fire. If you see smoke in the air and you think it is just there, it just happens to be there, you are not thinking straight. It is not just there in the sky. There are people at the bottom. That is where it has come from."

He pauses, but he is not finished.

"Somebody must have made AIDS. Maybe it went out of control. Maybe this is not what they wanted. But somebody made it."

"Fires start for many different reasons," I say.

"Tell me. You have never told me your explanation of where AIDS comes from."

I tell him of a virus called SIV that has been endemic in beasts of the central African jungles perhaps for centuries. I tell him that human beings entered these forests in large numbers for the first time during the last century, perhaps in the 1930s, that the virus was transferred and mutated into a form that could be spread from person to person. By the early 1980s, I tell him, there were cases of AIDS on every continent, but it is here in southern and eastern Africa that conditions permitted the virus to spread far and wide: weak governance and poor public health programs, the sorts of inequality that cause people to travel far both for work and for sex, the sheer accident of whether a male population is circumcised, a combination of poverty and tropical parasites that have made the bodies of many Africans more vulnerable to sexually transmitted infection than most. I tell him that this is the story I have accepted for the moment, that it comes from a reservoir of knowledge I have passively inherited rather than chosen, something that is just in the air around me, as witchcraft is in the air around him, that I myself have next to no expertise in these matters, and that the story is by no means adequate, that almost everything about it is provisional.

He listens intently and nods from time to time, but I know that I am talking to myself, just as he was talking to himself when he told me about the smoke and the fire.

———————

We get up and stretch our legs and wander slowly over to the clinic. A young woman is leaning against the front wall sunning herself, her eyes half-closed. She greets us as we approach, and the three of us stand together and chat.

"You are a counselor?" Sizwe asks.

"Yes."

"So I can test?"

She perks up and smiles at him. "You want to test? We can go in right now." She pushes herself off the wall and makes for the clinic door.

He giggles nervously, peers into the murky corridor beyond the door, and shakes his head.

"I cannot test," he says.

She smiles at him kindly. "You're sure?"

"I'm quite sure."

"That's fine," she says. "You are not ready. It is no good testing before you are ready. You will let it sit with you for a long time, and one morning you will wake up and know that it is time."

She goes inside. He watches her disappear.

"I will never be ready," he says. "How can I ever be ready to hear that I am HIV-positive? If I test today, and the result is positive, I will have to call off my marriage. I will have to send Nwabisa and the child in her womb back to her home. I will not be able to marry because I will soon die. And even if I am to live a long time, my children might be born positive. No woman could be my wife. I would be like an ox: I would sweat in the fields for a while and then get sick and die."

What he has said is so simple, the fears he has expressed so clear. Yet his words come like a welcome shock of ice-cold water, for it is immediately apparent that they issue from a place he has until now chosen to keep silent; and I know right away that in the coming months I will be hearing much more. For the first time, I understand something of what he is doing when he searches Ithanga for a suitable Kate Marrandi. In his scheme of things, MaMarrandi's work will always be twilight work. Hers is to shepherd ruined human beings, discreetly and with little fuss, to and from the clinics, their ruin written into the fact that everyone knows where they are going but dares not say it to their faces.

Sitting with him outside the clinic, I feel that a very opaque man, one who has given me only the most oblique glimpses of his inner world, has opened a door.

PART THREE

Sizwe and Nwabisa

I had known Sizwe for some time when I met Nwabisa, the mother of his unborn child and the woman he was to marry. The circumstances of our meeting were awkward.

I arrived at Sizwe's spaza shop in the heat of a midsummer afternoon. Already, drinkers were spilling out of the front door, the speakers on his tape deck banging out Zulu Maskanda music. It was a song I knew well. The Maskanda artist Phuzekhemisi was singing about his dog Udlayedwa: "He-eats-alone."

I dodged and squeezed my way toward the counter. In the center of the room, three elderly women were dancing in precarious drunkenness, one of them crooning the song's lyrics in mock anger. She complained, along with Phuzekhemisi, of the dog tax she was forced to pay for Udlayedwa. She asked whether her dog would get a state pension when he grew old.

The spectacle of an inebriated old Mpondo woman singing in Zulu about her dog was too much for Sizwe's patrons. Some buried their faces in their hands and chuckled quietly. Others slapped their thighs and howled with laughter.

Sizwe was standing behind the counter with his hands on his hips, a broad smile on his face. He greeted me impatiently and shouted above the noise that Nwabisa was home, that I was finally to meet her.

He told me to go next door, to his bedroom, where I would find her. His enthusiasm was boyish and agitated, almost nervous.

I slipped out of the service door and made my way to Sizwe's living quarters. The door was standing wide open. I knocked and shouted hello. There was no reply. I tentatively stepped inside.

Nwabisa was fast asleep on the bed. She lay in a fetal position, her body cupping a young boy. He too was asleep. I knew from what I had been told that he was her eight-year-old son, here to visit her during his school holidays. One of his hands was tucked under his side. The other lay open-palmed on his mother's swollen belly; she was due to give birth in less than a month.

I turned to leave, but the shuffling of my feet disturbed her. She opened her eyes and rolled them around the room in disoriented fashion. As they fixed on me, they widened with surprise. She sat bolt upright, waking her son, and buried her face in her hands.

"I'm sorry," I said, "I will come back a little later."

"No," she replied bravely, her face still in her hands. "We have waited a long time to see each other. You will stay and you will sit down."

I fetched a plastic chair from the corner of the room and sat on it. We smiled at each other a little sheepishly.

"You look just like Sizwe said you looked," she remarked quietly. "He has been speaking about you for a long time."

It struck me as she said this that I had given little thought to what she might look like. Seeing her now for the first time, I found myself, oddly, comparing her face to that of her future husband's. They were not alike at all. While his eyes were set wide apart, as if opening his face to an engagement with the world, hers were set close together, as if in defense; they were cautious and a little sad.

She sat uncomfortably on the edge of the bed, her body turned away from me; to make eye contact, she had to twist her head and look at me over her left shoulder. Despite her awkwardness, though, she was curious. She asked whether I was married, if I had children, whether my parents were alive, and if they lived close to me.

As I answered her questions, the sound of a commotion came to us from the other room. There was laughing, shouting, the thud of a heavy glass bottle hitting the floor, then more laughter.

"This is Sizwe's work," she said, nodding in the direction of the noise.

"He is doing well."

She shrugged. "It is a shebeen. A tavern. It is hard. You must have drinking people around your home."

There is a sense in which our meeting consisted of a mutual eyeing out. When I asked Sizwe whether I could write about him, he took more than a month to say yes. I knew that he consulted extensively with Nwabisa during that time. The decision was as much hers as it was his. Now, perhaps, she was judging whether they had made the right call.

As for me, Nwabisa was my subject's wife-to-be, and I was growing increasingly aware of what her presence in his life might mean for the book I was writing. Sizwe's remarks when he declined the offer to test for HIV at his local clinic still lay in the future. He had not yet told me that were he to test positive he would have to call off his marriage, send Nwabisa and the child in her womb back to her home, and live his remaining days like an ox. But I did already know him well enough to see that he had made his impending marriage the very kernel of his identity, and that it was not the sort of identity, nor the sort of marriage, that could withstand the presence of the virus in its midst.

THE STORY NWABISA and Sizwe tell of their courtship is one of forbidden love. They came together slowly, secretly, and chastely, over a period of two years. There were times when months went by as one crafted a move and the other responded. It was such an admirable tale—one of such dignity and patience—that I was immediately suspicious of it.

They met at a high school athletics meet. It was the summer of 2000. Both were in their next-to-last year of school.

Sizwe was with a friend. The friend pointed Nwabisa out in the grandstand and told Sizwe that she was a Mabaso. His interest was immediately piqued. The Magadla and Mabaso families were in the depths of an ugly feud. A cousin of Sizwe's had married a brother of Nwabisa's; the marriage had ended on bad terms, there had been a dispute over the return of bridewealth, and the two families had been volleying threats at each other ever since.

Sizwe made his way to Nwabisa's seat in the stands and asked if he could join her. She agreed, if a little hesitantly. They sat side by side all day and spoke guardedly to each other. When the races were over, Sizwe offered to walk with Nwabisa to the taxi rank. It was a long way. Neither remembers what they spoke of, only that Nwabisa was cautious. After some forty-five minutes of walking, she instructed him to turn back; she would walk the remaining distance herself.

During the course of the following year, Sizwe's soccer team twice went to Nwabisa's village to play against the local side. She would come to watch. After the game, the Ithanga team would walk home, and she would accompany Sizwe to the bank of the nearest river, a signal that she was enjoying his courting.

He was growing increasingly frustrated. He was more than infatuated with her; he found himself preoccupied, daydreaming, scheming. She lived under her parents' roof in a village Sizwe had no excuse visiting—he had no relatives there, no friends. And if her parents discovered their courtship, they would surely try to end it.

On their third post-game walk to the river, Nwabisa told him that since she was finishing school at the end of the year, she would soon be looking for work; she'd be grateful were he to find something for her. He took this as an invitation to seek a way to get her away from her parents and into a relationship with him.

And so he scouted the countryside for a job suitable for a young woman. In early 2002 he found one. There is a state forest not far from Ithanga. Some of the workers live on-site in clusters of two-room cottages. A handful of people are employed to keep the grounds and common areas clean, to maintain the communal kitchen, and to cook meals. The job Sizwe found for Nwabisa was in the kitchen. He sent word to her village for her to come.

She didn't.

"I was not sure what to do," Sizwe told me. "I put some money in the pocket of a young boy from Ithanga and told him to go to her village to fetch her. He came back without her. A few weeks later I sent a second boy. He also came back without her. The man who ran the kitchen at the forest was getting frustrated.

"He said, 'I cannot wait forever for the lady. Why don't you go and fetch her yourself?'

"I said, 'No, I can't do that.'

"Nwabisa has relatives in Ithanga. Eventually, I went to a young boy in that family and I said, 'Go and fetch your aunt. Do not come back without her.'"

This time she came.

She took up the job at the state forest and moved in with her relatives in Ithanga. Shortly thereafter, she and Sizwe slept together.

But there was soon trouble in the Ithanga household into which Nwabisa had moved. She was deeply unhappy there, and decided that she could not stay any longer. She was faced with a choice: she could return home and give up her job, or she could keep her job and move in with Sizwe. She chose the latter. In the same week that she began sharing his bed, Sizwe did the three-hour walk between Ithanga and Nwabisa's village, sat down with her family, and asked their permission for her to live with him. To the couple's surprise, Nwabisa's parents had heard rumors of their relationship months ago, and had already digested the idea and accepted it. Their need for secrecy, it seems, had been fueled as much by their fear and excitement as by a real threat.

Nwabisa's parents demanded a payment of three goats in exchange for their permission to have their daughter live under Sizwe's roof. He assented. He was a poor young man from an impoverished family; it was the most he had ever paid for anything.

———

ON A LATE-SUMMER afternoon I asked Nwabisa if I could accompany her to the river to fetch water. Soon after we set out, I told her teasingly that I did not quite believe the story she tells of her and Sizwe, that it seems to come more from a storybook than the world. I wondered about its seamless and graceful construction. Sizwe was twenty-four when he met Nwabisa, and by his own reckoning had slept with more than a dozen girlfriends in recent years. She was two or three years younger than him and the mother of a small child. Their long and deliberative period of chaste pursuit seemed not to issue from their world. I wondered whether the fact that their relationship was culminating in marriage had not caused them to tinker somewhat with the tale of its beginnings.

She laughed shyly. "You don't understand. He was forbidden to me because our families were fighting. If my father knew I was seeing a Magadla there would have been big trouble. So when he became interested in me, I thought to myself maybe I don't need this complication. But even while I was pushing him away, I felt I was falling in love.

"I confided in my sister. She was shocked. She said I mustn't tell anyone, and I didn't. That is why it was so slow and cautious.

"It was only after I started living in Ithanga that things came out. People saw us together and told my family. They were shocked. But he presented himself to them immediately and soon they were okay."

I ASKED SIZWE to explain the eccentricity of their courtship. I expected him to tell the same, bare-boned yarn of forbidden romance Nwabisa had given me. Instead, he offered an opaque, unexpected story, one that I struggled to make sense of at first.

"You waited patiently for two years before you consummated your relationship with Nwabisa," I commented to him.

"Yes," he replied blankly.

"But when you tell me other stories from this time in your life, it is a different world. You and Jake are moving from girl to girl. You are sleeping with several people in the space of a few months."

"Yes."

"But no sex with Nwabisa."

"No."

"It sounds like you were always chasing her and she was running away."

He nodded his head approvingly; he clearly liked the formulation. "Yes, in our culture you have to chase the lady. If you need a lady you need to chase her until you get her."

"Even if she loves you, she will make you chase her?"

"Yes. You have to chase the lady from far away. You go several times to propose but she runs away from you. Until eventually her parents ask, 'What is this man always doing coming here?' And then you, as the man who is after the lady, you wait for that moment when the parents are asking questions, and then you tell a member of the family, a parent or a sister, of your intentions. Those people will convince the lady that this is a good man. 'You must marry him. He has been here many times.'"

"But your other girlfriends you did not chase for two years."

"No."

"So what was different about Nwabisa?"

"In our culture," he replied obdurately, "you must chase the lady."

I gave up. He was giving me a version of the old Madonna-versus-whore story, and that was familiar enough. He had been young and foolish, sowing his wild oats across the villages of Lusikisiki; now he was settling down to a woman, and to a life, of substance.

And yet if he was telling an old-fashioned sex-versus-love tale, he had chosen an intriguing way to tell it. This is how things are done in our culture, he kept saying stubbornly, as if his relationship with Nwabisa came from the depths of a hallowed tradition, the relationships that preceded it from flotsam. It is an *Mpondo* lady one must chase, he appeared to be saying; deracinated girls come easily to one's bed.

I WAS ABOUT to abandon these thoughts and move on when an experience with Sizwe gave me cause to stop and think some more. It so happened that at the time he told me how one must chase the lady, slowly accruing allies among her family, we were interviewing Ithanga's octogenarians about their youth. As we moved from one interview to the next, listening to the old people remembering their courting days, it came to me that Sizwe was borrowing bits and pieces of their world, and cobbling them into the story he told about himself and Nwabisa. The young man's serial journeys to his sweetheart's father's homestead, her seemingly ceaseless refusals, his endeavors to make himself noticed among the members of her family, to win sympathizers—these were not memories of his own: they were idealized, recrafted episodes we had heard from the mouths of the old people.

The story Sizwe told of how he and Nwabisa met, of how one must chase the lady until her parents consent for you to take her, was an act of retrieval, or conservation. From the midst of his quintessentially 1990s sexual debuts, he had, in modified form, resurrected the idea of a traditional Mpondo courtship. Whether he did it just for my benefit, or whether it was a story he himself valued, I did not know at first.

Of Oxen and Men

By the time I set foot in Ithanga for the first time, I had begun to learn a great deal about love, sex, and courtship among Sizwe's grandparents' generation. It so happens that one of the finest ethnographic monographs ever penned in South Africa was researched in these parts in the early 1930s, and I had lapped it up greedily in preparation for my research. The anthropologist was a young woman named Monica Hunter, and the book she published was titled *Reaction to Conquest: Effects of Contact with Europeans on the Pondo of South Africa.*

Hunter did her fieldwork between 1930 and 1932. She never visited Ithanga, but she did spend a three-month period in several of Lusikisiki's villages. When she began her research she was twenty-three years old and fresh from Cambridge University, where she had studied history as an undergraduate. A daughter of one of Eastern Cape's more famous missionary families, she was reasonably fluent in Xhosa. She came to Pondoland as the guest of a white trader and his wife. She would settle in to the trading store in the morning, and listen to the gossip of the women who came to buy.

"A store serves as a club for the district," Hunter writes, "the people gathering there to meet friends, gossip, flirt, and beg tobacco . . . Sitting in the corner of the store I listened to the gossip and joined in the conversation . . . I heard about the latest *affaires;* who had been beaten by their husbands, and why; who were pregnant; what sort of crops had been reaped; who was sick, and who had bewitched them. I kept a bag of tobacco which helped the conversation along."

Hunter's book is written in the fashion of its times. The ethnographer views herself as a scientist: she seldom draws attention either to her place in the world she describes or to the relationship between her feelings and her observations. But one can of course tell a great deal about a writer by what her eye fixes upon and what it sees. And Hunter is clearly taken aback by what appears to be a paradox: Pondoland's premarital world is sexually permissive in the extreme and yet sexual relations are highly ordered.

Girls as young as eight, and boys nine, she comments with muted astonishment, begin to attend the weekend gatherings of the unmarried. "The young people of one small local district . . . gather in the evening in a secluded spot in the veld or in a deserted hut. They dance and sing, then pair off to sleep together. The couple lie in each other's arms, but the hymen of the girl must not be ruptured. If it is, the boy responsible is liable to a heavy fine."

Hunter cannot shake off her surprise at how young the children are when they begin to partake in these sexual adventures. She repeats the point in the following paragraph. "It is certain that boys and girls [sweetheart] before puberty. One overhears such remarks as, 'It is awfully good to have a girl to cuddle into these cold nights' from boys of 12. By 14 boys are complete young bloods, cutting their hair in fancy patterns, sporting snuff spoons, and wearing their sweethearts' beads."

A little later, Hunter notes that these childhood and teenage couplings are seldom kept hidden from the young lovers' parents. On the contrary, she writes, "it has always been customary for young men to spend nights with girls in the girls' own homes. This relationship . . . is marked by an exchange of gifts between his group and hers . . . The first gift from the man to the girl's father is usually a couple of goats, now sometimes one pound, then comes a beast, and if the relation lasts for more than a year, sometimes another beast . . . The girl is supplied with beads and blankets by her father, embroiders a loin-cloth and sometimes also another blanket, and makes necklaces and anklets, and a snuff-box, for her lover."

The young age of sexual debut, and the openness of youngsters' relationships to the gaze of adults, is not all that catches Hunter's eye. So too does the alacrity with which teenagers play the field. " 'A boy may be loved by as many as six girls,'" an informant of Hunter's tells her. " 'If he has many he cannot pay for them all, and then fathers will not have him . . .' A girl may also have a number of lovers, and her father may receive [gifts] from them all. 'A girl may have 12 or 13 boys come to her hut every evening. She will send away all but two or three, and then talk to one and send him, talk to another and send him, and remain with the third.' Her rivals may call her *isifebe* (a voluptuary), but it is no disgrace to her to accept several lovers at the same time. The more skulls the better."

I HAD MET seven Ithangans in their eighties, including both of Sizwe's grandmothers. Most were in their early teens when Hunter did her fieldwork. I set about to interview them all. At the beginning, I used Sizwe as an interpreter.

At each encounter, Hunter's book was vivid in my mind. I looked for discrepancies between her accounts and the ones I was hearing now. And of course they were there. It was not just the fog and nostalgia of the three-quarters of a century that lay between then and now. The respective contexts were different. Hunter listened in as young women gossiped freely. I was conducting formal interviews with elderly people in the presence of their grandson. Their narratives were sanitized and inhibited. Sex was discussed with heavy, awkward innuendo.

I found opportunities to interview old people without Sizwe, using more appropriate interpreters. I hired a middle-aged woman and a stranger when I interviewed grandmothers, a middle-aged man for the grandfathers. In these new circumstances, the old people were transformed. Nothing stirs the vanity of an octogenarian like an invitation to discuss the days of his or her sexual prowess. Their narratives grew raunchy, their accounts of their sexual pasts suspiciously exhibitionist. Some told me that today's youth were frigid, impotent, sexually shy, that they had lost the arts of love.

But it was the discussions in Sizwe's presence that remain most vivid in my mind. Here, the sex itself slipped into the shadows of innuendo and what came to the fore was the strict organization, and, above all, the strict *visibility*, of premarital sex. Hunter laid emphasis on the fact that penetration was strictly forbidden. But equally forbidden was secrecy, invisibility. There seemed to be a presumption among the old people we interviewed that the liaisons of those who stole away and coupled beyond the gaze of their peers or parents would end in intercourse, either by consent or by force.

"At the weekend party," an elderly Ithanga man named Peter Madikizela told me, "it is very important that the girl chooses her boy in front of everybody, and that everybody sees them go off together." He spoke animatedly and in the present tense, even though the events he described were seven decades past. "And where they go is also important," he continued. "Not behind a closed door. They must be in the forest, where the other couples are, so that if the girl feels uncomfortable she will shout and the others will hear."

And, of course, the sexual encounters of the "young men [who] spend the night with girls in the girls' own homes," as Hunter puts it, were monitored with equal scrutiny.

"In those days," Peter Madikizela told me, "all unmarried members of the household slept together in the kitchen. So a teenaged girl could not slip away for the night; it was noticed. If a boy wanted to spend the night with her, he must present himself to her father, and the three of them must all together choose the hut where the couple will sleep."

All of this monitored sexual adventure moved toward a fixed end: almost everyone was to marry. The young man who approaches his sweetheart's father to spend the night hopes one day to tell the patriarch that his daughter has agreed to wed him. What begins as a parental monitoring of sex becomes a bridewealth negotiation between two families.

The day before Sizwe first told me of how he and Nwabisa got together, we interviewed his maternal grandmother. I asked how her husband had courted her.

"It took a lot of time for me to agree to marry him," she began. "He had to visit several times to my homestead to ask me to be his wife. It took two years, maybe one and a half years, so that I could believe that this person needs me."

"Was he patient?" I asked.

"He tried not to be patient," she laughed. "At first he told me he needed me to come to visit him outside, at his home. I said no, I am a virgin. You need to come to my home, to my parents. So he came, and I made him go to a small rondavel and wait there. My father was already dead by then, so my mother and one of her brothers came to see him. He said to them, 'I am here because your daughter invited me. She agreed that I am her lover.' And then they nodded and said it's okay if you pay us a goat."

It was into this rubric that Sizwe wanted to fit his relationship with Nwabisa. "You need to chase the lady from far away," he told me when I asked why the first two years of their relationship were chaste. You must wait around long enough to gain allies among her relatives.

Of course, it did not happen quite this way with Nwabisa. But as he told the story he maneuvered it as close to the grooves of the old rubric as it would go.

The moment it was clear that Nwabisa was going to move in with him, Sizwe made the trip to her village to announce himself and to pay three goats. "I went to her place, to her family," he told me, "because they must know me very well. Not meeting me in the town and knowing nothing about me, only hearing rumors I am staying with their daughter. I must come. I must announce myself. That is how it must be done."

It was, of course, just a proxy, and a forced one at that, of how things were done in his grandmother's times. For Sizwe came of age long after the organized visibility of premarital sex had vanished. The trip to Nwabisa's village and the payment of the goats constituted no more than the faintest echo of what transpired between Sizwe's grandparents. And yet the continuity is what he emphasized. "That is how it is done in our culture," he told me stubbornly. "Things must be done properly."

When did young Ithangans begin sleeping together in secret? When did it start becoming customary for unmarried people to have penetrative sex beyond the gaze of their peers and parents?

Most of the elderly Ithangans I interviewed told me that the tradition began to crumble in earnest some time between their courting days and those of their children. Surveys done in other parts of Eastern Cape bear that out. Hunter herself led a team of researchers who conducted a census in Keiskammahoek, about two hundred miles southwest of Lusikisiki, in 1950. She found that just over half of women between eighteen and forty-five had children out of wedlock, compared to 20 percent of women over forty-five.

When I asked elderly Ithangans why the young started sleeping together in secret the answer I got puzzled me. For me it is surely a question of political economy. Three generations ago, life in places like Ithanga was organized around productive land. The pinnacle of adulthood was proprietorship of a peasant homestead, and a homestead unit consisted of a patriarch and his dependents. To live the life to which he aspired, an Mpondo man had to inherit land, cattle, and infrastructure from his father, and he would not inherit if he did not marry. The whole world thus arced into marriage, and in producing heirs within marriage; that is where everything was headed.

When the economic basis of that world began to crumble, so too did the relationships it sustained. Today, most young men in Ithanga will not inherit productive land or find a steady job. Nor can they afford to marry. The very foundation of the world in which it made sense to save penetrative sex and procreation for marriage has long vanished.

The old people I spoke to were of course acutely aware of such change. They told me incessantly that, unlike them, their grandchildren do not work the land and do not find jobs. But they refused to attribute the erosion of the visibility of premarital sex and the prohibition on intercourse to this. No, they say, it isn't because the children could not find jobs or work the land. What happened, quite simply, was an explosion of unbridled desire; the young could no longer contain their sexual greed. So they rebelled. They broke every rule and stricture and ran off to have penetrative sex behind closed doors. And nobody could stop them.

I asked Peter Madikizela, the elderly man who said that young men and women could only couple at parties if they remained in earshot, why youngsters started having sex in secret.

"It happened because boys started deciding they were men," he replied. "Girls decided they were women who can sleep with men. It happened when they stopped going off to the forest together and instead started coming inside. The young woman would secretly come to the young man's room and knock on the door. So even if she screamed nobody would hear. She knew that. To get herself into that situation, it means she wanted to have sex with him."

"For generations and generations," I said, "the youngsters went to the forest. Why did it change when it did?"

"Because young boys started demanding their own rooms," he replied. "They refused to sleep in the kitchen anymore. They wanted a door to close behind them, a door their parents were not allowed to go through."

"But why did this change?" I asked.

He shrugged. "We were defeated. The kids took over. They became ungovernable. They would just commandeer a room, move a bed in, and declare that it is their room."

———————

IN THE STORY he tells of his coming of age, Sizwe began his sexual life as a typical young man of the 1990s, losing his virginity long before the prospect of marriage, moving from one girl to another. Then he meets Nwabisa. The 1990s narrative disintegrates and vanishes. He plunges into the depths of a world that died long before his birth and emerges with another story of himself, damp and old and somewhat disfigured, but good enough. It is the story of a young, virginal Mpondo man in pursuit of an old-fashioned bride.

Why does he do this? What is his purpose?

I put these questions to him. I told him that when I listened to him talking of himself I heard two stories, a modern and then an olden one. I did not think, I told him, that it was merely a question of "settling down," of youthful exuberance giving way to adulthood. It was much more than that. He was sifting through the artifacts of his cultural inheritance in order to chart a course through the world. What was that course?

It was a Saturday morning in late summer. We had taken my car to a deserted field. I had just given him a driving lesson, one that had left us both feeling a little fragile. We were now sitting on the grass, our backs leaning against the car. He listened intently, and said nothing for a while.

"Yes," he offered finally. "When Nwabisa moved to Ithanga I had other girlfriends, and at first I carried on with them. You know the word *isishumane*? The *isishumane* is afraid of girls. A man in Ithanga who has only one girlfriend, they say he is *isishumane*. He is scared of the women.

"But then two things happened to make me stop sleeping with other girls. Nwabisa got so upset when I was cheating her. It was more than upset. She got thin. She got sick. I saw that there was this person I

was making so unhappy. I could not be happy while she was so unhappy.

"And then there is a second reason, maybe as important. It is about
Jake. It is about that Jake has died and I have not.

"I have noticed that these are very bad times if you have many
girls. If, by this time, you are not HIV-positive, you are lucky. And so
you must stop. At this very moment, if you are one of the lucky ones,
you must stop to mix with so many people. I stopped."

We talked no more of it that day; the powerful clarity with which
he had spoken had an unassailable air about it. It seemed rude to per-
severe.

Yet as his words sat with me, so they bothered me, for they were
not quite enough. That he had chosen monogamy because he lives in a
time of AIDS and because he feels the pain of his loved one spoke
powerfully of a man in whom little darkness resides, the sort one
would wish all young men to be in the midst of a plague. But there was
so much about him that his words had not explained. They did not, for
example, account for why he chose to describe his beginnings with
Nwabisa as an exemplar of a long-vanished style of courtship. The
Mpondo men of the past may have abstained from intercourse before
marriage, but, once they were wed, monogamy was not a virtue to
which they aspired. Sizwe's father and grandfather both had many ex-
tramarital lovers, as was expected of men of their times. His decision
to be monogamous was thoroughly modern, and without pedigree in
his world.

As so often happened, he finally provided a satisfying answer
almost by accident.

We had gone to town. Pension day was around the corner, Sizwe's
busiest time, and he had a great deal of shopping to do. In the aisles of
one of the large warehouse stores on the main road, hemmed in by
wide shelves of potatoes and mealie meal that rise almost fifty feet into
the air, we bumped into a young woman from Ithanga. She and Sizwe
chatted for a while and I wandered.

When I returned, the woman was gone, and there was a gray pallor
about Sizwe's face. He was struggling to conceal his irritation.

"What's the matter?" I asked.

"It is nothing," he replied, "but it is also not nothing. Nwabisa's
brother was in Ithanga looking for me this morning. I wish he had not
come."

He paused for a while, his eyes wandering around the store, then looked at me again.

"It can only mean one thing. He came to tell me that his sister has been living with me for a long time and still there is no *lobola*. He came to say it is time for me to get off my ass.

"It is bad timing. I have been saving for a long time. I am nearly ready to marry. Now the people see that the brother has to come to demand. It is a disgrace that the people see that."

Bridewealth, or *lobola,* is frighteningly expensive. Formal negotiations between Sizwe's and Nwabisa's families had not yet begun, but he could reasonably expect to be asked to pay an initial installment of cows and cash to the value of about twenty-five thousand rand. Few Ithanga men of Sizwe's generation had full-time work. Of those who did, only the most fortunate earned the value of bridewealth in a year. Sizwe's shop was doing well. He had been slowly accumulating his bridewealth. He had just bought two cows. He was almost ready.

"Disgrace?" I said. "That's a very strong word. Maybe a little too strong?"

"It is not too strong," he replied firmly. "In these times, the young people are living badly. A woman comes to stay with you a long time. You have one child. Then another. Then a third child. Still, she stays. You are not married. The children are not yours, they do not have your surname. They will not inherit your kraal or your rondavel. You are surrounded by people, but you are nothing, you are by yourself.

"It is a disgrace. You are like an ox, or like a bull who has hundreds of calves that all belong to other herds: you are a beast who pushes the plow all day and then one day drops dead. You will leave nothing behind you except your corpse in the field."

He gripped the handlebar of his heavy cart and began pushing it down the aisle. I stood and watched him, a hunched, laboring figure. He had spoken from the depths of his gut, from a place that does not usually find expression in words.

He had likened himself to an ox once before, outside the clinic, when he said he could not countenance the thought of the virus in his veins. Then, as now, he conjured an ox as a metaphor for a castrated man: castrated not in the sense that he cannot father children, but in the sense that he cannot father children he can claim as his own—a man without descendants and thus without permanence, a man who will leave in this world only his rotting corpse.

Today, he meant precisely the same thing when he spoke of an ox, but his words were more powerful. Back at the clinic, the oxen were young men with AIDS. Now he was speaking of his entire generation, and perhaps the last one, too. The erosion of marriage, which followed the decline of working land and jobs, had spawned lives without meaning or permanence. He and his peers risked living like animals who labor and then die. When he skipped two generations in his search for material with which to model his adulthood, he had in his mind an epoch when men were homestead patriarchs and left a lasting mark on the world.

I guess there is nothing remarkable in this. Pondoland was battered and shaken and gutted during the course of the twentieth century. It is unsurprising that among its heirs are young men of conservative bent who scour the recent past for better times: men intent on shoring up as unscathed an image of patriarchy as they can muster.

Yet for me it was a moment of revelation; it helped me make some sense of a person with whom I had spent a great deal of time, and over whom I had puzzled. Among the things I learned was that Sizwe was investing the profits of his shop in something at once material and metaphysical. Most men his age could not afford to marry, could not afford to sire children who would bear their names. Sizwe could follow the trajectory he imagined because he was lucky or smart or single-minded enough to earn a reasonable living. He had invested his profits in a proper marriage, in children who would be born Magadlas, and in a growing bundle of assets that they would inherit. He had, with his profits, begun to fashion his own permanence in these Transkei hills.

I think I understand a little better now what Sizwe was feeling that day outside the clinic when he refused the invitation to test for HIV. He was, of course, feeling many things, some of which I have yet to explore, others that I will never know. But whatever else it meant to him, being HIV-positive was a curse that one carries in one's semen and thus that one might transmit to one's children. He believed a diagnosis of HIV-positive would entail putting off his impending marriage, to Nwabisa or to any other woman, and sitting out a life that produced no more Magadlas. The corrosiveness of AIDS was expressed in the wasting away, not only of one's body, but of one's lineage, and, thus too, of the lineage of the dead ones who walked this earth in years gone by.

I wonder, then, whether at one level AIDS ought to be understood as a metaphor that describes the fate of the men of Sizwe's generation. Their fate is to fail to procreate as patriarchs do. AIDS represents this failure as a disease. In retrospect, once the epidemic has come, it perhaps brings with it the illusion that it was destined for these people in these times.

Progeny

The maternity nurse at the clinic had told Nwabisa that she would go into labor on or around January 18, 2006. On the morning of the 12th, Nwabisa packed a small bag and walked out of Ithanga with Sizwe. They caught a taxi to town, and then another to Nwabisa's mother's village, where they were met by members of her family and by the traditional midwife who would deliver the baby. Sizwe stayed long enough to chat, and to receive a light meal. Then he and Nwabisa said farewell shyly, and a little stiffly, the expression of their emotions inhibited by the gathering around them. He got into a taxi, went home, and waited for news.

Among the precolonial Mpondo practices that weathered the twentieth century is the banishment of fathers from the births of their children. The mother returns to her parental home to prepare for labor. The child's father can only begin visiting on the eighth day after the birth. Even then, he is to cover his entire body, save his head, for the duration of his visit, to speak only in hushed and deferential tones, and to stay as briefly as possible. He certainly cannot spend the night. His wife and child return to his home a month or two later.

Sizwe waited longer than he had expected. On the 21st, a hand-delivered note brought him news that he had a son, and that mother and child were both healthy. During the days that followed, a succession of windswept and hungry children arrived at his door, each clutching a note that bore more news. The second letter informed him that while the infant was not gravely ill, he was not quite well, either. He had a fierce rash on his skin, and it was making him miserable; he spent much of his waking time crying.

Nwabisa's family was poor. They would gratefully receive advice and herbs from their traditional nurse, but no more. Sizwe shoved a wad of banknotes into an envelope, wrote a letter asking Nwabisa to take the boy to a general practitioner in town, and handed his package to the child messenger who was gulping down a plate of food at Sizwe's table. He watched the child leave, then closed his door and paced his bedroom.

Beside himself with worry and impatience, he decided on waking the following morning to break ranks with custom and to see his child. He went into town, made his way to the doctor's rooms, and found Nwabisa in the waiting room, clutching a bundle. He would discover, during the course of the morning, that it weighed about seven pounds.

ON THE EIGHTH morning after she had given birth, I drove Sizwe to Nwabisa and his son, Mfanawetu—"Our Boy." It was a long drive. As the crow flies, Nwabisa's family's village was eleven miles from Ithanga. By car it was nearly four times that.

The gravel road ended about a hundred feet from the entrance to the Mabaso homestead. I turned off the ignition and we sat and watched. When his child is but eight days old, a father does not casually wander into his wife's parents' homestead. He waits to be invited.

It was an unforgivingly hot late January day. The radio weather report had put the temperature at equal to ninety degrees Fahrenheit. In the car, with the sun pummeling our roof and no trace of a shadow, it was much hotter than that. The homestead was still; not a soul was to be seen. To pass the time, we spoke of Ithanga's dogs. Sizwe said they were all devoted to him, even the dogs of his enemies. His grandfather had taught him a secret. Wipe your face with a towel, squeeze the sweat in the towel onto a dog's bowl of food, and then feed him. He will be yours forever.

The better part of an hour passed before a young girl, seven or eight years old, appeared from one of the Mabaso huts. She spotted our car and came over. Sizwe began speaking with her, and as I listened, I was struck by his tone. He addressed her with the deference he usually reserves for an elder, his chin bowed, his eyes lowered, his voice a cautious murmur. Watching him perform thus for a young child, I began to appreciate for the first time the full weight of the journey we had just made.

The girl went inside, reappeared a moment later, and signaled for us to come. As we got out of the car, Sizwe donned a heavy, thigh-length winter's coat, an ostentatious observance, I thought, of the stricture that a father cover his body at his infant's birthplace.

I walked several paces behind him. Watching him make his way to Nwabisa's hut I was struck by an odd thought. Just a few years ago Sizwe strolled through young women's homesteads with the confidence of a youthful hunter, his primary thought the prospect of seducing his target from her parents' home. Now he made his way furtively to Nwabisa's hut, his body concealed in a greatcoat and stewing in the heat, his countenance one of splaying humility in the face of a timeless tradition. I was struck by the immense disciplining power of the respectable patriarchy to which Sizwe had attached his worth. It had the power to tame libido, to dampen exuberance, to get a man to sublimate the substance of his being into the pursuit of a distant horizon.

———

YET IF SIZWE was emulating his grandparents inasmuch as he needed to marry, to command a patriarchal homestead, and to have descendants, his identification with them was by no means whole. In some respects, the marriage he was erecting with Nwabisa scorned the men who came before him.

Walking through the river basin at the bottom of Ithanga early that morning, Sizwe began talking of Vuyani, the grandfather whose corpse he believed to have been brained in the morgue.

"That man was crazy for his love potions," he said. "He was always spending a lot of his money on the medicines that make the women want to have sex with you. And then with his medicines in his bag he would go traveling. Even in my time, when he was already old, he would go traveling very far.

"He would leave Ithanga one morning and head south. Days later he would come back from the north. He had slept with so many women. That is why he had five wives. He liked sex too much. And maybe that is why we are poor, why he could not leave us more money—life was too expensive with all of his women."

It is an accusation Sizwe has also made against his father. When the family was slipping into penury, Buyisile's interminable training as a diviner was one reason. Another, according to Sizwe, was his many lovers, and the cost of maintaining them.

"If AIDS had come during your grandparents' generation," I asked, "would it have been worse than now?"

"Yo! So much worse. They all would have been dead. You sit down with an old man, any old man, when he is drunk, and he will tell you that the young generation are *isishumane,* we are scared of girls compared to them."

"You are consciously living your life in the opposite way to your dad and granddad," I said.

"Yes. They needed many women. I need one woman."

"What makes you different to them?"

"Two things," he replied crisply. "The first is AIDS. It has terrified us. My grandparents were lucky to live in those times. They got sick from the sexually transmitted infections, but they were not killed by them. Us, we die.

"The second is education. An educated person does not sleep with everybody and lose his money. He learns to save, to think of the future, to invest in his family. Look at me. If my father and grandfather had thought of the future, maybe I would have had a proper education. Maybe I would be a schoolteacher now."

It was a damning indictment of Vuyani and his generation. On the one hand, they were the real patriarchs, fathers of true descendants, investing their living years in their futures beyond the grave. And yet they squandered their assets and left their progeny destitute because they could not keep their pants zipped. It is the sort of paradox that makes for satire.

By the time we reached the edge of Ithanga it was about 7:30 A.M., and the sun had scaled the tallest of the hills on the village's eastern flank. We passed Simlindile's new spaza shop. It was boarded up and deserted. Sizwe nodded his head at it.

"That one," he said, "he is like the men from my grandfather's time. He will never be successful because he is spending at least half of his time making new children for this village. Look at his place. The sun is up, the people are walking past his shop to get the transport, and he is too tired from all his activities to wake up and open his shop."

YET IN OTHER respects, Sizwe's idea of a marriage was one his forebears would have recognized and approved of. About six weeks before the day we went to visit Nwabisa and her new son, as she entered the eighth month of her pregnancy, the question of maternity leave from her job at the forestry station arose. She had told her employer that she wanted a month's paid leave. He demurred. He said that if she left work for a month, she would not be paid. If she stayed away for more than a month, she would lose her job.

"It does not really matter," Sizwe told me when I asked whether the impasse had been resolved. "We will be married soon, and after we are married she will not work."

He said it so matter-of-factly that I simply took it for granted, and when I saw Nwabisa the following day I asked her casually whether she was looking forward to putting the forestry station behind her.

She looked up in surprise. Momentarily, her brow creased in anger.

"It has not been decided that I am leaving," she said evenly. "It is a difficult decision."

Uncomfortable with the rising tension, I began to talk to her of other things.

When I saw Sizwe the following day he told me that he and Nwabisa had quarreled after I left. We were driving to Nomvalo to see Kate Marrandi. A forty-five-minute car journey lay before us.

"She did not like that I told you it had already been decided she was leaving her job," he said.

"I guess she is worried," I replied. "She has a mother to support, and an eight-year-old son. What if you turn around one day and tell her you will not pay for her child? What will she do if this time next year you are divorced?"

He nodded slowly. "I know. I know that is what she is scared of. But she cannot work after we are married. It is not right."

"Why?"

"There are several reasons." He shifted his weight in the passenger seat and leaned forward uncomfortably. "First, if we are to be married successfully, she needs to spend a lot of time with my parents. They must get to know her very well. And the child must spend a lot of his time in the home of his grandparents, where he is close to his ancestors, where they will come to know him well. If Nwabisa is working, she and the child cannot spend much time there.

"Second, I am earning money, not just for myself, but for the whole family, and for the people she supports. It is for all of us. If she was earning a lot of money it would be one thing, but she is earning very little.

"Third, my parents are not educated people. They do not understand a woman going to work. They understand that a woman stays at home and looks after the home. A man goes out to work. That is what they know.

"She must understand that I am serious about marriage. I am very serious. She has seen too many people get married young and then get divorced. It happens with almost everyone who gets married these days. She must understand that this is different. I am not fooling around. I am now of an age where it is a problem if I am not getting married. I cannot be around my parents' place living with a woman indefinitely. They cannot keep seeing me have one child after another with her when none of these children are their children. I am becoming a respected person. I must get married. The one in Nwabisa's womb will not be my child because we are not yet married. It is the next child, the one who is born first after we are married who will inherit my homestead and my cattle if I have any cattle."

I left Lusikisiki the following day and did not return for about two weeks. Sizwe and I spoke several times on the phone. He told me, among other things, that Nwabisa would not be returning to work after the birth of her child. He said it was a joint decision, and that they were both at peace with it.

I returned to Ithanga on a Sunday. Sizwe's parents had come for lunch. I had brought steaks and boerewors, and Nwabisa fried them in a pan over a gas burner. She did not cook for herself, but saved a piece for later. Nor did she sit with us. She settled in a corner on her own, and took no part in the conversation.

It began to rain heavily while we were eating. We closed the door and spent the afternoon talking and laughing in Sizwe's small room; our voices mingled with the chatter of the rain on the corrugated iron roof. Buyisile, whose mood always set the tone of any occasion, was full of levity and play. The afternoon passed warmly and intimately.

When the rain stopped, Sizwe saw his parents out, leaving Nwabisa and me alone. She was washing dishes in a large, plastic tub. I was sitting at the opposite end of the room.

"Are you relieved that you are not going back to that job?" I asked lightly.

She continued with her washing, her back turned to me.

"Did Sizwe not tell you our agreement?" she asked.

I said nothing.

"He is paying me." She paused, took a dishcloth off her shoulder, began to wipe a plate, and turned to look at me. "The salary I was earning, plus 15 percent. Did he not tell you that?"

I nodded and gave her a colluding smile, one that signaled that I understood the significance of her victory.

She did not return my smile. She turned her back to me and plunged her hands into the dishwater.

THE YOUNG GIRL who had spotted our car outside the Mabaso homestead left us at the front gate. Like thieves, we stole gingerly toward the hut in which Nwabisa had given birth eight days earlier. Sizwe knocked cautiously on the door.

"*Ngena,*" we heard. "Come in."

It was a small, bare room, its only furniture a single bed. Nwabisa was sitting on it, her son cradled in her arms. She looked very tired, but at the sight of Sizwe the weariness in her face quickly gave way to pleasure. She held Sizwe's gaze for a long time, without blinking, and handed him his child. He drew very close to her, scooped his hands under the bundle, and lifted it up to his chest with exaggerated care, as if it were made of fine crystal, as if he did not trust his hands with this burden, his eyes moving quickly between Nwabisa and his son. I excused myself and left them alone.

Some ten minutes later, Nwabisa emerged and told me to join Sizwe inside. I went in to find him sitting on the bed, holding Mfanawetu in his arms, his face both proud and frightened.

Even in here it was hot, and Sizwe had unswaddled his son's blankets, leaving him naked. His body was covered in daubs of clay, which the doctor had said would soothe his rash. The rash itself was dying: it had left red-brown flakes and scabs all over his body.

Sizwe ran a finger uncertainly over a flake on his son's forehead. Then he began picking at it, gently, experimentally. It offered little resistance, peeling off at the lightest touch. Mfanawetu dozed peacefully. Sizwe turned his attention to another scab, then another still. Once he had started, it seemed that he could not stop. He moved from his son's forehead, to his chest, to his arms, working intently, never looking up.

I was fairly sure I knew at least one of the thoughts close to the surface of his mind. Eight months from now, Sizwe, together with seven or eight male relatives on his father's side, would drive four cows from Ithanga to Nwabisa's village. Sizwe would have five thousand rand in his pocket, the value of a fifth cow. A feast would await them at their destination. A goat would be slaughtered and there would be enough *umqombothi* beer for everyone to drink his fill. Sizwe himself would remain on the margins of the event. He would sit quietly in a room with boys and unmarried men. He would not make a showing at the main rondavel.

On the party's return to Ithanga in the evening, Nwabisa would be Sizwe's wife. She would move into her in-laws' home, perhaps for as long as two months, to be trained by her mother-in-law in her wifely duties.

But this was all eight months into the future. Here and now, the couple was unmarried and the child in Sizwe's arms was thus a Mabaso, not a Magadla. To make him a Magadla, Sizwe would have to pay the Mabasos a great deal of money, almost as much as bridewealth itself. A few days ago, I asked Sizwe what he would do.

"He must be a Magadla," he replied emphatically. "I must pay." He paused and frowned, and then sighed deeply. "But it is not as simple as that. It is a lot of money. If the Mabasos promised that they would keep that money for his education, then it would be fine. But they won't do that. So why must I give these people so much money, when the money should be invested in the child? It is hard. I am not sure what to do. Maybe we must wait. Maybe this one's younger sibling will be the first Magadla."

Now I watched him gently picking the flakes off Mfanawetu Mabaso's skin, and I felt quite sure that I knew the decision he would make. To pay for the possession of a first descendant would be greedy, precipitous, self-defeating. One cannot invest in one's own eternity by robbing from the ones who will bring that eternity. This boy would not bear Sizwe's name, but Sizwe would love him and bind himself to him nonetheless, and he would give him the best education he could afford. As for the next generation of Magadlas, there was time, and Sizwe was a patient man.

He had thus begun living the life of a young man who had skirted a plague. Holding his child in his arms, eight days after the little one's birth, the afternoon quiet of his in-laws' homestead about them— these were emblems of a future untouched by AIDS and by the sterility and futurelessness it embodied. He had drawn a line: he himself was on one side, the victims of the epidemic on the other.

And yet he was not prepared to test that assumption. He did not want to know for sure on which side of the line he stood. He would not test for HIV. This image of father and child he now enacted was not one in which he fully believed. It could be snatched from him any-time. It may already have been taken—by a virus in his blood.

From whence did Sizwe's fear come, this fear that at any moment he could be robbed of everything? Sitting next to him on the bed, I knew that I would not have finished writing his story until I under-stood why he would not test for HIV.

Leaving

The next patient to walk into Hermann Reuter's examination room stopped my breath. His eyes were certainly alive: they were large and moist, and they glistened in the room's fluorescent light. But the rest of him seemed borrowed from a corpse. His flesh was all gone, even his cheeks mere sunken hollows. Where he once had round shoulders, his body now ended in the lump-like protuberances of skin-covered bones.

It was his neck, though, that drew me. It was very long and wrist-thin, and it sported a tightly bound, clean white bandage, one that covered only his throat, his Adam's apple disappearing under it every time he swallowed. Momentarily, I was struck by the bizarre thought that his neck dressing was a rude and deliberate aesthetic, as if he was to take his place that night in the chorus of a cabaret of the macabre. Later, I would recall this odd image as the prelude to a series of dark, wounding thoughts.

Hermann looked up from behind his desk, took in the sight of the skeletal man, and smiled cheerfully.

"This woman is very pleased to see you," he said, pointing at my interpreter, whose name was Phumza. "The last five patients were all women. She wanted to know why we don't see any men."

The patient stared at Hermann blankly and began to unbutton his shirt.

"I am coughing," he said in Xhosa, Phumza translating for Hermann. "My throat is very bad. I have an injury on the neck. I was operated on there. Where they operated, my throat is now leaking pus." His voice was strained, his words slurred by a thick and heavy tongue.

"When was the operation?" Hermann asked.

"Three weeks ago."

"Where?"

"Kroonstad. I am in policing college."

"Did they say you had TB?"

"No. I just injured myself."

"You've never had treatment for TB?"

"No."

Watching Hermann hovering over his patient, a sensation began leaking into my body. It brought shame and discomfort, but I resisted the urge to expel it. The man sitting on Hermann's examination table was already dead, a walking corpse: he was no longer one of us. I felt indignant: why is Hermann standing over a dead person? Why is he investing precious time and resources on this corpse when these ought to be spent on the living?

More than aggression, there was triumph in these questions: my insistence on his deadness affirmed the fact that I was alive. I no longer had time for him.

"And here at the clinic," Hermann continued, "have you done the spit test and the blood test?"

"I did the spit test today. The blood test last week."

"And what was the result?"

"Positive."

"What was that?"

"I am HIV-positive."

"Good," Hermann said. "It is good that you can say it like that. You must practice saying it."

He carefully unwound the patient's white bandage and put it down on the examination table.

"There is another problem," the patient said. "Inside the throat. Whenever I swallow."

"Yes, I can see," Hermann replied. "It is the same problem as the outside. The pus is dripping inside, too."

"When I eat rice," the patient said softly, "it comes out the hole."

Hermann raised his eyebrows. "Well then you must go straight to the hospital," he said emphatically. "I thought we'd try with the medicines for a week, but no, I think you must go straight to the hospital.

"How did you get this wound in your throat?" Hermann asked.

"I don't know. I got high on ganja, and then I don't know what happened."

"It looks like a knife," Hermann remarked, almost to himself. "It's a stab wound."

A nurse came in and asked Hermann to help her with a diagnosis. He excused himself, leaving me, Phumza, and the patient to await his return.

Hermann's fan hummed and rattled. Phumza stared at the patient's throat.

"How did you get that wound?" she asked quietly in Xhosa.

He bowed his head and replied softly. "I tried to kill myself."

"When you tested HIV-positive?"

"No. It was before that."

"Then why did you do it?"

He did not reply. She asked again, and he turned his head away.

None of us spoke. The feelings I had toward this man had shamed me and I felt agitated and uncomfortable in my skin. I tried to will a sense of empathy. Instead, a passage came to me, quite unexpectedly, from Isaac Bashevis Singer's childhood memoir. Singer watches a group of mourners walking through the streets of 1920s Warsaw. They are following the coffin of a man named Mordecai Meir. "Their manner," Singer writes, "seems to say: 'Mordecai Meir is Mordecai Meir, and we are we. He's a corpse, but we're alive. He's about to be buried, but we must pay our rent and our children's tuition. We no longer have anything in common.'"

IN THE LATE afternoon, after the last patient of the day had gone, I began to share with Hermann the ugly thoughts I had when I watched him examine the skeletal man. I wanted to tell him that what I had felt was a variant of something universal; that we sniff out death and triumph over the dying in order to validate a deep-set belief that death does not happen to us, only to others. I wanted to ask him how a movement that aims to forge solidarity around the HIV-positive confronts that fact. I began speaking of the feeling that came over me that the patient was already a corpse.

"I am pleased you noticed that," he interrupted breezily. "It is one of the two main causes of stigma. The family sees the patient is getting thinner and thinner and soils his bed and can't eat. They think, He's dead anyway. Why waste our time?"

"And the other main cause of stigma?"

"Money. The patient is a financial burden on the family. 'We don't have sugar because of you. You are killing us all.'

"And the thing is that both these causes of stigma are easily addressed. The financial burden is addressed by the government disability grant. And the other cause of stigma, the one you noticed today, it is taken away by the drugs.

"You saw that man today and you saw death. For me, it is exactly the opposite. He is my favorite kind of patient. I know that in twelve weeks he will be back to his ordinary weight and his skin will look healthy. That is the power of these drugs. And people see that power. There is no hiding in these villages.

"I have only one worry for that man we saw today." He looked at his watch. "It is ten to five. Less than an hour ago, at the hospital, the doctor will have walked through the OPD deciding which patients to admit to the wards for the night. There are a lot of patients, much more than the number of free beds. Maybe the doctor looked at our patient's card and thought, Oh, this is Hermann Reuter's patient from the clinic. We don't have enough space for all these clinic referrals. I'll send him home."

It was indeed as simple as that for Hermann. The problem was never the people, always the state. What was happening in villagers' heads was secondary. What was happening in the health-care system was what really counted. If the drugs were accessible, the treatment good, the clinic lines short, the hospital beds free, people would come, and they would heal. Both their bodies and their minds would heal. Like death, stigma was a function of poor health care.

"From your perspective," I told him, "my book is irrelevant. I am exploring the health-seeking behavior of ordinary people. You're telling me that's worthless."

"Yes," he replied. "Not to discourage you, though."

How CLOSE DID Hermann Reuter and Médecins Sans Frontières come to proving the point that took them to Lusikisiki in the first place? When MSF established its Lusikisiki project, it said it wanted to show that any health system, even the most rickety and dysfunctional, could be made to provide everyone who needed it with antiretroviral treatment. It said that any population, even the people of a remote, poverty-stricken place debilitated by AIDS stigma, would come and get treated.

MSF arrived in Lusikisiki in early 2003. Exactly three years later, it began to meet the most important of its self-imposed measures of success. The best available actuarial model of the rate of the South African AIDS epidemic suggests that between 100 and 110 people fall ill with Stage IV AIDS in Lusikisiki every month. By the end of the first quarter of 2006, about 110 people a month were beginning ARV treatment in Lusikisiki. The rate of treatment had finally caught up with the rate of illness; it was now time to accelerate further and begin catching up with the long backlog.

As for whether patients stayed on treatment, the figures were particularly pleasing to MSF. When the South African government began, belatedly, to roll out a national ARV program in 2004, it did so through hospitals, not clinics. MSF disagreed. The South African AIDS epidemic was too extensive, shortages of medical personnel too severe, to restrict treatment to hospitals, the organization said. Programs would quickly bottleneck. The ill would either die waiting, or they would not even bother to come.

Besides, MSF argued, patients were far more likely to adhere to treatment at a clinic than at a hospital. The average hospital patient has come from some distance away, usually at great expense. She is counseled and briefed, she is given a supply of pills that she slips into her bag, and then she vanishes. The personnel who treated her hope to God that she takes her pills and comes back the following month.

But if you roll out through the clinics, the patient lives perhaps five hundred yards from the nearest community health worker, perhaps a mile or two from the head nurse. Everyone knows her name. If she does not turn up for her next batch of pills, clinic layworkers will find her.

And so it proved in Lusikisiki. At the HIV unit in Saint Elizabeth's Hospital in the center of town, 17 percent of patients had been lost to follow-up by early 2006. In Lusikisiki's twelve clinics, the figure was 2 percent. Both in getting people on treatment and in keeping them there, the clinics were clearly the superior of the two institutions.

Only the churlish could deny that MSF's achievements were considerable. More than half the nursing posts at Lusikisiki clinics remained vacant. Aside from Hermann and an MSF colleague, no doctor had set foot in a Lusikisiki clinic in years. And yet 110 people a month were signing up to treatment and most were coming back. It seemed a vindication of MSF's vision at its most idealistic.

To HERALD THE program as an unmitigated success, however, would be very hasty indeed. The system may have been absorbing 110 new patients a month, but it was groaning under the strain. The sight of the lines outside the clinics in the morning took one's breath away. The daily workload of clinic nurses had more than doubled since MSF came to town. The beds in the hospital were full, with critically ill patients being sent home to die.

MSF was scheduled to hand the ARV program over to the Eastern Cape Health Department in October 2006. The real test would come after the organization's departure. They had said that ordinary, overworked nurses could put people on ARVs across the country. If a solitary program in Eastern Cape failed the moment it was left to itself, the organization would have failed spectacularly.

The truth is that by mid-2006, nobody could say for sure what would happen to the program after MSF left. The nongovernmental organization had wanted to show the South African government that investing in clinics as well as hospitals was the only way to treat the casualties of the AIDS epidemic. And yet it was precisely government's underinvestment in clinics that posed the gravest threat to the program after MSF's departure. In district after district, hospitals, not clinics, were being accredited to administer antiretroviral treatment. And since it was the accredited site that courted the lion's share of new resources and posts, the clinics became AIDS medicine's stepchildren.

The Lusikisiki clinics were victims of this syndrome. Not only were they more than 50 percent understaffed, they had not advertised a single vacant nurse's post during MSF's last year in Lusikisiki. A Lusikisiki nurse looking for a promotion would have to leave the district and go elsewhere, probably to a hospital. It was quite conceivable that the entire cohort of nurses Hermann Reuter had trained in AIDS medicine would soon disperse to all corners of Eastern Cape.

That was just the first of several worries. Another concerned the management of the program. The primary health-care district under which Lusikisiki fell was run exclusively by former nurses. The South African nursing profession has been referred to as a "feminized military." Professional nurses take instruction from chief professional nurses. Chief professional nurses do nothing without the say-so of a doctor.

And yet there were no doctors in Eastern Cape primary health-care districts. And so if the nursing profession is indeed a militarized hierarchy, in Lusikisiki it ended at the rank of lance corporal. The district manager seldom acted without instructions from above, especially in the political minefield of AIDS medicine.

It was impossible to say how the nurses who ran the system would cope without Hermann Reuter. They were exasperated by him, at times they resented him, but he brought a flexibility and capacity to solve problems for which they were grateful. MSF was donating its two vehicles to the district, but would their licenses be renewed every year, and would they keep getting gasoline? At some point, patients would begin developing resistance to their drugs and would have to go on to second-line treatment. Would managers develop a sound treatment protocol, and would they disseminate it across the district? Or would they instead wait for an instruction that never comes? These were some of the known uncertainties. There would be many others nobody had thought of.

Then there was the fate of the young laypeople and activists Hermann had distributed into the clinic system on MSF salaries. There can be little doubt that their work had animated the ARV program. When MSF set up camp in Lusikisiki, the two gravest problems in the clinics were drug supplies and staff shortages. It was the young men and women Hermann recruited as pharmacist assistants who brought the drugs flowing to town, bombarding the Mthatha medicine depot with volleys of calls and demands, clearing blockages between the local drug reception center and the clinics, and monitoring nurses' supply requests for signs of logistical errors.

As for nurse staffing shortages, it was the adherence counselors Hermann had recruited who made it possible for nurses to withstand the workload the ARV program had placed on them. They were the ones who took each new patient on the long, time-sapping journey from testing to treatment, who monitored adherence and followed up on those who did not return to the clinics to replenish their pills, who collected and analyzed each clinic's growing archive of patient data.

What would become of them after MSF left was uncertain. The local district did not have money to pay their salaries. MSF formed a new nongovernmental organization to support the work of the adherence counselors, but with limited funding that the new organization itself would soon have to replace. As for the assistant pharmacists, the provincial government said it would consider paying their salaries from a special fund, but nothing was certain.

Yet even if they did remain, their futures in the clinic system were insecure. If the nursing profession is indeed a quasi-military hierarchy, young and assertive laypeople have no place in it. Their assertiveness offends. While Hermann was around, they did their work under his authority. Nurses did not dare throw them out of their clinics, for if they did, they would have to answer to Dr. Hermann. With Dr. Hermann gone, the laypeople would have to fend for themselves. And if nurses obstructed their work, it would not take much for them to pack their bags and leave; Hermann had trained them well, they had transferable skills now, and so they could move to more satisfying jobs.

MSF's rebuttal to this unhappy prognosis was both simple and expected: the people, the ARV users themselves. The activists Hermann placed in the system were merely the vanguard of a phalanx, MSF argued, a 2,200-strong phalanx of ordinary Lusikisiki residents whose lives were saved by the drugs, and who would fight to keep them coming. That, indeed, was the article of faith animating the entire treatment movement that had grown out of South Africa's AIDS epidemic: that as bearers of the rights to life and to bodily health, ordinary citizens would force their health-care system, with all its decrepitude and its lethargy, to deliver.

Whether they were right I truly did not know. Hermann had told me jokingly that the book I was writing about Sizwe was irrelevant. And yet when I spoke to him about my travels with Sizwe, it sometimes seemed that I was bringing him news from another planet, that Hermann himself lived in a charmed circle of activists and converts. Out in Sizwe's world it was not clear at all that people would fight for ARVs. And my own reactions in the presence of the ill, such as the man with the neck bandage whom I had estranged with a force that shook me, had given me an inkling of why creating solidarity in the face of this epidemic is not a simple task.

I WOULD BE doing Hermann Reuter himself an injustice if I did not press home the fact that even while MSF was in Lusikisiki, with all its will and its efficiency, with its proud claim of 110 new ARV users every month, people died horrible deaths every single day because the clinics were under-resourced, the hospital beds full, the medicine inferior.

In late 2006, shortly before he left Lusikisiki, Hermann witnessed one of those deaths in the rawest and most brutal circumstances.

He had gone to one of Lusikisiki's remoter clinics, Bodweni, with Mrs. Sapepa, the manager in charge of HIV treatment in the district, for a supervision visit.

"There was no nurse when we arrived," Hermann told me a few days later. "There is one professional nurse in that clinic who moonlights, and she was on leave. The assistant nurse was on a training course. The counselors had kept four or five of the patients who'd turned up that day because they knew there would be a supervision visit with a doctor.

"When we walked out to leave, there was a family waiting outside. They had heard a doctor was in the area. Could we visit the daughter? She was very sick and could not speak anymore. It was raining hard, but we went anyway.

"I looked at her, and she was very, very sick. She looked to have TB. I picked her up, put her in the car. There was also another patient I had agreed to transport to the hospital. She was psychotic. We had a small car, a Toyota Tazz. In the front seat was me and Mrs. Sapepa. In the backseat was a psychotic patient with her mother, and a dying patient with her mother.

"As we were about to drive off, an argument started among the woman's family. Should they actually take her to the hospital? She will probably die, and if the patient dies in hospital, the undertakers charge a lot of money for fetching the corpse, and they don't have money.

"There were negotiations for about half an hour. I was the doctor: I took the position of, you know, if we can help we should try. I was also uncomfortable about having the conversation in front of this person. She was probably still hearing: that is the last of the senses still functioning in a dying person. In the end, the family decided to trust the doctor and take her to hospital.

"When we arrived at the hospital, she was dead. She had died in her mother's arms in the backseat. So we unloaded the psychotic patient and took the dead patient to the mortuary so that the family would not have to pay for that: me and Mrs. Sapepa in the front, the dead woman and her mother at the back."

It was late at night when Hermann told me this story. We were conducting the interview in his bedroom. My Dictaphone lay on his bed between us. The noise of a DVD, which his housemates were watching in the lounge, joined us in spasms.

"So, ja," he continued, "they say eight hundred people die of AIDS in South Africa every day. That was the one I experienced. You know, I looked at the clinic card . . ." He meant to interrupt himself with a giggle, but what came out was a hollow snort, a mixture of sadness and disgust.

"What was on the clinic card?" I asked.

He stared at my Dictaphone. "You know . . . Ja, um, she had been to the hospital twice that week. Discharged both times. I told Dr. Thomas, the hospital superintendent, about it. I got so sad telling the story and he was getting sad also. He said every day he sees people discharged from the hospital who cannot walk home, going home on a stretcher. He said the hospital doesn't have beds, and you cannot keep people with a poor prognosis. But it's still sad when you see people with HIV considered people with a poor prognosis, especially when their problems were treatable and no proper diagnosis was done."

He paused for a long time and stared past me. "One can hardly blame Dr. Thomas," he finally said. "If the government were investing in its clinics, that woman would not have had to go to the hospital in the first place. She should have been treated at the clinic because there should have been a drip and an x-ray machine at the clinic. If she had lived in Cape Town she would never even have gone to a hospital. Think of the Bodweni clinic you know: a queue around the building in the mornings. Half a nurse running the show. Think of Bodweni with polished floors, a computer at the front desk to clock your patients in, pot plants. If that's what Bodweni clinic looked like . . ." He waved his hand dismissively and fell silent.

Good-Bye,
Dr. Hermann

In June 2006, some four months before Médecins Sans Frontières's scheduled departure, the National Health Department in Pretoria began to enforce, without warning, a rule barring nurses around the country from prescribing ARVs. They had always been Schedule Five drugs, prescribable only by doctors, but until now the stipulation had not been enforced.

It was a crushing blow for the Lusikisiki program. Nurse-initiated treatment at clinics, rather than doctor-initiated treatment at hospitals, lay at the very heart of MSF doctrine. Nurses at all twelve Lusikisiki clinics had been initiating patients onto ARV treatment since the earliest days of the program. Hermann was leaving in four months, and no other doctor came to the clinics. The national instruction threatened to end ARV treatment in Lusikisiki in one fell swoop.

Hermann was incensed. "It is a definite attempt to block access to treatment," he told me. "It is always convenient to say there is a law stopping this, but, I mean, last year there was a new pharmacy law that was supposed to come into effect in June saying only hospitals and clinics with dispensing licenses can dispense any drugs at all. Ten days before the new law was passed, the director-general of health issued a memorandum saying that in the government sector we will not penalize nurses who prescribe. So here is a postapartheid law that can be ignored, and yet this old apartheid law is suddenly so important. This is a way of blocking access to drugs, of putting a bottleneck in the system."

After a relay of meetings between the local district and the provincial health department, two doctor's posts were advertised for the Lusikisiki clinics. It would be the first time in its history that the Lusikisiki primary health-care subdistrict would employ doctors at all, and it would save the ARV program.

The posts were filled in the late winter of 2006, one by a Congolese doctor, another by a local man. Hermann began to withdraw from the clinics. The two new doctors took his place. For patients and staff, the change was a rude awakening to how spoiled they had been. Instead of Hermann's sixteen-hour-a-day dedication, they were confronted by two ordinary work-to-rule doctors both new to ARV medicine. They sometimes arrived late, sometimes left early. They made mistakes. When a drug was out of stock, they did not give the head nurse a mouthful; they shrugged.

At the clinic support group meetings I attended during that period, ARV users complained volubly. They were getting their first taste of ordinary, state-delivered medicine, and they didn't like it at all.

"I'm lucky I started treatment while Dr. Hermann was still here," a woman remarked casually. "There were complications. I had peripheral neuropathy. If it had been during Dr. Freddie's time, I would have died."

No sooner had the two doctors arrived than both left, one after the other, the first at the end of September, the second at the end of October. The problem was simple. The posts the district had made available were Grade 10, the lowest grade for a doctor in the state sector. Both new recruits began looking for better posts the moment they arrived, and with doctors in short supply all around the country, neither had to look very hard. The Grade 11 posts they found were, of course, at hospitals, not clinics. After they left, both their posts remained vacant. Once again it was the government's underinvestment in clinics, the heart of MSF's complaint, that threatened the future of MSF's own project.

Lusikisiki's district management approached the superintendent of Saint Elizabeth's Hospital, Dr. Thomas, cap in hand. They asked him whether he would lend them his ward doctors. It was not a light request. Of the twenty-four doctor's posts at the hospital, only nine were filled. But Hermann had built a good relationship with Dr. Thomas over the past three and a half years, providing the hospital with ARVs before it was accredited to receive them, for instance. And Dr. Thomas obliged. Doctors from the hospital would visit two clinics once a week, and another five clinics once a month.

It was hardly ideal. The founding principle of the program was decentralization to the lowest level, ARV drugs within walking distance of everyone's home. Now some clinics would have to begin referring patients to other clinics. Bottlenecks would develop, waiting lists grow, despondent patients explore other remedies.

I met during this time with Mrs. Sapepa, the manager in charge of HIV treatment in the district, the one who had been in the car with Hermann when the young woman died in the backseat.

"Don't you feel sorry for us here?" she asked. "Aren't we pathetic? We can't run this place without doctors. What if the ones Dr. Thomas releases to the clinic are stubborn or lazy doctors? What if they are not cooperative? Then what do we do?"

In October 2006, the month MSF left Lusikisiki, the clinics put fifty-three new patients onto ARV treatment. The monthly intake of the first quarter of the year had halved. It seemed the program might die an unceremonious death.

"Why does government continually underinvest in its clinics?" I asked Hermann shortly before he left Lusikisiki. "It is not wickedness or evil. It is surely a blind spot."

"Why did the Israelites spend forty years in the desert?" he replied. "Doesn't that story strike you as odd? You read the Bible and you just take it for granted—oh, the story says forty years in the desert. But why didn't they just leave? Nobody told them to stay in the desert. It was a mental block.

"Same with our health administrators. They have a mental block. They think if you put resources in the clinics they will not be used."

"Because?"

"Because they don't trust that nurses can do anything proper. Because our health managers come from a hospital-based system. They see a mess at the hospital, they say that is what we must fix."

"What produced that prejudice?"

"There is this thing that health care must need technology. There must be an x-ray. There must be machines and specialists, otherwise it is not proper medicine."

"And that's when paranoia about African inferiority comes into play," I said. "Health administrators say to themselves: In Europe they would never have laypeople and nurses dishing out these drugs from prefabricated buildings in villages. They would have proper doctors."

"You do not need doctors for this," Hermann said, repeating his oldest mantra. "You don't even need nurses."

———————————

ON THE MORNING of October 12, 2006, a crowd of some two thousand people gathered in a community hall on the grounds of the Eastern Cape Department of Health's offices in Lusikisiki. The vast ceiling of the building had been draped in red and white cloth, and a deejay pumped music from outlandishly large speakers. Outside the building, a motley collection of the town's street vendors had set up shop, selling everything from goat meat to bananas. The billing of the event had been filtered through the fraught and sensitive politics of the provincial health department, and MSF was barely mentioned in the program. Instead, the posters invited all and sundry to join the government in celebrating eight years of partnerships with NGOs in the fight against HIV. Among the list of advertised speakers was "Dr. Herman, MSF—an example of a partnership."

Various visiting dignitaries and local figures spoke—the provincial health minister, the chief director of HIV/AIDS in the province, a founding member of the Lusikisiki branch of the Treatment Action Campaign. Then the master of ceremonies called Hermann Reuter to speak, and before he could get to the podium some two dozen young people materialized from the crowd, beaming and giggling, and made for his chair. They surrounded him, obscuring him from view, a swarm of benign and hungry bees launching on their honeycomb. When he finally emerged he was dressed in traditional Mpondo garb, a kerchief around his head, baggy, multicolored trousers, a white cape of raw cotton with the word HERMAN hand-stitched across it in red thread. It was a fine honor indeed to bestow upon a white man.

The ones who had outfitted him now led him to a raised platform below the stage where he was joined by a troupe of Mpondo dancers. The deejay turned up the volume until the music drowned even the roar of the large crowd, and the dancers danced around Hermann in a frenetic rhythm, their arms and shoulders glistening with sweat. Suddenly they all came to a standstill, turned their backs, and jumped off the platform, leaving Hermann alone. Now the crowd was louder than the music; they were calling for him to dance. His face reddened with embarrassment. He took two or three uncertain steps, then fled to the stage to deliver his speech.

Amid the crowd, I spotted Kate Marrandi. I waved to her, my arms stretched above my head, and I finally caught her eye. Opening her face into the broadest of smiles, she raised a clenched fist into the air, threw her head back, and laughed without inhibition. There and then, she seemed to me an emblem of that moment, of all the people in that hall. They had come to pay tribute to a man they had grown to love, a man who had come among them to fight like a single-minded maniac against death.

At the VIP luncheon after the event, held in an enormous tent outside the hall, I caught a glimpse of Hermann in earnest conversation with the district health manager, a woman with whom he had fought bitterly for nearly four years. That was the last time I laid eyes on him. He had fallen in love with an MSF colleague from Ethiopia; come November, he was going to get into his car and drive north, arriving in Addis Ababa in January, just in time for his wedding.

New Year

I returned to Lusikisiki two weeks before Christmas. It has an odd feel about it at that time of year. It is at once fuller and quieter than usual, fuller because thousands of migrant workers have returned home for Christmas, quieter because fewer people are at work. As one moves from place to place the air seems to hum.

I had set up appointments with about a dozen people, all of them in the health-care system, about half of them adherence counselors, pharmacist assistants, TAC activists—Hermann Reuter's people.

Just before he left South Africa, Hermann had attended a national workshop on AIDS medicine in rural settings. At that workshop, the chief director of the HIV programs in Eastern Cape, Nomalanga Makwedini, who had invited MSF to the province and had been the Lusikisiki program's staunchest supporter, announced that she would countermand the national instruction prohibiting nurses from prescribing ARVs. Where nurses had been initiating treatment successfully, she said, they would continue to do so.

Now, two months later, I arrived in Lusikisiki to discover that nurses were still not initiating treatment. Mrs. Makwedini, I was told, had not come to town to instruct nurses in person to resume initiation, and the district health manager would never carry out a decision like that on her own.

"But senior personnel from the district were in the meeting when

Mrs. Makwedini announced that nurse-initiated treatment would resume," I said.

"Yes, but the district manager needs Mrs. Makwedini to come and say it here."

"When is she coming?"

"I don't know."

"Why can't she just write the instruction in a memo?"

"I don't know."

When I spoke to one of the senior district officials who ran the HIV program, it was clear that she had long ago resigned herself to a world in which nurses no longer prescribed ARVs. Indeed, she had talked herself into believing that it was right.

"You know," she told me, "I don't want to put nurses down, they do a great job, but the truth is that there are even opportunistic infections they have been misdiagnosing. So maybe they must be patient with ARVs. Maybe they must first go on a course, a long and thorough course, on antiretroviral medicine. We must stress quality: quality before numbers."

This was the manager whose job it was to support the work of her medical personnel. If the nurses who ran Lusikisiki's clinics had been listening in on our conversation, I wonder whether they would have bothered ever to treat a case of AIDS again.

It seemed to me that a prophecy from on high was in the process of fulfilling itself. Pretoria sent down an instruction saying nurses were not up to the task of treating AIDS. They were taken off the job, and it was not long before their managers told themselves that they were indeed not up to the work, that they never had been. And so, almost overnight, Lusikisiki threatened to fall backward through time and settle once again into the first quarter of 2003, when nurses were indeed incapable of treating AIDS. I wondered whether it was possible that the reservoirs of self-belief in this place were really that shallow. An image came to me of the Lusikisiki ARV program as a giant hot-air balloon, its furnace coaxed and fed and nurtured until the colossus finally took to the air, only for a pinprick to penetrate its fragile skin and bring it down to the ground.

―――――――――

THE ASSISTANT PHARMACISTS and adherence counselors I spoke to were despondent. They told one gloomy story after another. An adherence counselor had been forced to surrender the room he had always used to prepare patients for treatment. "This is a government clinic," he was apparently told, "and you are not a government employee. We don't have space for you."

The previous week, I was told, a patient arrived at a clinic near town a week before she was due to receive her new batch of ARVs. She did so because she was suffering from chronic headaches. The nurse who received her warned that if she ever came to the clinic again outside her monthly appointment, she would be taken off ARVs and left to get sick and die.

And, to complete the picture, another horror story, also from one of the MSF-trained laypeople. When she arrived at work the Monday morning after Hermann left, she said, the nurse at her clinic took her aside and had a quiet word in her ear.

"I have been waiting to tell you this for a long time," the nurse reportedly said. "And now that your Dr. Hermann is gone, my tongue is free. You are not welcome in this clinic. You have *toyi-toyi* [a militant dance crowds performed during the uprisings against apartheid] on the mind. You are here only to make trouble. And you have been influenced by that white man. He was a bad influence. He was pushing black people to work like slaves. I am nobody's slave."

I did not doubt that any of these stories were true. But I wondered about the tone and the spirit in which they were uttered. The young laypeople Hermann Reuter had trained in Lusikisiki were perhaps his finest accomplishment. Meeting them one after the other, I was struck by how well he had chosen: each of them ingenious and clever, each overflowing with will. Before they met him, their futures had been deeply uncertain. They lived in a place with few jobs, and they were not sufficiently educated to find good work in South Africa's cities. Hermann had changed their lives. He had lent them his powerful moral purpose, and had trained them in invaluable skills. Above all, he had shown them the art of the possible; it was their collective agency that had resurrected their district's health-care system, and they knew it.

But listening to them now, I began to wonder. Many referred to Hermann, from time to time, as the father of Lusikisiki's treatment program, and it seemed now that they were not so much agents of the possible as abandoned children. Perhaps, I thought, they had taken nothing from Hermann after all; perhaps they had only borrowed. With him gone, they were once again the sons and daughters of Transkei peasants, fated forever to be on history's receiving end. They were the Israelites wandering the Sinai, their Moses lost to them.

Perhaps that is unfair, I thought. Hermann has only been gone two months. They are in shock. When I return next year, they will have found their feet once more. But as things stood, the story they conjured rendered them helpless bystanders in the face of an immovable drama. The image they painted of the health system was that of a wretched monster. Hermann had force-fed it an ARV program, and it had churned the thing around in its great mouth while he was there to watch. The moment he turned his back, it spat his food out.

And each nurse, in this story, was a monster writ small, a personification of the beast itself. It seemed to me, as I drove away from Lusikisiki, that from the district officials to the adherence counselors, each had her own story of the program's decline, and the nurses were the demon of every tale. They had become the repositories of everybody's sense of failure.

I STAYED AWAY from Lusikisiki for a full six weeks, speaking to few people there, save Sizwe, for whom the fate of the program was a matter of concern somewhere on the periphery of his life.

I returned in the first week of February. It was apparent from the moment of my arrival that something was different. My first meeting was with Bavuyise Vimbani, the head of the new organization of adherence counselors. There was a lightness in his step as he moved about his office, a palpable sense of relief in his voice.

"What is it?" I asked.

He smiled at me quietly over the top of his monitor. "I've just calculated January's uptake figures," he said. "Between the hospital and the clinics, we put more than a hundred new people on ARVs."

"How?"

"Ah," he sighed. "That is a long story."

It is also a story that is difficult for me to tell. For it involves a range of people across Lusikisiki's health system breaking innumerable rules. In my last interview with Hermann before he left, I asked him what would have to happen, at a minimum, for the program to keep flourishing after MSF's departure.

"Nurses need to find ways to quietly keep doing what they did before the order came for them to stop initiating," he replied. "They need to cheat. No, *cheat* is the wrong word, but nurses need to find a way to get their folders to doctors to sign for them. Nurses don't want people to die, and they see that if ARVs aren't initiated, people die.

"Whether they will be allowed to cheat depends on the district management. If our district management has enough backbone and says we will find proxy ways of people initiating treatment, I don't foresee a problem. If they start acting as a policeman and start threatening nurses and demotivating nurses, and saying you are not allowed to do it, you don't have a doctor anymore, you must stop, there will be big problems."

I do not know whether district management turned a blind eye, or whether they just didn't know; they denied it vociferously when I tentatively raised it. But by January 2007 a system of small-scale cheating had instituted itself in pockets across the district. It always emerged from particular relationships between individuals. Doctor X, who saw clinic patients every week, would develop an understanding with Nurse Y. In the straightforward cases, the ones she'd been handling with confidence since the beginning of the program, she'd give the doctor the folder, not the patient. When confronted with cases that stretched her, the sort of cases she once referred to Hermann, she would send both folder and patient to the doctor.

And so a host of invisible pathways opened up between the clinics never visited by a doctor and the clinics the doctors staffed every week. Sometimes these pathways conveyed folders, sometimes patients; the logic of the system was fluid, established and reestablished by relays of trial and error.

Often, though, the initiator of the new relationship was neither the doctor nor the nurse, but one of the laypeople. "I went to the head nurse," an adherence counselor told me, "and I said you either get these folders to Doctor X or we throw the folders away because the people they belong to will soon be dead. Do it. Doctor X is a good man. He does not want people to die, either."

When I had visited before Christmas, I saw now, I had come to a place in a state of shock. The shock was receding. In the sobriety of the new year, people were feeling their agency return to them, they were beginning to act.

It was, in a sense, the most gratifying of my trips to Lusikisiki, and the more I learned, the more curious I became. I wanted to know more about how these informal networks of understanding worked, who knew, who didn't know, who didn't want to know. But few people were prepared to say much. I was here to write things down, and this was about rule breaking; I was not the sort of person with whom a prudent rule breaker is candid.

I should not exaggerate. The program's future remained fragile, its present a far cry from perfect: awful stories still abounded. There is, for instance, a particularly remote clinic, some twenty-five miles from town, its roads in poor condition, its surrounding population dirt-poor, even by the district's standards. On the day in January its batch of ARVs were meant to travel, there was heavy rain, and the district's transportation department refused to use any of its vehicles. Three months earlier, MSF would have averted the problem. They would have taken the drugs in one of their vehicles, or hired one, or made another plan, but ARVs would never, ever be delivered late: they were sacrosanct.

When the head nurse at the clinic responsible for dispatching the drugs heard the news, she shrugged and went back to work.

"We must make a plan," an adherence counselor told her.

"The patients can make a plan," she replied. "They can come to town to collect their pills."

"They are too poor to come to town. They can't afford it."

"And what do they think is more expensive," the nurse retorted sharply, "a trip to town, or a funeral?"

And so the vehicle never left town, and a batch of ARV users out in the sticks defaulted on their treatment.

There were other awful stories. Clinics would not pay attention to their inventories and thus fail to order new stock in time, sometimes leaving gravely ill patients without drugs. Or a pharmacist would notice that nurses were not increasing the dosages of drugs when their patients gained weight, rendering their drug intake dangerously out of kilter. When she raised the alarm, she was told to mind her own business. The system had lost its center of authority, it was clearly suffering for it, and the price would be paid in ill health, in death, and, no doubt, in the emergence of drug resistance among some of Lusikisiki's ARV users.

Nor was the future of the program certain. An American NGO, University Research Corporation, had just arrived in town to fill some of the gaps left by MSF's departure. They were to pay the salaries of two pharmacist assistants and two senior nurses. The nurses were to form mobile units, supervising and supporting their colleagues' work at clinics across the district. The two doctor's posts were being advertised again, and the new NGO was to subsidize their salaries to make them equivalent to Grade 11, thus keeping incumbents in their jobs. The clinics would soon stop borrowing doctors from the hospital.

In eighteen months or so, University Research Corporation would pull out, too. Like MSF, its task was to facilitate the building of a sustainable health-care service, rather than become a crutch for an inadequate service—and it was impossible to say whether the district would have sufficient budget by then to fill the gaps they left. So it could be that fatal systemic weaknesses were merely being masked for a while.

Nonetheless, the spirit that began trickling through the system in January 2007 without doubt represented a moment of redemption. If the clinics had indeed spat out the ARV program as a foreign, undigestible object, the only tale to tell would have been macabre beyond the saying of it. It would have been the story of an institution and its people so lacking in self-belief as to be unable to maintain a lifesaving machinery. It would have been a tale of collective resignation in the face of mass death, the protagonists telling uglier and uglier stories about one another as they stewed in their sense of failure. Instead, a myriad scattered people were coming together quite organically in a quest to give the gravely ill the medicine that was their rightful due.

WHEN I RETURNED to Johannesburg, I was tempted to write to Hermann in Addis Ababa to give him the news of the January figures. I resisted the impulse. Nobody in Lusikisiki had heard from him since his departure the previous October. I do not know whether he had found a discreet channel of information, but he had clearly deemed it best, both for himself and the program, to absent himself entirely. If he wanted news, he knew where to find it.

As time passed, my perspective on his work shifted a little. I had kept my head down and told a narrow story, the tale of one ARV program in one rural town. As I write now, in February 2007, more than a quarter of a million people have started ARV treatment at public health-care institutions in South Africa. That is hundreds and thousands of people short of the target, a shortfall measured in death on an unspeakable scale. But it nonetheless represents a great deal of work. I have told a story about 2,200 ARV users. Where does their story fit in with the other two hundred fifty thousand? In the absence of any clarity of purpose from the central government, in the context of failing drug supplies, chronic nurse shortages, and local managers congenitally incapable of self-assertion, who put a quarter of a million people on ARVs?

In late 2005, when around eighty thousand people were on treatment at South African government facilities, the public health systems scholar Helen Schneider wrote a paper that asked similar questions. She noted that growth in the numbers of people on ARV treatment was unevenly distributed across government-accredited ARV sites. The areas doing well were those where "HIV care initiatives had existed prior to the start of the formal rollout. These sites emerged spontaneously across the country in response to falling drug prices from 2001 onwards."

In other words, where people were getting drugs it was in spite of national government; it was because the hope inspired by the availability of treatment had quite spontaneously given birth to pockets of will across the country. Sometimes it was large, rich NGOs that went to work, sometimes local community-based organizations with a few cents to rub together, sometimes just a charismatic manager in the government health system itself. But every case was animated by local people mustering ingenuity. By force of will, people learned to cheat a little, as Hermann put it, learning which corners of the health system were dead and useless and thus ought to be skirted, which corners were alive and ought to be milked for all they were worth.

The MSF program in Lusikisiki is perhaps best understood as just one of these innumerable instances of localized will. It took the form of a famous NGO, a charismatic project leader with a budget to pay three dozen salaries, a voice loud enough to attract people like me to come to write and record. Most of the other instances are quieter, more modest, less successful. But together they represent two hundred fifty thousand people and counting.

In a remote place in the Transkei called Madwaleni, I met a doctor and a lawyer, Richard Cooke and Lynne Wilkinson, who left their lives in Cape Town and took up government jobs at a forlorn district hospital. When they arrived, it had five doctors on its staff, a quarter of a million people in its catchment area. Within two years they had an

ARV treatment program up and running, not only at the hospital, but also at surrounding clinics. When I met them, their program had put six hundred people on ARVs. They had little outside money, just a massive quotient of determination and ingenuity.

Perhaps, in the end, that was Hermann's gift to Lusikisiki. After MSF had gone, what was left was a network of people who had come to see, through the potency of their own deeds, that the horizon of the possible stretched further than they had ever imagined.

MSF's PROJECT IN South Africa was to show the government that universal ARV treatment is most likely to be achieved when the service is as decentralized as it possibly can be; when treatment is available at each of the country's roughly three thousand clinics; and that one does not need a doctor at every one of these sites, nor even a nurse, to succeed.

Hermann Reuter believed that the government would eventually offer a universal service under the force of popular pressure.

"All these people on drugs," he told me, "their relatives all see that their lives have been saved, the word spreads. Soon millions of people know. They start coming for treatment. The hospitals are too full so government starts using the clinics under the sheer force of the pressure. One day the drugs are in every clinic in the country."

I was not so sure. What I saw in Nomvalo and Ithanga told me that the mass, unequivocal embrace of the drugs Hermann envisions would never come, that by its very nature, a mass outbreak of dying does not yield crispness of action, still less unalloyed solidarity. My time with Sizwe had shown me that in spades.

And yet a few months after Hermann left Lusikisiki, the prospects for his prophecy unexpectedly rose. South Africa's health minister, the living symbol of the government's ambivalence toward antiretroviral medicine, fell very ill. As she lay in the intensive care unit of a private hospital, her deputy secretly met with Zackie Achmat, the pioneer of the South African social movement that had arisen to demand AIDS treatment. President Thabo Mbeki, embroiled in and weakened by a bitter succession race for the leadership of his party, remained silent. A momentous change was quietly slipping in under the radar. In March 2007, the government announced a new plan to combat HIV/AIDS.

Among its goals was to bring treatment to three-quarters of those who need it, by 2011. By then, the plan envisaged, 70 percent of people beginning treatment would do so with nurses in clinics, not doctors in hospitals.

I read these words in a newspaper report at dawn on a February morning in my apartment in Johannesburg. I rubbed the sleep from my eyes and read the words again. Nurse-led treatment at clinics: what MSF had fought and scrapped and screamed for now stood casually on the page of a health department press statement, as if it were the most natural idea in the world. That it was now in the heartland of government policy was a direct result of MSF's Lusikisiki project.

And so, finally, very late in the day, MSF's view of matters was reflected in the South African government's most important policy document on the epidemic. Whether this commitment would be momentary or lasting was an open question. So too was whether the country's health-care system would prove capable of delivering the service envisioned in the policy document. And whether Sizwe and thousands like him across the country would come forward to test—that was also an open question.

"Sizwe Magadla"

On the first Monday of April 2007 I boarded a dawn flight from Johannesburg to Mthatha. An hour and a half later, the plane sank gently into the morning fog and deposited its twelve or so passengers in the old Transkei capital's miserable little airport terminal. I hired a car and began the ninety-mile drive to Lusikisiki. Making my way through Mthatha's rush-hour thicket of schoolchildren and minibus taxis and those outlandishly long 1970s-era Mercedes-Benzes one seems to find only in the old Transkei, the mist lifted off my windshield and evaporated into a clearing sky. By the time I hit the coastal road from Port Saint Johns to Lusikisiki I was driving through a crisp autumn day.

I met up with Sizwe outside the Metro Cash & Carry warehouse store on Lusikisiki's main street. For the rest of the morning and through to the early afternoon, I followed in his trail as he went about his business. Then I drove him home to Ithanga, my car filled to the brim with supplies for his shop.

I had phoned him a few days earlier to tell him of my intention to come, and to ask whether he had a morning and an afternoon to spare for me. He said that he did. He did not ask why I was coming. He regarded such inquiries, I had learned by now, as rude. It is for a person to tell you in his own time the reason for his journey and the nature of his business.

I had come because I could not finish writing my book. I had resisted making this journey for some time, trying to shape the closing chapters with the material I had. It was futile.

I had arrived in Lusikisiki in the first week of October 2005 and met a man too afraid to test for HIV. Nineteen months later, pretty much to the day, he was in the same position, too afraid to test, and despite some progress I had made in understanding his world, he still had not revealed to me, and perhaps not to himself, either, the deeper sources of his fear. I had come in the hope that he would take me to a place inside him he had not shown me before.

FROM THE VERY beginning of this project, I knew in the back of my mind that my own experience of AIDS prefigured Sizwe's in ways that were astoundingly obvious. I noted this idly, in the way one registers the humming of an electrical appliance or a singing cricket: something that is just there, something that deserves no attention. And yet, as I struggled to finish this book, so I began, with some reluctance at first, to give the connection its due. As I did so, I started to notice, with some alarm and embarrassment, that the crickets had been singing very loudly all the while, that their noise was indeed so deafening I could barely hear myself think. They were singing about a portion of my own history that I had long ago chosen to forget. It was the history of my testing for HIV, and it was deeply troubled.

Over the following weeks, events from my past began gradually to return to me, not so much in increments as in deeper sweeps of emotion. The more I permitted myself to remember, the more difficult and anxiety-ridden my memories of testing, and of trying to test and failing, became. I grew familiar once again, after a long period of forgetfulness, with something of a nightmare.

The more I thought about it, the stronger my suspicion grew that the history of my own and Sizwe's respective anxieties might resemble each other in the way the chins and noses of relatives do. That the faces are related to one another is as clear as the fact that they are also very different. It would be through the route of the common chin or nose, I began to believe, that I would come to understand better the things Sizwe does not share with me. For his anxiety is obviously modulated by cultural and political forces that are of his world, not mine. But that is precisely what I hoped I would come to understand better by drawing out what we had in common.

So I left home that Monday morning in early April with a story in my head, one about my own forgotten history. My intention was to share it with Sizwe. I hoped that his response would help me to finish my book.

WHEN I WAS fifteen or sixteen—about as old as Sizwe was when this book picks up the thread of his story—few people foresaw that AIDS would kill hundreds of thousands of young South Africans. We were living in the mid-'80s, the final years of apartheid, and our minds were on the body politic, not the human body. We knew dimly that the spread of AIDS had reached pandemic proportions in some African countries thousands of miles to the north of us. We knew too that, unlike in the developed world, it was being transmitted primarily by heterosexual men and women. Yet Cameroon, Uganda, and Zaire were faraway places, not only in miles, but in our imaginations. Under apartheid, South Africans, both black and white, grew to think of ourselves as exceptional Africans, indeed, as exceptional human beings, a hubris the world's fascination with us only quickened.

Back then, less than a tenth of a percent of the population was thought to be HIV-positive. As in the developed world, AIDS was considered a ghettoized disease, one that primarily afflicted middle-class, homosexual men.

I am gay, middle class, and entering my late thirties. When I became sexually active in the mid-1980s, I was considered to be at the heart of the epidemic's highest risk group. In Lusikisiki, the word *AIDS* had yet to pass into popular currency. Teenagers who had unprotected sex were believed to be at risk of pregnancy, not death.

When I drove into Lusikisiki for the first time in October 2005, our respective positions had been turned inside out. The prenatal HIV prevalence rate at Lusikisiki's clinics was nudging at 30 percent. I doubt whether a single young person in the villages had not witnessed the death by AIDS of someone she had known since childhood. I, on the other hand, had lost nobody. Among the friends I had made in my late teens, none, nearly two decades later, had fallen ill with AIDS. The epidemic's center of gravity had shifted from my world to Sizwe's.

I was as sexually adventurous during my late teens as Sizwe was during his. From his perspective, I was probably more so; unlike him, I slept with people whose names I never learned, and whose faces I would not remember for long. And I was at least as careless as Sizwe about using condoms. Sometimes I did, sometimes I didn't. When I did, it was usually at the insistence of my partner. If Sizwe is lucky to be strong and healthy today, I am as lucky as he.

————————————

My first HIV test was little short of catastrophic. I was eighteen or nineteen, I don't quite remember. Three and a half months earlier, I had had unprotected sex with a man I knew well. I thought nothing of it for a week or two until suddenly, while taking notes at the back of a lecture hall, I was overwhelmed by the conviction that he had infected me with HIV. I lost the thread of the lecture, felt my pen become slippery with sweat in my fingers, put it down, and stared ahead. By the time I walked out into the sunlight, I felt dizzy and nauseous, as if the virus had already started making me ill. I walked across a wide campus piazza. All around were students in jeans and t-shirts, absorbed in conversation, laughing, or walking in silence; they seemed menacingly indifferent to me.

As my sense of panic rose, I wondered, with some desperation, about the connection between my actions and my anxieties. Why had I not insisted at the time that we use condoms? Why was I now bathed in sweat, the thought of my impending illness and death drawing me close to tears, when all this could have been prevented by a simple decision?

These questions were more upsetting than clarifying. If you had asked me, under less troubled circumstances, what sex meant to me, I would have told you that it conjured mastery: being an adult, not a child; being desired, not humored; acquiring the force to be free, instead of being shunted and ordered about. What I felt now, above all, was deep humiliation; I had somehow robbed myself of my authority over my body, my health, my well-being, for reasons I could not begin to fathom. And this feeling of blindness and self-resentment attached itself to my thoughts about sex itself; I wondered whether the act of sex was for me not a groping toward a picture of myself I could imagine but never earn. I was very much a child again: I needed the protection of someone much wiser, saner, and gentler than I.

I understood that the virus was undetectable for three months after infection. I waited three months to the day, and then walked into the student health center at Wits University in Johannesburg, where I was studying for a B.A., and asked for an HIV test. I chose the campus health center for its anonymity; I wanted merely to be a face interchangeable with innumerable others.

It was 1988 or 1989, the final years of apartheid. The most outrageous of the dying regime's puritanical fears remained on the statute books, sometimes enforced, usually not. In law, sodomy between consenting male adults remained a crime so grave that the police were permitted to use lethal force to prevent those suspected of it from resisting arrest. South Africa in the late 1980s was hardly the best place to be dealing with the prospect of HIV infection. But Wits University prided itself on being a liberal, oppositional institution, one that spoke the discourse of human rights with great fluency. If there were places in Johannesburg that ought to deal well with a virus transmitted primarily by gay sex, Wits was surely among them.

The pretest counseling did not make for a promising start. A prudish nurse looked at me with what I could only interpret as squeamish distaste and asked whether I slept with men. I shrugged and asked her to test me. She looked down at her clipboard, put the tip of her pen to the page, then thought better of it. She glanced at me again with a thin, distracted smile, one that seemed to express the magnitude of her professional burden: I have chosen to work at a place crawling with eighteen- and nineteen-year-olds who have come from God knows where and get up to God knows what, her thin smile said. But mine is to keep my head down and do my job.

I went to get my results a few days later. The waiting room at the health center was full. A long and jagged line started at the door and ended at a reception window being worked by three staff members. When I got to the front, I found myself jammed up against the bodies of those waiting alongside me.

The young woman attending my section of the line asked me what I wanted. She had to make herself heard above the noise around her and spoke in a loud, hurried voice. I told her my name, and that I had come to get test results. A little impatiently, she asked what the results were for. That is a private matter, I replied.

She picked her head up sharply, showing me her chin. Looking at me very carefully, she asked me to repeat my name, and wrote it down. She turned her back, went to a filing cabinet in the recesses of the room, and spent some time searching through it. She returned to the reception desk with a folder, and opened it. As she read, her brow furrowed.

"Ah," she said, looking up at me: "You are here for the results of your HIV test." The expression on her face and the tone of her voice communicated a dense package of messages. Her eyes were furtive and quick: she was embarrassed to have ignored my request for privacy. Her voice dropped a note or two, as if she knew that what she should have done was lower her voice, but could not, because of the noise around us, and thus spoke deeper instead, a quite useless substitute.

I nodded coldly. Her eyes noted my hostility and threw back a reciprocal anger; her silent apology had given way to the indignation of one who stands accused.

She dug her hand into the bottom of the folder. It emerged a moment later holding a folded sheet of paper. She unfolded it, glanced at it, then put it back in the folder.

"There's no need for counseling," she said, her voice now soft and sympathetic. "You tested negative."

I turned around, put my head down, and walked away. I did not look around to see whether anyone had taken interest in our exchange. I simply needed to leave.

Out in the open air, I discovered that my forehead was wet with perspiration and that my cheeks were burning. I needed to shake off the unpleasant feelings as much as to flee the health center itself, and so I did not pause to reflect on what it was that had upset me. I just kept walking, the health center and my experience of it behind me.

Some months later, I began talking casually of what had happened with a cool smile on my face; I had turned the episode into a light anecdote about a prudish nurse and a thoughtless receptionist. I no longer remembered that there had been sweat on my brow, never mind what had put it there.

But looking back now, the scene I was rehearsing in my mind as I walked briskly away from the health center is vivid and unmistakable. I was imagining that the people around me had overheard the entire exchange. I put myself in their shoes and thought their thoughts. Comeuppance. That is what they were thinking. He has been gallivanting around town with the hubris of a nineteen-year-old fool, and now he is paying for his excesses. His dick is humbled and shriveled up in his pants, and there are beads of worry on his forehead. We have nothing but contempt for him.

Their accusation was one I had put to myself over and over again without ever having heard it clearly: he has been trying to take more than his due.

REMEMBERING THAT MOMENT now, I am struck by how fluently my experience describes the architecture of shame. Neither the nurse who took my blood nor the receptionist who announced my results was overtly hostile. And as for the crowd in the health center, there is no evidence that anyone overheard the exchange between the receptionist and me, let alone cast any judgment. And yet I felt I was walking a gauntlet of sniggers: that was the very heart of my experience, its sine qua non.

And that is also the sine qua non of shame. At its root lie myriad watching, judging eyes that look at one and see a disgusting and gluttonous figure. They are the eyes of others, but one has internalized them. They are strangers' eyes whose watchfulness is nonetheless experienced in secret on the inside. When one stands in a crowded room and a person shouts "HIV," the very name and embodiment of one's shame, the secret opprobrium expressed by the strangers inside heads for the real strangers on the outside like electrons in a force field. You are suddenly struck with the sickening feeling that the contemptuous eyes have always been on the outside; that is their natural home.

I SHARED THESE memories with a friend who practices as a psychotherapist. From some remarks she had recently made, I knew that she was preoccupied at the time with understanding shame among her patients.

I recounted as simply as I could my memory of the scene in my mind as I escaped the clinic. "It was a hallucination," I said. "It was as if the feelings of scorn I had toward myself had always been searching for a bunch of strangers, as if the proper place for this scorn was always on the outside. As soon as the three letters H-I-V were enunciated, they grabbed the scorn and placed it in every pair of eyes in that room."

"You call it hallucination," she replied, "but it is quite real, quite shared. And the proof that it is real is in a thousand social conventions. If you look for it, you'll find analogues of your experience all over.

"The simplest one I can think of is the prohibition in force three or four generations ago on pregnant women appearing in public. Pregnancy was referred to as confinement; the pregnant woman literally had to be confined. She could not be seen in public in her bloated state; it would have been a source of huge, huge shame.

"What was at the root of that shame? What was it that had to be concealed? It is not the fact that she has had sex. Everyone knows she has. It is the external manifestation of the sex she has had that must be hidden. The bulge in her stomach shouts out: what you have done is manifest now, what you have done is known; your guilt is now on public record.

"The letters H-I-V were your bloated stomach, your public record, only far worse, for HIV is a virus. The scorn you felt inside not only became manifest, it became manifest as a deadly disease."

"But what guilt is now on record?" I asked. "What am I and the pregnant woman guilty of?"

"Of being gluttonous," she replied. "Of being disgustingly greedy. Of being shameless. The closest analogy I can think of is having an audience watch you while you sleep. You are snoring raucously and lines of spit dribble down your chin. You are grotesque."

It was an arresting image, but it did not quite answer my question. Why should an external manifestation of sex be a sign of such disgusting greed? I can only answer in terms of my own experience: in the sneering accusations I had imagined emitting from the crowd at the health center. What is it they were accusing me of taking that was not mine?

Quite simply: sex. That I had come with my tail between my legs to test for HIV, they said accusingly, that I had done something I feared was making me sick, affirmed that I was a child trying to take things that only adults are licensed to have. I had stolen into an arena in which I had no place. It is as if the marital bed one spends one's childhood nudging and disturbing and edging one's way toward, is forever off limits.

AT THE TIME I went to the campus clinic to test for HIV, half of my university fees were being paid by a scholarship, the other half by my parents. My fee invoices came quarterly, and were addressed to my mother. Some six weeks after my visit to the campus health center, she opened an invoice from the university to find an eighty-rand charge for a blood test.

"What was it for?" she asked with concern.

"I didn't know I'd be charged for it," I snapped irritably. "It is my business."

The moment they left my mouth I understood that my words were unacceptably cruel; I could not possibly leave her with this half-knowledge indefinitely.

"It was for HIV," I continued. "I'm fine."

She bowed her head in embarrassment, then looked up at me briefly and smiled. "That's a relief," she said cheerfully, and emitted a forced chuckle. We shuffled around each other for a few moments before she left the room.

I had told her a year or two earlier that I slept with men, but I had always studiously revealed nothing to her about my sex life. In retrospect, it is quite clear that my secrecy was in part an attempt to court her attention; I wanted her to wonder about me a great deal. And now her imagination would certainly follow me as vividly as it ever had behind the doors I closed, but not with the inquisitiveness of one who is curious or jealous. Rather, she would be imagining a son who cannot look after himself, who goes out into the city seeking pleasure and returns with trouble and anguish and pain.

When I enrolled at the university in February 1988 I dived headlong into the antiapartheid student movement. At the time I went for my HIV test, I was spending a good six or eight hours a day at the offices of the National Union of South African Students. I was reading Marx and Lenin with the hunger of a young convert. Among the debates I had with my peers was whether a shopping mall full of the rich and bejeweled beneficiaries of apartheid was a legitimate target for a bomb blast. I believed I was part of a movement that was going to rout the state and overturn the economic order.

And yet not once did I consider raising my ire against the campus health center. The possibility of approaching the Students Representative Council to tell them that there was something wrong with the way the university dealt with HIV was not something I entertained. The meanness that had been cast at me was utterly indistinguishable from, was indeed entirely parasitic upon, the meanness I felt toward myself. Even if I had found a way to express my anger, I would not have known whom to fight.

"I'VE COME BACK to Lusikisiki because I can't finish my book," I said to Sizwe.

Some three or four hours had passed since we met up outside the Metro Cash & Carry. In the interim, I had traipsed after him as he moved about town accumulating a mountain of supplies for his shop. They were now crammed into a minibus that was driving ahead of us, and into the tiny car I had hired back at Mthatha's airport; it was complaining volubly of the unexpected burden.

He turned to me and nodded and then looked ahead again, waiting to discover in precisely what form I wished to shake him down.

"I still don't know why you won't test for HIV," I said. "I've just spent the last few weeks trying to figure out for myself why you won't test, and it got me thinking about my experiences. I started remembering how difficult I have found it to test in the past, and I thought to myself, If I can relive my own experience, maybe I can understand yours better."

I began to tell him of what had happened in the campus health center some eighteen years ago; of the moment the letters H-I-V crossed the lips of the young woman receptionist; of how a roomful of people, their thoughts in all likelihood consumed by their own business, became, in my mind, an audience of naked hostility.

Sizwe listened very carefully. He did not interrupt. But the moment the story reached its first natural pause, he spoke.

"It is not the same for me," he said quietly. "I have thought about it a lot and it is not the same. A little bit of me is worried about what other people will think, but that is not the main reason why I won't test."

He cleared his throat, wrapped his fingers tightly together in his lap, and stared ahead.

"If I know I am HIV-positive," he said, "I will no longer be motivated to do the thing I am doing now, I mean the thing I am doing right now, what I have spent the morning doing here with you—putting all my energy, every moment I am awake, into my shop. It will all be meaningless for me. I will stay in bed in the mornings."

He said nothing more. It was senseless asking a question now, so we drove on in silence for some time.

"I am doing all of this for my children," he finally said. "If I have AIDS, then all this work is no longer for my children."

"Because you will die before you have accumulated enough wealth for them?"

"Because if I die while my children are too little to take what's theirs, my money will end up going to people like my father and my brother. These are people who do not help me to earn my money now. They are not interested in helping me with my business. My dad did not educate me. That's fine. I do not blame him for that. Now, I support him, and when my brother needs money for the doctor it is to me that he comes. But they do not help with the business.

"So that is my first reason. If I die of AIDS, Mfanawetu will not get my money. Some others will get it. That is why I will not test. If I test positive, I will no longer get up in the morning to work."

Of the emotions his brief soliloquy transmitted the one I felt most was love: a fierce and restless love for Mfanawetu, and for his brothers and sisters who are not yet born. His love is of course selfish: it is his progeny, and no one else, for whom he wakes up in the mornings. But what fiery and desperate love; he must be omnipotent, it is all up to him, like the last man on the *Titanic.* If the virus has found his blood and he dies a young man, the entire ship that is him and his descendants will be ripped apart by hostile storms.

In a sense, what he was telling me now was not so different from the things he had expressed during the first months of our acquaintanceship. I had met a young shop owner who was anxious that envious people would destroy his nascent success. He worried of Simlindile the gangster arranging for young men to hold him up at gunpoint; of demons who would come to him in his sleep and infect him with untreatable illness; of other demons who would slip into the interiors of his customers and make them wild and crazy and tear his place to pieces. And Sizwe and I had both watched in muted horror the aftermath of Brian's death: Brian the wealthy spaza shop owner whose assets his own uncle Charlie and cousin Simlindile had quite literally dismembered, selling them off one by one, and using the proceeds to start a shop of their own.

But Nwabisa was not yet his wife then, and Mfanawetu was invisible in her womb. Now the entity he needed to defend had taken life and was there in front of him every day: it was not his flesh-and-blood corporeal self, but a line of Magadlas he loved with all his might. And the menace that threatened them was not a gangster with a gun; it was the most primordial of rivals—fathers, brothers who would take one's children's inheritance and spend it on themselves.

"You assume," I said to Sizwe a little later in our car journey, "that if you test positive you will die soon. If I tested positive, I would go to the opposite extreme. I would instinctively tell myself I have another three decades to live at least."

"No," he replied. "That is in fact the biggest reason for me not to test. If I know that I am positive, I will die quicker. Once I know the virus is inside me, it will take me over very quickly. Knowing that my blood is dirty, feeling it every time I wake up in the morning, it would not be long before I'm dead."

"And the pills?" I asked. We had, just an hour earlier, bumped into a woman we both knew was among the first people in Lusikisiki to start ARV treatment. Once we had chatted and she was walking away, I had remarked, and Sizwe had agreed, how stunningly beautiful she was, and how healthy she looked. "We have both just seen what the pills have done," I said.

"I do not like those pills," he replied. "To take them every day is a reminder that your blood is dirty. Especially that big yellow pill, that huge rugby ball pill. If I had to take that pill every day it would be close to the end for me. It would just remind me that I am dying."

"You would choose not to take the pills?"

"I would take them because they would be the only thing left to me. But I would not be happy."

I SPENT THE early evening in Ithanga with Sizwe, Nwabisa, and their son. Mfanawetu was fourteen months old now. With his toddler's unsteady gait, he marched between Sizwe and his mother and me, his face very serious, his voice very loud, demanding to be cuddled and cooed at and made a fuss of. We each obliged him in turn.

After dinner, at about eight o'clock, Sizwe walked me back to the outskirts of the village. It was the night after a full moon. As we crossed the river, our socks and shoes in our hands, the pebbles on the river's pedestrian crossing appeared and disappeared in the pale moonlight.

"I think a difference between me and you," I said, "is that the times I thought I felt the virus in my blood have been momentary. Over the last twenty years, on an average day, I have not felt that there is this thing in my blood. I think it is the opposite for you. I think you believe deep down that it is in your blood."

"There are so many different symptoms I feel," he replied, "that it is hard to know whether it is AIDS. I do not have a desire for sex as much as I used to. My hips ache. My body feels weak and it aches. The same thing is happening to Nwabisa. It is possible that we both have AIDS. And Mfanawetu."

"Because of a demon?"

"More likely because I got it, or Nwabisa got it maybe, before we were together. Maybe it was there all this time, but it was quiet for a while. Maybe it was hidden in Nwabisa that time she tested for HIV.

"Or maybe a demon. I don't know. Both of us have recently experienced demons having sex with us in our sleep. It is probably the same demon. It is a woman when it is with me, a man when it is with Nwabisa."

"A part of me is so frustrated," I replied. "If you are HIV-positive, I know at the bottom of my heart that you would embrace those pills as a life force. You would swallow them and they would invigorate you because they would represent life. You would feel the virus getting weaker in your blood and your thoughts would make you stronger.

"I think that the certainty with which you feel you will not survive the knowledge of your illness is a lie. The trauma you are imagining, it is something you have already experienced; you have already survived it."

"Maybe you are right," he replied. "But it's not worth the chance."

"You have seen Jake's brother every day since he started taking the pills," I said. "Do you not see life returning to him?"

"He looks better if you just glance at him," he said evenly. "But if you look at him very closely, he is not right. He is much thinner than he should be. And if you look at him around the eyes, he is not right. There is something around the eyes."

"You look at him and you see death?"

He did not reply. One does not say it out loud; one does not will-ingly coax the evil eye.

I MET SIZWE at half past six the following morning on the outskirts of Ithanga. He had asked me the night before whether I would drive him to Mount Ayliff, 125 miles away, to book an appointment for a driver's license test. He was desperate for a four-by-four of his own and for a license. Hiring transportation to carry his stock from town was his largest expense and his most burdensome dependence on others. In recent months, the prospect of a vehicle of his own had begun to consume him. He craved it, but feared too that it might be a poisoned chalice: in the eyes of Ithangans it would be the first categorical symbol of his wealth. He would have to erect a tall fence around his property, buy several dogs, and park his car outside his front door.

Driving from Ithanga, I picked up our discussion from where we had suspended it the previous evening.

"Just think of the relief," I said. "You go to the clinic, you test nega-tive, and you are free. This whole burden lifts from your shoulders."

He laughed out loud. "This is not a disease you go and look for," he said. "You wait until it comes to you. And then you deal with it. If I start getting sick with AIDS symptoms, then I will go and test.

"In any case, if you go and look for it, maybe you will find it. Maybe the nurse who does the test is someone who is very angry with you. And she gives you the disease in the needle."

So many things were condensed into the thoughts he had shared over the last fifteen hours. The first was quite simple: as much as he knows he will die one day, at bottom he does not believe in his own death. That is something we all share. One sees it every day. It is there in all of our lives. Some weeks ago I attended the funeral of a middle-aged man. Two years ago, he felt a throbbing in his head and wished it away and wished it away until he collapsed, a tumor the size of a golf ball strangling his brain. It was there in the colleague with whom I had coffee yesterday morning; he smokes three packs of filterless Camels a day, and knows, but does not at bottom believe, that he will die young and badly.

Sizwe also expresses a fear that, paradoxically, belongs to a person who believes that he is in grave danger of dying. He said that he has aches and pains and he thinks that they are symptoms of AIDS. He has had intimations of what it feels like to have dirt in his blood and he believes it is a feeling that will kill him. What is this dirt, this contamination?

When Sizwe says his brother and father will snatch his worldly possessions from his son Mfanawetu, he believes he has sinned against them. When he says his community will tear him down for doing well, he fears that he has taken too much from them. When he says his premature death will rob his progeny of their inheritance, he feels he has stolen the progeny of his peers. I think it is these feelings that have taken the form of dirt in his blood.

This book has been awash with examples of a contamination that elides the boundary between the physical and the moral. It was there in the rigid prohibition on drinking and smoking that Lusikisiki health-care workers imposed on ARV users. It made little medical sense, but users understood it intuitively and latched on to it with fervor. It was as if, along with the pills, they had been given the chance to cleanse their bodies and their beings of dirt.

It was there when I interviewed Edwin Cameron in his study in Johannesburg. He had not known, he said, that in the eleven-year period between testing positive for HIV and starting antiretroviral treatment he had all the while felt that his blood was contaminated; that the contamination was at once moral and physical, a self-reproach that ran through his bodily fluids. "I only began to understand these things," Cameron told me, "when I realized that the drugs were working. Once the viral activity had been stopped in my body, I stopped feeling contaminated."

It was there too in me as I left the campus health center through what I imagined to be a gauntlet of contempt. My blood test had made it public that I had taken too much. And in Sizwe's blood too, I believe, is the feeling that he has taken far too much, that he has been contaminated by his choices.

How do I know these things when he has not told me himself? I don't. I have only felt it, intimated it, and I can only share these intimations as best I can.

Periodically, I asked Sizwe how business was going. Well, he would invariably reply. Long may it last, I would say.

"But it will not last long," he would always reply. "It is only a matter of time before my customers leave me."

"Why are you sure they will do that?"

"One day I will bring home a car, and they will see this. Then I will build myself a big rondavel, and they will see that. At some point one of them will say out loud, 'Whose money is making him so rich? It is ours. Every pension day we come here to him to pay our debts, and there our money is in his car and his rondavel.' And then they will all leave to go and make some other spaza shop owner rich, leaving me with nothing."

Sometimes he would say it in the spirit of a wry joke, sometimes as a superstitious precaution, as if by prefiguring it he would chase the actual event away. Nonetheless, it is a fantasy he has rehearsed incessantly. Over and over again he tells himself that his success will not last because it wasn't his to begin with: he has triumphed over the people around him and they will get their revenge.

Is an entrepreneur who has taken more than his due from his community also a man who has taken more than his due from sex? Shadowing us in the background during every step of our journey was the question what he was doing with his body. He was sleeping with one woman. He was saving his worldly possessions for her bridewealth. His intention was to produce children who would bear his name.

What does it mean to do this in a village where practically every other man of one's generation is unable to do the same? What does it mean to tell one's peers that one is now *isishumane,* a man who has given up sexual conquests, and yet who, paradoxically, grows more powerful than them every day? In having sons and daughters he can claim as his own, is he accosted by the sense that he is stealing their progeny?

From the very beginning, getting ahead meant pushing another aside. Going to school, learning to read and write, that in and of itself was a victory, the outcome of a silent struggle with his father.

These are my questions at any rate. I asked Sizwe why he could not test for HIV. He told me of a boy he loved called Mfanawetu, and of a fear that the boy would be robbed of his patrimony because of the dirt in his father's blood. This is what I have made of his reply.

WHEN SIZWE AGREED that I could write about him, it was understood that I would use his real name. I advised him to take care. He had spoken to me candidly about his relationships with other people—

with his parents, with ex-lovers, with those whose presence in Ithanga he found threatening. We agreed that he would read everything I wrote, and that he should look out for trouble. "For instance," I told him, "I want to write about you and your father. But the thoughts you share with me about him are obviously not necessarily thoughts you would want him to hear. When you look at the draft, you must take it as given that somebody will tell your father what is in the book. There must be nothing in it you would rather he didn't know."

Sometimes he seemed to take this advice to heart, but mostly he could not take it seriously at all. In all his years, he had seldom seen anyone in Ithanga reading a book, nor, with the exception of novels and plays teenagers studied at high school, had he ever heard a single conversation about one. I tried to impress upon him that this book was different: it was about Lusikisiki and would thus be read in Lusikisiki, and news of its content would come to Ithanga.

"Maybe," he would reply. "But I don't think so."

His nonchalance about privacy ended abruptly when he told me about Thandeka, a loved one with AIDS whose condition was a secret, and whom I would reveal were I to write of Sizwe's own relation to the epidemic. There and then we decided on two things. We would give both Sizwe and his village pseudonyms. And, since those who really want to discover his identity could do so simply by approaching people whose real names do appear in this book, we disguised Thandeka's identity, such that no one would find out precisely who she was unless Sizwe himself were to tell them.

That is how things stood during much of the period in which this book was researched and written. Officially, we were using pseudonyms to protect Thandeka.

But there was obviously more to be said than that. Whatever the official reason, Sizwe was now collaborating with me undercover. And the question that ought to have arisen, but that did not until the last days of our collaboration, was what, precisely, this cover was permitting us to do.

During one of my last trips to Lusikisiki, in February 2007, I put a suggestion to Sizwe. If we could agree among ourselves, I said, that Thandeka's identity was sufficiently hidden, would he consider dispensing with his pseudonym? Would he allow me to name him and his village?

"If somebody who reads this book really wants to find you," I said, "it won't be too hard. The reason was to protect Thandeka, and I think she is protected."

He thought about it for a moment or two. He had nothing to hide, he said. There is nothing in his views about AIDS of which he is ashamed; they are reflective of the views of many black people. Even in the things he has revealed of himself, there is not much that would surprise those who knew him. Despite all that, he said, he wanted to keep his pseudonym.

Why? He gave me a hundred reasons during my two-week stay in Lusikisiki that February, but none rang true. He trusted blacks to understand the things he expressed in the book, he said, but not whites; they would make trouble. Or he trusted whites, but not Indians. He was babbling, filling up space: he did not want to say.

The closest he came to expressing his real fears was on the last afternoon of my trip.

"I would be accused of giving away black people's secrets," he said. "It is like what you are accused of when you act as a guide. When Graeme and the bird-watchers were there at their cottage, and I was showing them around the forest, my cousin and I organized a cultural tour for them. We took them to see a sangoma, an inyanga, to see traditional dance, to see the floors of the hut being cleaned with cow dung. They watched the ritual when a goat is being slaughtered.

"After they left, some people in Ithanga were very angry with us. They said, 'You go around showing the white people our culture, but they show us none of theirs. You are giving away our secrets to put a few cents in your own pockets. But it is our secrets you are making money off, our culture.'

"I am afraid that I would be accused of the same thing."

"Doesn't that argument have some power," I asked.

"No. I don't think the whites are going to use our secrets. It is we who keep borrowing the culture from the whites. And anyway, these people who get angry, if they had money to travel to other places, they would also want to know about the people they met there. It is just that they are too poor to travel."

"I'm not sure," I replied. "Maybe they are saying two things. First, that the tourists are given their secrets for nothing. But the second is different. Maybe they are saying that when the whites come here on holiday it is like they are going to a game reserve to look at the animals. They are interested in your culture in the same way they are interested in the fact that the leopard sleeps alone in a tree and the lion with his family on the ground."

"Yes," he nodded, "they are making that point, too."

"And that is humiliating. It is an unequal relationship."

"Yes, it is."

"So why are you cooperating with me if you think that these people who will be angry with you might have a point?"

He grinned widely, insouciantly, a little irritably, as if to say, You asked for it, now you'll get it.

"You know Botha Sigcau," he began, "the Mpondo chief during iKongo?"

"During the 1960 Pondoland uprising," I replied, "in which many men from Ithanga were thrown in jail."

"Yes, iKongo. The whites put in front of Sigcau a bag of money and a bag of soil. They asked him to choose. He chose the money and gave away his land, the land on which his people farmed. And when the people rebelled against the theft of their land, the whites took Sigcau up in a helicopter, and they asked him to fire the first shot. He did: he shot at his people."

"So you are Sigcau," I said. "You are selling your people's culture and their secrets to me?"

He shook his head and laughed. "I'm not selling you anything so valuable. As I said, it is us who are stealing your culture from you."

"But what is the exchange? You agreed to do this for nothing."

"I did it to make friends with the *umlungus*," he beamed. "We know that if you make friends with the *umlungus* now, you gain something later."

"Like the stooge Botha Sigcau?"

"Yes." He laughed loudly. "Botha Sigcau and Sizwe Magadla are the traitors of Lusikisiki."

———

ON THE MORNING I drove Sizwe to Mount Ayliff to book an appointment for his driving test, I took up the issue again.

"Is your fear that people will accuse you of giving away your culture's secrets the real reason you are keeping your name disguised?" I asked.

"No," he said softly. "Well, it is a reason, but it is not the main reason. The main reason is that I would look stupid for talking about private things. Like that I went to school behind my father's back. This is not something about your life that you share with people. They read it in the book, they see it is me, and I will get embarrassed."

"Then why are you doing this?"

"I bumped into Phumza a few days ago," he said by way of reply. Phumza is a woman I hired as an interpreter early in my research. I once asked her, in Sizwe's presence, whether she would consider allowing me to write a chapter about the time I spent with her. She said she would think about it. Some six weeks later I heard from her. We spoke about this and that, but she did not raise my request, and so neither did I; from her silence it was clear that she had decided against it.

"I asked her," Sizwe continued, "why she didn't want you to write about her. She said, 'I'll never let him. He'll get rich doing it, and I'll get nothing. I will have given him private things about my life and I will look stupid.'

"So what people will maybe say about me," he continued in a calm, even voice, "they will say I have sold something that is not for sale."

The heaviness of what he had said sat with us in the car.

"I do not think that I have," he continued. "But there are others who might think so. It is not such a big thing. It does not matter so much what they think. If we had been using my real name it would have been okay. But since I was given the opportunity to use a different name, I would like to take that opportunity."

Outside the window, I noticed, the landscape had changed considerably since the beginning of our journey. The sharp hills and deep valleys of the Lusikisiki district were beginning to make way for a magisterial landscape; we were driving toward large mountains.

A feeling of unhappiness settled over me. Sizwe was trying to be reassuring, to wish away something painful. But his attempt only caused it to linger. In his recurring nightmare about the ruin of his business, which he talks of as a joke or a warding off of the evil eye, the wool is suddenly lifted from over his customers' eyes. It dawns on them that all the things he has sold them were never for sale, that he has been getting rich with their money under their very noses. There is something similar in the unease he had just expressed to me now. Here too, he stands accused of selling that which is not for sale. In order to get close to the world of the *umlungu*s, he is bartering his privacy. To have this sale revealed to the world would be embarrassing, he said.

Yet perhaps it is a good deal more than embarrassing. He is a black man selling his interior to a white man. There is a special transgression in this sale, one as powerful as it is hard to articulate. It is something you know because you feel it deep in your bones: it has grown out of generation upon generation of racial hurt.

You do not sell your interior to whites, for what is inside you is an instance of a shared, black interior. What you are offering to the white man is not yours, it is everybody's: a collective sphere of privacy bounded by race and politics. You do not hawk a piece of that interior to people who have spent generations trying to extinguish your spirit. That is what he was saying when he likened himself to the stooge Botha Sigcau, a man who sold his people's birthright because he believed it was his to hawk to whites.

Sitting in the car with him on the drive to Mount Ayliff, I thought I glimpsed the high-water mark of his moral doubt. I saw something of the burden he carries in his quest to give his children the future he has dreamed for them. I understood as well as I ever will his feeling that his blood might be polluted, and his suspicion that Mfanawetu's blood might be, too.

THE BUBBLE OF a tiny car is an intimate space. I do not know whether Sizwe felt the full extent of my unease, but he certainly sensed my change of mood. When he spoke again, his voice had taken on a colder, more distant quality.

"I have said this to you before," he began, "but I will say it now. My generation, and the generation before mine, are dying younger than the last. In the old days, only the very old would die, and even then, only occasionally. Now there are funerals every weekend and it is young people who are being buried.

"Partly, it is diet. We are eating things our ancestors never ate: *amafuta* [saturated oil], rice, coffee. Even the children are drinking coffee now. In the old days, the elders would throw the dregs of the pot out, fill it up with water, and the children would drink that water. The coffee was hardly there anymore.

"And as for AIDS, the *umlungu* definitely have a cure. I know absolutely for sure that they do. And they are holding it back. The *umlungu* are so clever. It is not possible that they don't have a cure. They want the blacks to die so that life can be more comfortable again. Tell me, why did people start dying of this thing after democracy came in 1994? And why does it only affect the blacks?"

"It started in other countries long before 1994," I replied. "And as you know it hit countries very hard in which the white rulers had left long ago—for Britain and Belgium and other European countries."

"Exactly," he said. "Why only in black countries?"

"America was just about the first country in which it was detected," I said. "And it killed thousands of young, white, middle-class people."

"Yes, but they stopped dying, didn't they? They got better. Why did they get better when we didn't?"

That is Africa's great question about AIDS: why has the epidemic been uniquely terrible here? Sizwe answered this question from his vantage point in a village in the old Transkei. He also answered it from his place in a conversation in my car. We had spent some of the last fifteen hours talking of our fear of testing. He did not want to test for dirt in his blood, he said, because the knowledge would kill him. And from there we had discussed the selling of things that are not his to sell. He was expressing guilt, guilt that his life's quest was poisoned because it would entail triumphing over people around him.

And then the mood in the car changed, and when he spoke again, it was still about AIDS, but he was no longer guilty, no longer a wrong-doer. The source of the hostility was outside him now, far outside. He was now a black man among other black people, and together they were the victims of a gruesome conspiracy. He had freed himself of the guilt he was feeling just moments before, but at a heavy price. For he was now a man facing a pernicious and invisible onslaught, a man who must not trust whatever comes from the outside. An anti-entrepreneur, really: one who retreats in the face of the new.

The switch from one to the other had happened at lightning speed.

Sizwe and Hermann

S ome eight or nine years after my first HIV test, I entered a state of anxiety about my health similar to the one I had experienced at the back of the lecture hall in Johannesburg. This time I was a doctoral student at Oxford University in the United Kingdom. I was twenty-seven. I still hadn't had a lasting sexual relationship, and if the criteria established by my last bout of anxiety held, I thus remained suspended, despite my age, somewhere between childhood and the grown-up world.

My anxiety came in a very different form this time. It did not crash down upon me in a single moment, but accumulated quietly over time. One by one, I went over in my mind the sexual encounters I had had since I last tested. They had all, I thought, been reasonably safe. And yet the more I reflected on it, the more the boundary between safe and unsafe seemed to blur. I could not be absolutely certain unless I tested. Whenever I brooded upon it, I felt dizzy and nauseous in the way I had nearly a decade earlier, as if the virus itself was in my body and had decided to make its own contribution to my internal dialogue. I was tormenting myself; I needed to test.

I made an appointment with my doctor, Andrew Rutland, the same word-shy man whose benign, authoritative presence had helped me give up smoking, my memory of whom had been stirred as I watched Kate Marrandi and her patients. His consultation room was about the safest space in Oxford I could imagine in which to be tested for HIV. I would be in his hands.

When I told him what I wanted he shook his head. He would take blood from me if I really insisted, he said, but he felt he should tell me that it was not in my interests to be tested here. He could not guarantee that the results would be confidential. They would enter my record where they might be accessed by a host of institutions that could one day use them against me: life insurance companies, medical insurers, prospective employers. It would be better if I went to the nearest public facility, the Radcliffe Infirmary, not far from the center of town. The service there is good, he said, and I could be sure that no record would remain of my having tested there.

I left Dr. Rutland's consultation room puzzled. Something was not right. A hundred questions flared up in me that I should have asked him moments earlier. Do insurance companies have a right to demand to see a private practitioner's patient records? Prospective employers? And if not, how on earth would they get their hands on them without the doctor's permission? Had this island become a totalitarian state? Had I missed it in the newspapers?

I held no ill feeling toward Dr. Rutland himself. On the contrary, he remained the paternal figure in whom I took comfort, looking out for my interests, steering me from a danger that in my ignorance I had drifted toward. But I was nonetheless enraged. I was twenty-seven now, not the fumbling nineteen-year-old who had walked into the Wits health center in a cold sweat. Back then, the prospect of disapproving strangers barging into the rooms in which I had sex to take notes and keep records and write to my mother bore some sort of symmetry to the child I was. I was an adult now. I had earned my privacy. When I closed my door it ought to remain closed.

Now, to hold on to my privacy, I would have to take my place at the end of the line at the Radcliffe Infirmary: small, reduced, cap in hand. What came to mind was another crowded room, like the one at Wits, another hurried, indifferent person managing the line. This was a violation of my adulthood, I thought to myself, an insult to the integrity of my genitals themselves, as if they were still those of a prepubescent.

Looking back now, it is hard not to view the advice Dr. Rutland gave me as terribly destructive. As with the young woman at the reception window years earlier, he was either woefully ignorant of the workings of shame or, unconsciously, only too aware. For if shame is an internalized voice of opprobrium, one in search of an echo from the outside, Dr. Rutland gave my shame all the echo it could ever have hoped for. Of course an HIV-positive person in 1997 had a great deal of cause to fear the prejudice of insurers and future employers. But the point is that they could not get into Dr. Rutland's consultation room. They could not pore through his patient records. He had in effect told me that the virus that may be in my blood carried an accusation so vicious and penetrating as to threaten a right to confidentiality established by generation upon generation of common law; that the very prospect of recording it, even here, in a consultation protected by doctor-patient privilege, was too dangerous.

If I had been clear-sighted I would have seen at once that what Dr. Rutland said could not possibly be right. But since I was a person living with a great deal of shame, a feeling I had never reflected upon with any measure of insight, his words instinctively rang true. Of course there were powerful forces out there and in here seeking to damage me; I knew the feeling of their presence all too well, since I had been living with them inside me my entire adult life. And so I turned my rage against these forces. And since I could not distinguish whether they were inside me or outside, I confused the object of my rage. Unwittingly, I pointed my venom at myself.

A few days after my visit to Dr. Rutland, I cycled to the Radcliffe Infirmary, which most residents of Oxford knew was on Woodstock Road. Quite bizarrely, I could not find the front entrance. I had it in my mind that the infirmary was on Walton Street, a block behind Woodstock Road. Indeed, I was absolutely convinced that the entrance was there; I would have bet my life on it. And I did find a sign to the Radcliffe Infirmary on Walton Street, but it was to a back entrance, an asphalt alleyway that turned sharply to the left and disappeared behind a building.

I sat on my bicycle, one foot on the ground, the other on the pedal, and stared down the alleyway. Several thoughts accosted me at once and I knew within a second that I would go no farther. The first was that I lived more than a mile away from here. The second was that I had no way of getting home except on my bicycle or by foot. (The prospect of hailing a taxi did not cross my mind.) The third was that having blood taken from my arm would make me dizzy and weak, and I would have no way of returning home. In that moment, I forgot entirely that I had never felt remotely faint at the sight of blood. I imagined myself in the wake of the test, stumbling around and disoriented, my legs weak and unsure. I mount my bike and fall down on the pavement on Walton Street, and my residence room, its work desk and laptop waiting for me, remains empty and silent.

I turned around and rode my bike quickly back to my college, lonely, triumphant, and angry. At the time, I was as fit and healthy as I had ever been. I either ran or played squash or went to gym almost every day, and on weekends a friend and I often explored the surrounding countryside on bicycles. I turned the corner into Little Clarendon Street. As I began ascending the hill, I stood up tall, dug my left heel into the pedal, felt the quadriceps in my thigh flex, felt their strength, and celebrated it. The sickness lay in the Radcliffe Infirmary; that is where the taking of blood from my arm would make me weak and unsteady, leaving my thighs unable to carry me. I was cycling away from sickness, and toward my continued health.

Looking back, it is as clear to me now as it was opaque then that I had scooped up the aggression and hostility that had been hurled at me—that of the insurance companies and the prospective employers, whose toxic message had been delivered to me via the mouth of the trusted Dr. Rutland; I had scooped up their dark hostility, mistaken it for a friend, and hurled it with all my might at my own will to live.

It is among the most disturbing and pitiful images I have of myself: a terribly lonely, terribly angry man on a bicycle, riding as fast as he can from self-care.

IN MARCH 2007, about a decade since I had last laid eyes on him, I wrote to Andrew Rutland, told him of the book I was writing, and asked whether he could comment on the advice he had given me back in 1997. Two days later, he e-mailed a clipped reply of unadorned candor. He said that while he had followed the established protocol of the time, the protocol itself was "rather precious," and "in retrospect rather silly."

"There was guidance at the time that HIV testing was best conducted in specialist centres with people who were trained to give pre-test counselling," he wrote. "This was always a rather precious approach to the issue and has disappeared as HIV testing has come to be accepted as just another medical test."

As for the question of my test results being used against me, he wrote that people "working in practice settings" had been concerned, at the time, "about access to test results . . . Again, this was in retrospect rather silly and treated HIV as an exceptional case. Of course, all medical data should be treated with complete confidentiality by practice staff and HIV shouldn't be treated any differently."

I CAN'T BE entirely sure now, but I think I forgot that I had ever gone to the Radcliffe Infirmary to test. I certainly gave little thought to the fact that I had not tested at all.

Two years later, I found myself sitting in a blood laboratory in Johannesburg. I had just returned from a malaria zone and I was coming down with the flu; taking a malaria test was a responsible precaution.

As the nurse prepared her needle, she gave me a folder to sign. On it was a printed list of some forty blood tests. She had ticked two of them.

Casting my eye down the list, I saw "HIV." It came as something of a revelation.

"Can I tick this one, too?" I asked. "Can this blood sample also be tested for HIV?"

"Of course," she replied.

I sat on the bed, rolled up my sleeve, turned the inside of my arm up, and bunched my fingers into a fist. She inserted the needle so gently I did not feel it.

"Damn," she said calmly. "I should have asked you to do this lying down."

"Why?"

"Because you're going to faint, and I won't be able to break your fall. Please lie down."

"I've never fainted when someone's taken blood from me," I replied cheerfully.

"Well then this is your first time."

The next thing I remember I was feeling grotesquely nauseous. I felt the starched pillowcase scrape as I turned my head.

WHEN MY MEMORY began returning to me and I recalled the morning I had hurtled away from the Radcliffe Infirmary on my bicycle, I thought immediately of Sizwe. I thought of him standing outside the school in Ithanga on the Saturday when the counselors and nurses came to conduct voluntary testing.

I went to a testing site at the heart of the developed world. Sizwe went to a makeshift site in an old apartheid Bantustan that had never known decent medicine. And yet on the face of it, the HIV program he encountered was far more sophisticated than the one I did. At the sites I went to test, a university health center and a doctor's practice, the personnel at hand were clueless of the workings of stigma. Sizwe, in contrast, had Médecins Sans Frontières. They had thought of little else but how to conquer stigma. Was there nonetheless something they failed to understand? Did the scent of hostility reach Sizwe's nose because there was something MSF had not thought through?

Of course there was hostility outside the school that morning. It was so thick Sizwe could almost touch it. Back at the campus health center in the late 1980s, I had felt my cheeks flame when my test results were announced in a room crowded with strangers. Afterward, I had imagined them assembled into a sniggering gauntlet, giving me my comeuppance. Sizwe did not need to leave so much to the imagination. The hundreds of pairs of eyes watching the school had known him since he was knee-high; there was not a stranger among them. That they would have sniggered triumphantly was no paranoid fantasy, but a plain truth, for he had heard the sniggering with his own ears when the day was done.

Those who designed the treatment program of course knew of that hostility. They knew that the testing sites they erected in the villages were amphitheaters filled with uncharitable audiences. Their message to those who walked into their testing centers was this: Yes, there is ill feeling out there, but it doesn't matter. Yes, your community will know your status, but you will be okay. Once you realize that the hostility will not hurt you, you will have walked through an invisible barrier. You will have shaken off an unspeakable burden and an intolerable pain. Come with us, there are many of us, we will protect you.

As Hermann Reuter had put it to me soon after I met him: "Your friend Sizwe, if he goes to test and he tests positive, then yes, the people in his community will know, and he will make some enemies. But the friends he makes will be more important than the enemies. The people testing positive develop meaningful relationships, the sort of relationships they have never had. Before, they were sitting around and doing nothing. Now, their lives become meaningful."

To Sizwe, it smacked of a cult. The beseeching sincerity, the invitation to jump out of your world and into another: bands of proselytizers had been wandering in and out of Ithanga since he was a small child. They all came heralding a cure. He had, he believed, seen it many times before.

When I pushed him on it, he stood up and cleared his throat and showed me what it was he had seen that Saturday morning at the school. He stood with exaggerated erectness. His eyes glazed over. And when he spoke, what came from his mouth was the high-pitched, fervent voice of a Sunday preacher.

"I am living with this virus," he said in his shrill, insistent voice. "I am living with this virus and I am healthy, I am strong. With these pills, the virus is dormant inside me. It cannot hurt me now. It cannot make me sick."

He sat down, a little sheepish from his performance. "It sounded like the Zionists," he said, "like a new Zionist church had come to town. How are they so different from the Zionists? They say they have come to heal, they have a new cure, but you must join them in their rituals if you want to be cured. It is the same."

And as with the preacher who tells his audience that he was mortally ill before his epiphany cured him, Sizwe simply did not believe it. He had to wait more than a year, when evidence that the pills did good work was too apparent to ignore, before he knocked on Jake's brother's door and took him to the clinic to test again for HIV.

I do not think that Sizwe believed the nurses and counselors at the school to be hostile. But he did think them dangerous. For the choice they were offering was unacceptable to him. Come in and test, they said, and if you test positive, you will either walk out alone into a world of ridicule and condemnation, or you will come into our circle where we will protect you. He did not believe them capable of protecting him: not from the sense that there is dirt in his blood, not from the theft of his children's inheritance. He still does not believe that the pills can shelter him from these things. He lives in a space the MSF program has not penetrated: he is the embodiment of the program's limits.

If there was ever a moment Sizwe came close to believing that

ARVs might be for him, it was during our time with Kate Marrandi. Instead of holding up a mirror to his shame, she spurned it with love and acceptance. That is indeed her magic: her capacity to show a face that is ineluctably benign.

I INTERVIEWED HERMANN Reuter for the last time on a Sunday morning in September 2006. It was about two weeks before his farewell event at the community hall in town. We sat in the sun on a small patch of lawn outside his front door. He clutched a bowl of milky breakfast cereal and ate from it noisily. Inside the house, a colleague of his sat alone at the dining room table waiting for him; they were to spend the day preparing MSF's Lusikisiki exit report.

He asked how the book was going. I told him I doubted whether he'd like it. Instead of being about his program it was about the people and places beyond its margins: places like Ithanga and Nomvalo, people like Sizwe and Kate Marrandi.

"The things at the periphery are very important," he replied. "I have no doubt it will be a very good book."

We did not often talk about Sizwe, but when we did our conversation fell into a familiar pattern. He listened very attentively, even hungrily, I thought, as if I were bringing him intelligence from a murky and ill-defined zone that lay beyond the boundaries of his world. And yet the expression that would come over his face was both troubled and unimpressed, as if the intelligence he was receiving was compromised, his task to separate the nonsense from the useful. For my part, I was childishly titillated by the ambivalent interest he took in the news I brought him. Watching him make sense of it, I imagined, was to watch him take down an invisible guard.

At the time of our conversation, the woman Sizwe had approached to become Ithanga's Kate Marrandi had been on the job about six weeks. Sizwe and I had just learned that she was trying to pass herself off to her patients as HIV-positive. I told Hermann this. I also told him of Sizwe's belief that she had been instructed to lie by the counselors who trained her, that the program itself was encouraging the people it sent out to the villages to deceive.

"He still doesn't want to use his real name?" Hermann asked.

"Yes."

"For me, that is the one reason I won't like your book. I think it will ruin your book."

"Why do you feel that strongly about it?"

"Because of the things that are said about people living with HIV. That they are just pushing a line, that they are lying. We need to say where we stand in our society. We need to be able to stand with who we are. This man is so quick to talk to you about this and that. But when it comes to putting his name to his thoughts, he says no."

"There are people around him who have not disclosed," I said.

"Yes," he replied, "and the family needs to acknowledge who they are and what is part of them. Disclosure is linked to acceptance of your reality. If your book perpetuates secrets it becomes part of that mystic kind of mentality that is so damaging: the mentality of witchcraft."

"It is not for him to disclose on behalf of members of his family," I replied.

"It is. He must disclose on behalf of his family. That is the beginning of healing. It will heal them."

Perhaps it was defensiveness on my part, for Hermann had certainly jabbed at a raw nerve, but I felt my distaste rising. What came to mind was the radical gay practice of outing. Those in the closet are tracked down, hounded out into the sunlight, and healed, through violent humiliation, of their homophobic self-hatred. I found myself sympathizing with Sizwe's wariness. This is a cult, I thought to myself; that a delicate tissue of privacy surrounds everyone, holding their dignity, keeping them sane, is something this cult has forgotten. Salvation through confession: that is its trade.

"This is a person," I said to Hermann, "who has shared with me thoughts about his father, his wife, his own body, thoughts that are by rights private. That I am writing of them at all—"

"I see myself as a psychologist," he interrupted. "I want to heal people. You just report about it, you don't need to change his life. I wouldn't be able to hear anything about his life without wanting to change him. That's me. I'm a doctor. I want to heal. I think not wanting to disclose a name is part of a big pathology."

"It is pathological that he—"

"I just don't understand. If anyone from his village reads this book, the story can be about no other person but him. Anyone who doesn't know won't know. It's that simple. By you saying we have to keep the name secret, blah blah blah, I don't know, it creates such a, I think it destroys the story. It is like . . . think of it: people who know him will recognize him in the book. But they won't be able to talk to him about it because his name is not there. They find it interesting. They want to engage him about it. But he is denying them that. That for me is the worst kind of disclosure: hidden disclosure. People come to me and say they are not disclosing to anyone, but everyone in the community comes to me and says this person is HIV-positive, you must help them. That is terrible."

"You want me to convince him . . . ?"

"Don't try to convince him. Try to heal him. Point out to him how openness is part of the healing process."

He turned his head away and shrugged dismissively. "I don't know. I haven't engaged with him deeply. I rejected him quite early in my encounters with him."

"Why?"

"I decided not to engage with him. I don't have time to engage with everyone. He was too big-mouthed in a way."

"What do you mean?"

"I don't know. I don't know him."

"What do you mean by big-mouthed?"

"Yes, that's what disturbs me. He is attention-seeking, but then he wants not to disclose."

"How was he attention-seeking with you?"

Hermann laughed nervously. "I'm judging him unfairly. I . . ."

I stared at him. We both said nothing for a while. He sighed.

"Whenever a white person goes to that village, they come back talking about him. First it was a photographer, then an anthropologist, then you. They come back and talk about him and the stories he tells are so striking. Somebody who pours his life out the first time he meets people. Do you know of this man at Ithanga who is scared of his shop being attacked? If you're really scared you wouldn't pour it out to any white person who comes past. White people are distrusted. I didn't like that. I like people when one doesn't see what bothers them on a daily basis."

I was not sure what to say. I felt wounded on Sizwe's behalf. Hermann's musings were awfully close to Sizwe's most jaundiced thoughts about himself. Indeed, the doctor had found and was prodding at the very kernel of Sizwe's shame, the very thoughts that had contaminated his blood.

Hermann laughed nervously again, as if his desire was to say these things and retract them at the same time.

"I'm unfair," he said. "I don't know him. I'd probably enjoy talking to him. I'd probably like him very much. Because he has a lot of very interesting things to say. I'm probably jealous that I didn't get to spend time with him."

LISTENING TO MY recording of this conversation in my study, the birdcalls and children's shouts of Sunday morning Lusikisiki in the background, our exchange struck me as amusing. Two white men in conflict over whether the black man one of them has found is a genuine article or a trickster.

Hermann had both the grace and the intelligence to point out immediately that what he was expressing was sour grapes. You're telling the story of a person who won't test, he was saying, a person out of my clutches and thus an emblem of my limitations. But so what? You can have him. I washed my hands of him long ago.

Of course Hermann was "jealous," as he put it. The jealousy he was expressing was an activist's frustration with his limits. He was jealous of those he imagined had seen Sizwe's interior because it was a place he and his program could not reach, the interior of a man who will not test despite having lived within the boundaries of an MSF program for nearly four years. It is comforting to grow suspicious of him: it is self-justifying. Perhaps, you tell yourself, we cannot reach him because there is something wrong with him, because he is a fake. And so you divide the world into two: those you can heal, and those you scorn.

I wondered why Hermann could not see that people like Sizwe represented a victory, not a failure. Sizwe was the low-water mark of Hermann's achievement: a young man who simply refuses to test. Yet even Sizwe concedes that if he falls ill, he will go to the clinic, test, and take the pills. That this option is available to him at all, and that he will take it, is thanks to MSF. Indeed, so many of those who people these pages are Hermann's victories: Thandeka went to the clinic for a CD4 count via a failed attempt at a traditional cure. Xolela sat at home sick and in denial until his dead brother's closest friend insisted on taking him to the clinic. Vukani went onto treatment secretly, attended a support group, but tried to conceal it. These are the frail, imperfect ways of ordinary human beings in the teeth of a great epidemic. They have, according to their various signatures, chosen to live.

———————

DURING THE CAR journey to Mount Ayliff early on the first Tuesday of April 2007, I asked Sizwe what he thought of Hermann Reuter.

"What do you mean?" he asked. "In terms of him leaving Lusiki-siki? In terms of the health of the people?"

"Both of those things."

"Maybe he left because he was getting bored of living among the black people," Sizwe said. "That is fine, it is his choice. But the way he left was wrong. He should have found another white doctor to replace him. Or not even a white. Just somebody who is gentle with the people. Because the black nurses are so cruel to sick people. You go there with AIDS and they shout at you. Even Nwabisa is scared to go to the clinic with Mfanawetu. She went to take him the other day because he had worms. And the nurse shouted at her: 'How can you allow your son to get worms!' You come away from the black nurses and you are feeling ashamed of yourself.

"So it is okay that he left, but he should have found someone like him to replace him."

"You no longer believe, then," I asked, "that he is part of the conspiracy of the *umlungus* to kill the blacks? He is not one of those who knows of the cure for AIDS but holds it back?"

"No," he replied. "He wants to do good with those pills. He is not part of the plot. He doesn't even know about it."

———————

THERE IS NO particular reason why Hermann Reuter should stand as an emblem of the quest to heal a country of AIDS. Nor is there a special reason Sizwe's response should reflect that of ordinary people across South Africa. But these are the people I have found through whom to tell a story of AIDS treatment, and it is hard to stop myself from thinking of them allegorically.

On this stage, one I have erected, there are two figures. The doctor expresses his frustration with those who will not be patients. During moments of weakness, his frustration becomes an accusation, a rejection, a washing of the hands. As for the other figure, he has, despite his initial suspicions, come to see the doctor as a good soul and a healer. But a healer in the limited way of a Florence Nightingale, stitching and bandaging the victims for all his worth—while out of sight, in the war rooms of the powerful, more carnage is being planned.

Epilogue

Late one evening at the end of April 2007, I phone a woman named
Sharon at her home in the middle-class suburbs of Port Elizabeth.
We have spoken just once before, about a year ago. I had made contact
with her to ask about a bird-watching trip she, her husband, Graeme,
and a party of amateur ornithologists had done on the Pondoland
coastline in December 2003. I wanted to talk about the young man,
Sizwe Magadla, who had guided the party through the coastal forests,
and how it came about that they decided to capitalize his new business
venture.

She was pleased that I had called, and for the better part of an
hour she spoke warmly of Sizwe: of his breathtaking knowledge of the
forest and its fauna; of the attractiveness of his curiosity, at once penetrating and unobtrusive; of how for months after the trip nobody in
the party had been able to shake him out of their thoughts.

Now, a year later, she does not wait to hear why I have called
again.

"It is so strange that you phone now," she says. "Just last week I had
a long conversation with Sizwe, our first in ages. He kept me for nearly
two hours. He was very agitated. It was partly about you."

"What's the matter?" I ask.

"He said you came to see him a couple of weeks ago, and that you
needed to know why he would not test for HIV. Your conversations left

him disturbed. He told me he needed to test, that it was keeping him up every night, but that he was scared."

"What did you say?"

"Well, throughout the conversation, his wife was in the room listening. And I said to him, 'You are sharing all this fear with the woman in your life. You clearly love and trust one another so much. Your world cannot collapse around you. Nwabisa is there.' I told him that if he wanted, he and his wife and child should get on a bus and come; that he should test here, that they could stay with us for as long as they wanted."

"What did he say?"

"That he'd think about it."

———————

I PHONE SIZWE the next morning. We speak about this and that. We have never communicated well on the phone. Our stilted exchange seems a bad context in which to tell him about my conversation with Sharon. I am about to say good-bye and hang up.

"Wait," he says. "I went to Village Clinic in town last week. I went for them to test me."

He pauses a long time.

"And?"

"They had no electricity, no running water. It was so crazy there. I waited until after lunchtime. Then I went home."

"But you went back?"

"Yes. Two days later. It was still dark in there. I waited until after lunch again. They couldn't test me."

"The electricity is back now, surely?"

"I don't know."

"I'm sure it's back."

He chuckles, affectionately, but mockingly. He is laughing at my earnest concern.

"Maybe," he says. "We will see."

But the lightness in his tone suggests that the urgency of his need to know has passed. The restless fear that caused him to phone Sharon out of the blue and ask for help, the agitation that had taken him away from work for two days to sit in a clinic waiting room, these are things from last week; they are gone now. Mfanawetu's plaintive voice pierces our conversation.

"I am keeping you from your son," I say. "I can hear that he wants to play with you."

His laughter is even lighter this time. "No. He is playing with some other children, and with a dog. They are all together on the floor. They are all happy."

"And so are you."

"I am very well," he says. "Everyone here is very well."

I PUT DOWN the phone and think of Hermann Reuter. He is right. Sizwe went to test and couldn't. The problem was not one of demand for health care but of supply. "People arrive at a health-care facility frightened and unsure," Hermann told me a few months before MSF left Lusikisiki. "If you turn them away, they will not come back."

I discover subsequently that there is no electricity because the clinic has not paid its utilities bill and the municipality has cut its services. When Hermann came to Lusikisiki he fought bitterly to have electricity installed at the clinics. I cannot say for sure, but if he had still been around I doubt that the bill would have remained unpaid. The darkness is one of the many symptoms of a treatment program that has lost its champion. Perhaps other champions will come.

But Sizwe's failure to test is not simply a tale about health-care services: it is a tale about men.

ON THE DAY of our telephone conversation, some 262,000 people have begun antiretroviral treatment at public health-care facilities in South Africa. More than two-thirds of them are women. Why? Where are the missing men? Why are they so less likely to find their way to ARV treatment than women?

That is not a question I set out to answer when I began writing this book, but it has been hard not to notice it on almost every page. It is unlikely that Sizwe is among the missing men; in all probability, he has the immunity of a healthy thirty-one-year-old. But when he speaks of his reluctance to test and of his conviction that were he to fall ill and take the pills they would only remind him that he is dying, he is speaking not just for himself but also for the missing men. When he expresses terror it is their terror he is expressing.

The sociologist Deborah Posel has written that with the AIDS epidemic "sex itself has become the vector of death . . . [I]t is the very intimacy of the home—mother, father and children—which has become contaminated. And it is men particularly—the fathers and sons of the nation—whose moral credibility is most acutely called into question."

There are few men left in Lusikisiki who do not know where to go to be treated for AIDS. That is the considerable accomplishment not only of Médecins Sans Frontières but of the social movement for AIDS treatment that has arisen in postapartheid South Africa. Tens of thousands of men have benefited from this movement, but only a tiny minority will ever join it. Most will never make of ARVs a right for which they will fight, or of HIV the substance of their self-assertion. They are too ashamed. To embrace lifelong treatment, men like Sizwe need something else entirely.

On our car journey to Mount Ayliff in early April 2007, Sizwe told me that his relation to white people was mercenary. And yet the events leading to his attempt to test belie a far more complicated story. When he needed finally to confront the prospect of dirt in his blood, it was to the bird-watchers he turned, people whose place in his world is so unheralded and strange as to be ghostly. Why?

Perhaps precisely because they are of another place. By the accident of their social and physical distance, they had become equivalents of the benign figure Kate Marrandi so skillfully carved. Kate filed away at herself until she was no longer of and in her world—no sexual history, nothing to rival, nothing to envy, nothing to reflect hostility or shame back at you. For Kate, another person was only a life to hold and to preserve. The bird-watchers are not of Sizwe's world. Because of what they gave him, they are merely the bearers of an extraordinary gift, a wondrous embodiment of his life interests.

Perhaps Kate and the bird-watchers are a model of the place the missing men might dare enter to be treated; a place sufficiently detached from the thick of the world to have become absolutely safe; a place where one might find the means to stay alive.

Notes

PAGE

1   *"People are too scared"*: Edwin Cameron, *Witness to AIDS* (London: IB Tauris, 2005), p. 67.

2   *About 2.1 million people died:* UNAIDS, "AIDS epidemic update, December 2006," p. 13, http://www.unaids.org/en/HIV_data/.

6   *A new democracy is an era of resurging life:* This idea of AIDS as an attack on both the individual's and the nation's generative powers was originally made by sociologist Deborah Posel. See her "Sex, death, and the fate of the nation: Reflections of the politicization of sexuality in post-apartheid South Africa," *Africa* 75, no. 2 (2005): 125–43.

38   *"If when the dogs bark"*: Monica Hunter, *Reaction to Conquest: Effects of Contact with Europeans on the Pondo of South Africa* (1936; rept. London: Oxford University Press, 1961), p. 351.

38   *"The values they preach and largely practise"*: Philip Mayer and Iona Mayer, "Report of Research on Self-Organisation by Youth among the Xhosa-Speaking Peoples of the Ciskei and Transkei," Pretoria, Human Sciences Research Council, 1972, p. 127.

45   *"a strange, whistling kind of language"*: Jeff Peires, *The Dead Will Arise: Nongqawuse and the Great Xhosa Cattle-Killing of 1856–7* (1989; rept. Johannesburg and Cape Town: Jonathan Ball, 2003), p. 113.

149   *"They often incited whispers that the 'long needle' of the White man"*: Benedict Carton, "The Forgotten Compass of Death: Apocalypse Then

and Now in the Social History of South Africa," *Journal of Social History* 37, no. 1 (2003): 204.

150   *"The women say [the doctor and the anthropologist] have used our blood against us"*: Wulf Sachs, *Black Hamlet* (1937; rept. Johannesburg: Witwatersrand University Press, 1996), p. 210.

150   *In the Kenyan city of Mombasa, it was widely believed that the fire department captured Africans*: Louise White, *Speaking with Vampires: Rumor and History in Colonial Africa* (Berkeley: University of California Press, 2000), pp. 3, 102.

150   *"The authorities ordered vaccination"*: Joseph Roth, *Job*, translated by Dorothy Thompson (Woodstock, N.Y.: Overlook Press, 2003), pp. 8–9. (Roth's book was first published in German in 1930.)

151   *"Thousands flocked to the clinics from all over the southeast"*: Terence Ranger, "Godly Medicine: The Ambiguities of Medical Mission in Southeastern Tanzania," in Steven Feierman and John M. Janzen, eds., *The Social Basis of Health and Healing in Africa* (Berkeley: University of California Press, 1992), p. 264.

205   *"The gay past is not pure"*: Colm Tóibín, *Love in a Dark Time: Gay Lives from Wilde to Almodóvar* (London: Picador, 2002), p. 14.

264   *"Their manner seems to say"*: Isaac Bashevis Singer, *In My Father's Court* (1962; rept. New York: Farrar, Straus & Giroux, 2000), p. 186.

284   *The areas doing well were those where "HIV care initiatives had existed"*: Helen Schneider, "Reflections on ART policy and its implementation: Rebuilding the ship as we sail?" *Acta Academia Supplementum* 1 (2006): 27.

326   *"sex itself has become the vector of death"*: Posel, "Sex, death, and the fate of the nation," p. 92.

Further Reading

The following books and articles are here for one of two reasons: they helped me to shape aspects of this book, or they are my recommendations for further reading.

I know of only one general history of the African AIDS epidemic—John Iliffe's *The African AIDS Epidemic: A History* (Oxford: James Currey, 2006)—and found it extremely valuable. The question of why the AIDS epidemic has been uniquely terrible in Africa has produced many rival answers both reasonable and unreasonable. Iliffe's book contains an incisive commentary on the debate. Of the scholars who have weighed in on the debate, I have learned much from Eileen Stillwaggon, *AIDS and the Ecology of Poverty* (New York: Oxford University Press, 2006), and Helen Epstein, *The Invisible Cure* (New York: Farrar, Straus & Giroux, 2007). Stillwaggon and Epstein agree on almost nothing; their divergence tells a good deal about the scale of controversy.

On the coming of antiretroviral treatment to Africa: Anne-Christine d'Adesky, *Moving Mountains: The Race to Treat Global AIDS* (New York: Verso, 2004); Greg Behrman, *The Invisible People* (New York: Simon & Schuster, 2004); Stephen Lewis, *Race Against Time* (Toronto: House of Anansi Press, 2005). On the struggle for antiretroviral treatment in South Africa: Edwin Cameron, *Witness to AIDS* (London: IB Tauris, 2005); Nicoli Nattrass, *Mortal Combat* (Durban: University of KwaZulu-Natal Press, 2007); Steven Robins, "Long Live, Zackie, Long Live!" *Journal of Southern African Studies* 30, no. 3 (2004): 651–72.

As Hermann Reuter's various soliloquies at the beginning of Part Two of this book make clear, there is a lengthy debate in progress on the economic efficacy of ARVs in Africa. Can the continent afford to put and keep the ill on drugs? Would the money not be better spent on interventions that lower the rate of new infections? The literature on these questions is vast. To get a sense of the terms of the debate, see an exchange between Richard Cash and Nicoli Nattrass that took place at Princeton University's Center for Human Values in April 2006 at http://www.princeton.edu/~uchv/archive/2005calendar.html.

The most persuasive and articulate defender of Hermann Reuter's view that the demand for health care is a function of its supply is Paul Farmer. See Paul Farmer, *AIDS and Accusation: Haiti and the Geography of Blame* (Berkeley: University of California Press, 1992); Paul Farmer, *Infections and Inequalities: The Modern Plagues,* 2nd edition (Berkeley: University of California Press, 2001); Paul Farmer, *Pathologies of Power: Health, Human Rights, and the New War on the Poor,* 2nd edition (Berkeley: University of California Press, 2005). See also Tracy Kidder, *Mountains Beyond Mountains: The Quest of Dr. Paul Farmer, A Man Who Would Cure The World* (New York: Random House, 2003).

Barrels of ink have been spent on South African president Thabo Mbeki's views on AIDS. Two books tower above the rest: Mark Gevisser, *Thabo Mbeki: The Dream Deferred* (Johannesburg: Jonathan Ball, 2007), chapter 41; and Didier Fassin, *When Bodies Remember* (Berkeley: University of California Press, 2007).

On AIDS stigma in South Africa, the scholar I have learned from most is the sociologist Deborah Posel. Her work on stigma is part of and should be read together with a broader project on sexuality in postapartheid South Africa. See Deborah Posel, "Sex, Death and Embodiment: Reflections on the Stigma of AIDS in Agincourt, South Africa," paper for symposium on Life and Death in a Time of AIDS, The Southern African Experience, WISER, Johannesburg, October 14–16, 2004; Posel, "Sex, death, and the fate of the nation: Reflections of the politicization of sexuality in post-apartheid South Africa," *Africa* 75, no. 2 (2005); Posel, " 'Baby rape': Unmaking secrets of sexual violence in post-apartheid South Africa," in Graeme Reid and Liz Walker, eds., *Men Behaving Differently: South African Men since 1994* (Cape Town: Double Storey, 2005), pp. 24–63.

The historians Peter Delius and Clive Glaser have produced a wonderful survey of anthropological and historical scholarship on sexuality in South Africa. See Delius and Glaser, "Sex, disease and stigma in South Africa: Historical perspectives," *African Journal of AIDS Research* 4, no. 1 (2005): 29–36; Delius and Glaser, "The Myths of Polygamy: A History of Extra-Marital and Multiple-Partnership Sex in South Africa," *South African Historical Journal* 50 (2004): 84–114; Delius and Glaser, "Sexual Socialisation in South Africa: A Historical Perspective," *African Studies* 61, no. 1 (2002): 27–54.

On the political economy of sex in contemporary South Africa, Mark Hunter's work is unsurpassed. See Hunter, "Zulu-speaking Men and Changing Households: From providers within marriage to providers outside of marriage," in Benedict Carton, John Laband, Jabulani Sithole, eds., *Being Zulu: Contesting Identities Past and Present* (London: Hurst; Pietermaritzburg: University of KwaZulu-Natal Press, forthcoming); Mark Hunter, "Informal Settlements as Spaces of Health Inequality: The Changing Economic and Spatial Roots of the AIDS Pandemic, from Apartheid to Neoliberalism," Durban, University of KwaZulu-Natal, Centre for Civil Society Research Report no. 44, 2006; Mark Hunter, "Cultural Politics and Masculinities: Multiple Partners in Historical Perspective in KwaZulu-Natal," in *Culture, Health and Sexuality* 7, no. 4 (July 2005): 389–403; Mark Hunter, "The Changing Political Economy of Sex in South Africa," *Social Science and Medicine* 64 (2007): 689–700; Mark Hunter, "The Materiality of Everyday Sex: Thinking beyond 'prostitution,'" *African Studies* 61, no. 1 (2002): 99–120.

On mourning and the feeling of triumph in the living over the dead, see Melanie Klein's essay "Mourning and its relation to manic-depressive states," in Klein, *Love, Guilt and Reparation and Other Works, 1921–1945* (London: Hogarth, 1975), pp. 344–69. See also the two Freud papers on which Klein based her essay: Sigmund Freud, "Mourning and Melancholia," in Freud, *On Metapsychology: The Theory of Psychoanalysis*, trans. James Strachey, ed. Angela Richards (London: Penguin, 1991), originally published in German in 1917; and Freud, "Our Attitude Towards Death," in Freud, *Civilization, Society and Religion*, trans. James Strachey, ed. Albert Dickson (London: Penguin, 1987), originally published in German in 1915. In thinking about Sizwe's quest for permanence through generativity I was helped a great deal by Philippe Ariés's classic studies of death: *The Hour of Our Death*, trans. Helen Weaver (London: Allen Lane, 1981); and Ariés, *Western Attitudes Towards Death From the Middle Ages to the Present*, trans. Patricia M. Ranum (Baltimore: Johns Hopkins University Press, 1974). Closer to home, discovering the work of the South African anthropologist Hylton White was both validating and enlightening. See, in particular, Hylton White, "Ritual Haunts: The Timing of Estrangement in a Post-Apartheid Countryside," in Brad Weiss, ed., *Producing African Futures: Ritual and Reproduction in a Neoliberal Age* (Leiden: Brill, 2004).

On the questions of African belief, science, and medicine in contemporary South Africa, see Adam Ashforth, *Witchcraft, Violence and Democracy in the New South Africa* (Chicago: University of Chicago Press, 2005); Ashforth, "An Epidemic of Witchcraft? The Implications of AIDS for the Post-Apartheid State," *African Studies* 61, no. 1 (2002): 121–43. See also Isak Niehaus, "Witchcraft and the New South Africa: From colonial superstition to postcolonial reality?" in Henrietta Moore and Todd Sanders, eds., *Magical Interpretations, Material*

Realities: Modernity, Witchcraft and the Occult in Postcolonial Africa (London: Routledge, 2001). On traditional medicine and AIDS, a special edition of the journal *Social Dynamics*, 32, no. 2 (2005), edited by Nicoli Nattrass, is devoted to the subject.

Two extraordinary studies of Zulu traditional medicine are Harriet Ngubane, *Body and Mind in Zulu Medicine* (London: Academic Press, 1977); and Axel-Ivar Berglund, *Zulu Thought-Patterns and Symbolism* (London: Hurst, 1976). On the status and the use of traditional medicine in a postcolonial context I learned much from Murray Last's essay, "The Importance of Knowing About Not Knowing: Observations from Hausaland," in Steven Feierman and John M. Janzen, eds., *The Social Basis of Health and Healing in Africa* (Berkeley: University of California Press, 1992), pp. 393–406.

On Christian Zionism and its conceptions of health and healing, mentioned so often in this book but never adequately explored, see Bengt Sundkler's classic study, *Bantu Prophets in South Africa* (London: Lutterworth, 1948).

This book is set in Lusikisiki, once the capital of Eastern Pondoland, the last of the Eastern Cape's independent African polities to surrender to the British. Pondoland's best historian is William Beinart. See his book *The Political Economy of Pondoland 1860–1930* (Cambridge, U.K.: Cambridge University Press, 1982). Beinart has also written a thought-provoking essay on youth socialization in Pondoland: "The Origins of the *Indlavini*: Male Associations and Migrant Labour in the Transkei," in Andrew Spiegel and Patrick McAllister, eds., *Tradition and Transition in South Africa: Festschrift for Philip and Iona Mayer* (Johannesburg: Witwatersrand University Press, 1991), pp. 103–28. For some of Beinart's other work on Pondoland, see Beinart, "Pig Killings, Contagion and Purification in South Africa," paper prepared for Conference on Culture and Consciousness in Southern and Central Africa, Manchester, U.K., 1986; Beinart, "Worker consciousness, ethnic particularism and nationalism: The experiences of a South African migrant, 1930–1960," in Shula Marks and Stanley Trapido, *The Politics of Race, Class and Nationalism in Twentieth Century South Africa* (London: Longman, 1987), pp. 286–309; Beinart, "Transkeian Smallholders and Agrarian Reform," *Journal of Southern African Studies* 11, no. 2 (1992): 178–99; Beinart, "Environmental Origins of the Pondoland Revolt," in Stephen Dovers, Ruth Edgecombe, and Bill Guest, eds., *South Africa's Environmental History: Cases and Comparisons* (Cape Town: David Philip, 2002), pp. 76–89.

For a brilliant ethnography of Pondoland in the early 1930s, see Monica Hunter, *Reaction to Conquest: Effects of Contact with Europeans on the Pondo of South Africa* (London: Oxford University Press, 1961), first published in 1936. Hunter also wrote two seminal essays on Pondoland, the first on women, the second on witchcraft. See Hunter, "The Effects of Contact with Europeans on the Status of Pondo Women," *Africa* 6 (1933): 259–76; and Monica Hunter Wilson, "Witch-Beliefs and Social Structure," in Max Marwick, ed., *Witchcraft and Sorcery,* 2nd edition (Harmondsworth: Penguin, 1982), pp. 276–85.

Dunbar T. Moodie's book, *Going for Gold: Men, Mines and Migration* (Berkeley: University of California Press; Johannesburg: Witwatersrand University Press, 1994), contains a magisterial account of the masculine identities of Mpondo men that formed in the nexus between the gold mines and rural homestead economies of Pondoland; the book is something of an elegy to Buyisile's generation.

For a remarkable study of Mpondo engagement with the politics and power of Western technology in the 1920s, see the chapter on Pondoland in Helen Bradford, *A Taste of Freedom: The ICU in Rural South Africa, 1924–1930* (Johannesburg: Ravan Press, 1987).

For a study of livelihood strategies in two Lusikisiki villages very similar to Ithanga, see Flora Hadju, "Relying on Jobs instead of the Environment? Patterns of Local Securities in the Rural Eastern Cape, South Africa," *Social Dynamics* 31, no. 1 (2005): 235–60. See also Hadju's doctoral thesis, "Local Worlds: Rural Livelihood Strategies in Eastern Cape, South Africa," University of Linköping, 2006.

For Médecins Sans Frontières's own accounts of its Lusikisiki project, see Médecins Sans Frontières, "Achieving and Sustaining Universal Access to Antiretrovirals in Rural Areas: The primary healthcare approach to HIV services," October 2006, at http://www.msf.be/fr/pdf/lusikisiki_final_report .pdf; and "Siyaphila La Programme—Lusikisiki, Eastern Cape: Implementing HIV/AIDS services including ART on a rural resource-poor setting, Activity Report 2003-2004," at www.epi.uct.ac.za/ideufiles/Lusikisiki2004.pdf.

For a journalist's early assessment of the project, see Belinda Beresford, "Pioneering Treatment Access in a Rural Area of South Africa," *Development Update* 5, no. 3 (2005): 277–91.

I fear that I have written far too superficially and too coldly in this book about nurses. For an incisive account of nursing in South Africa before 1990, see Shula Marks, *Divided Sisterhood: Race, Class and Gender in the South African Nursing Profession* (New York: St. Martin's Press, 1994). Marks and others have also written of the pioneering, midcentury project of preventative social medicine established by Sidney and Emily Kark in the old province of Natal. The Karks' work was something of a spiritual precursor to MSF's Lusikisiki project and stands as testimony to the health-care system that South Africa might have built in the second half of the twentieth century. See Shula Marks and Neil Andersson, "Industrialization, Rural Health and the 1944 National Health

Services Commission in South Africa," in Feierman and Janzen, eds., *The Social Basis of Health and Healing in Africa,* pp. 131–61. See also Sidney and Emily Kark, *Promoting Community Health: From Pholela to Jerusalem* (Johannesburg: Witwatersrand University Press, 1999).

Acknowledgments

First thanks go to the health-care workers, activists, and administrators in Lusikisiki who gave generously of their time to share their perspectives on antiretroviral treatment with me. Former Médecins Sans Frontières staffers: Mfundo Fogobile, Nomzi Khonkwane, Nomini Mabena, Zikhona Majavu, Doli Mapungu, Lwazi Mfecane, Siphokazi Somhlahla and Bavuyise Vimbani. From the Treatment Action Campaign: Akona Ntsaluba. From Saint Elizabeth's Hospital: Drs. Thomas, Okito, and Hussein. From the Qaukeni LSA: Mrs. Nombulelo Mofokeng and Mrs. Tandiwe Sapepa. From the Eastern Cape Department of Health in Bisho: Nomalanga Makwedini and Thomas Dlamini. Many thanks too to the staff at Bodweni Clinic, Gateway Clinic, Goso Forest Clinic, Magwa Clinic, Malangeni Clinic, Qaukeni Clinic, Village Clinic, and the mobile clinic at Good Hope, who accommodated me in their working environment and answered my questions.

To the HIV doctors who took time out to help me understand something of their work: Hoffie Conradie, Richard Cooke, Eve Mendel, François Venter, Sabine Verkuijl, and, of course, Hermann Reuter, to whom I owe a special debt of gratitude, not least for having the foolish courage to allow a layperson to write about his work.

For invaluable discussions and exchanges on the material and ideas in this book: William Beinart and his graduate students at the African Studies Centre at Oxford University, Dhianaraj Chetty, Nomboniso Gasa, who helped me to understand Sizwe's relationship with his father a little better, Lungisile Ntsebeza, Deborah Posel, and Helen Schneider.

I am especially grateful to Hillary and Tony Hamburger and to Susan Levy, who, over many, many hours, gave me an education in the psychology of shame. Our discussions profoundly shaped the last two chapters of this book.

Many thanks to those who read and commented on drafts of the manuscript: Antony Altbeker, Edwin Cameron, Ben Carton, David Jammy, Nicoli Nattrass, Helen Schneider, Carol Steinberg, and Ivan Vladislavić, a masterful reader, from whose experience and perspicacity I have now benefited three times in a row.

I needn't have to add, but will nonetheless, that all errors of fact and foolishness of perspective are mine alone.

Mark Gevisser, my colleague, peer, and friend, gave more time and wisdom to this project than I could possibly measure. I am, as ever, deeply grateful.

Thanks to my agent, Isobel Dixon, and to my editor at Simon & Schuster, Dedi Felman, who has taught me a great deal about storytelling. At Jonathan Ball Publishers, thank you to Jeremy Boraine, Francine Blum, Tanya White, and to Jonathan Ball himself, whose warmth and loveliness are beyond any telling.

This book was funded by the Ford Foundation through the Institute for Security Studies in Pretoria. Anton du Plessis, former program manager at the institute, offered to facilitate the funding of the project before I had even begun to badger him. Many thanks for that. Anton's successor at the institute, Boyane Tshehla, has accommodated my work in warm and generous spirit. Busi Nyume handled the budgetary administration of the project without complaint. Many thanks.

Finally, to Lomin Saayman, who has not complained, either, despite having now seen two books through from beginning to end.

Index

About the Author

Jonny Steinberg was born and bred in South Africa. His previous two books, *Midlands* (2002) and *The Number* (2004) both won South Africa's premier nonfiction literary award, the *Sunday Times* Alan Paton Prize. Steinberg was educated at Wits University in Johannesburg and at Oxford University, where he was a Rhodes Scholar. He has worked as a journalist at a national daily, written scripts for television dramas, and has consulted extensively with the South African government on criminal justice policy. He is currently writing a book about immigrants in New York.